Thymic Hormones

Thymic Hormones

Edited by

T. D. Luckey, Ph.D.

Professor of Biochemistry
University of Missouri Medical School
Columbia, Missouri

University Park Press
Baltimore · London · Tokyo

UNIVERSITY PARK PRESS
International Publishers in Science and Medicine
Chamber of Commerce Building
Baltimore, Maryland 21202

Printed in the United States of America

Library of Congress Cataloging in Publication Data
Main entry under title:

Thymic hormones.

   Bibliography: p. 317.
   1. Thymus gland. 2. Hormones. I. Luckey, Thomas
D., ed. [DNLM: 1. Thymus gland. 2. Thymus gland—
Immunology. WK 400 L941t 1972]
QP188.T5T48   612′.43   72-8929
ISBN 0-8391-0705-6

Contents

**3   Thymus Replacement and HTH, the Homeostatic
       Thymic Hormone**

J. Comsa

4   Hormonal Interactions of the Thymus

J. Comsa

12   Perspective of Thymic Hormones
         T. D. Luckey

Preface

The thymus is a complex organ composed of a permanent stroma and a regenerating lymphoid tissue. The stroma accounts for about 10 per cent of the organ weight and is composed of a reticulum and epithelial cells; the lymphoid cells account for 99.9 per cent of the mytotic activity and are a mixture of thymocytes and transient bone marrow cells (Defendi and Metcalf, 1964).

From an embryological standpoint, the thymus is one of the first endocrine organs to appear and is the first organ to become lymphoid. The origin of the thymocyte is not yet clear. Lymphoid cells are transported to the thymus and other organs in early embryology and throughout life. In the embryo, these lymphoid cells populate bone marrow, which becomes the major lymphocyte production center (Sainte-Marie and Leblond, 1964; Nossal, 1964). The thymus continues to export lymphocytes and thymocytes, as may be deduced from the prolific reproduction of leukocytes in thymus, the difference in the total leukocyte count of afferent and efferent thymus blood vessels, and the genetic tagging of thymus implants. These cells and their derivatives comprise the major defense system of the body against undesirable microorganisms and certain foreign molecules. The thymus is both the progenitor and enabling organ of the lymphatic system. This system, together with its cellular components in lymphatic tissues, blood, bones, liver, and other organs, comprises 5 per cent of the body weight (Osgood, 1954).

The endocrinologic activities of the thymus may overshadow its morphologic contribution in postuterine life. It now appears that the parenchyma of the thymus produces a variety of hormones. The early endocrinology of the thymus was controversial because important experimental variables were not well controlled. These variables include the state of maturation of the thymus, the condition of the experimental animal, the amount of stress within the experiment, the role of wasting disease (infection), possible incomplete thymectomy, possible removal of other important tissues (parathyroid gland) during thymectomy, the presence of unrecognized accessory tissue such as the bursa in some species, the development of compensatory tissue (the so-called gut equivalent), and inclusion of factors not specific to the thymus. In the last category may be placed promine and retine, described by Szent-Györgi *et al.* (1963), the histones (Hnilica, 1971), and other factors. Despite the progress chronicled in this book, these problems have not been completely resolved in present research laboratories. They partially explain the sporadic nature of thymus research for half a century; the thymus has frustrated most researchers who were attracted to its siren call. Early reviews of classic thymic endocrinology were largely ignored; in 1938, Hammar suggested that thymectomy studies were clouded because they were performed too late in life.

One of the purposes of this book is to present the only complete review of the work of Jean Comsa, Stefan Milcu, and Isabela Potop, who individually bridged the gap between pioneer and current work. Beginning with Comsa's first publication in 1938, their combined years of thymic research approximate one century. Both Milcu and Potop had collaborated with Parhon, who worked on the thymus for four decades, beginning in 1927. During a lecture on germfree life at the Parhon Institute of Endocrinology in Bucharest, my incidental reference to our "early" (1964) thymic research led to a conference with Dr. Potop which revealed the significant progress made by Milcu and his collaborators, progress little known in the United States. The culmination of their work in the isolation of thymosterin matches that of Comsa's isolation of HTH (homeostatic thymic hormone); both efforts climax classic research efforts.

The different compounds reviewed here provide concepts of the thymus as varied as those alleged for the elephant by the six blind men. Although integration is attempted in the final chapter, the true dimensions of the thymus will not be comprehended until many more compounds are isolated and all have been tested in a single laboratory under precisely defined conditions. Critical experiments are needed for a complete reevaluation, with the research performed under clean and/or gnotobiotic conditions in which infection and stress cause no unprogrammed wasting disease or unwarranted involutions.

The first four chapters of this book present a thorough review of classic thymic endocrinology. Subsequent chapters provide a definitive review of thymic humoral factors important in the establishment of immune competence and elucidate compounds active in the stimulation and inhibition of leukocyte differentiation, maturation, and reproduction.

The present emphasis on the thymus as a central immune organ began with early studies by Klose and Vogt (1910) and Hellman and White (1930). These investigations indicated that thymectomized animals were susceptible to infection, the major component of wasting disease studied during the past decade. The humoral aspects of this phenomenon were first suggested by Metcalf (1956, 1959) and Gregoire and Duchateau (1956), and were amply confirmed early in the past decade by Osoba and Miller (1963) and others. The ontogeny and phylogeny of the thymus in immune competence have been reviewed by Hess (1969), Adinolfi and Humphrey (1969), and Good and Fisher (1971). No attempt has been made here to correlate the literature of thymic hormones with that of other compounds of importance, that is, nucleic acids or proteins (see Hnilica, 1971, for a recent review of histones).

The reports in this book of the identification of a variety of compounds with their activities and interactions establish new concepts of thymology. The thymus is more independent than other endocrine glands. The permissive role of the thymus toward endocrines is developed by Comsa in Chapters 3 and 4. Thymic hormone, cytocrines, or both confer immune competence to leukocytes. The thymus appears to be a master gland in the development and differentiation of leukocytes. The importance of these concepts to the development of endocrinology cannot be evaluated until the role of each compound has been determined for endocrine interactions and different aspects of cell proliferation, stem cell differentiation, and the maturation of individual lymphoid cells with resultant clones to provide immune competence. The medical importance of the activating compounds reported and the inhibitory compounds which will be isolated in the near future can hardly be overestimated.

Researchers in transplantation immunity are aggressively searching for new inhibitors; they must now consider inhibition by high concentrations of activator compounds and stimulation by minute quantities of inhibitors. Although inhibitors are the compounds of immediate demand, the activators will be of prime interest for the re-establishment of immune competence following the destruction of immunologic competence. The use of thymic hormones in combination with bone cell transplants will be an exciting development. The genetic immune diseases of man, reviewed in Chapter 2, will benefit greatly in having a source of pure inhibitor and activator compounds. Those diseases are the diseases of the newborn; thymic hormones will have greater significance over a wider population base in ageing man.

Although the size of the thymus relative to body weight is greatest in the newborn animal, the actual size and weight of the thymus does not begin to involute until puberty in most species. Following this involution, at a respectful distance in time, comes increased susceptibility to infection and to cancer. Future understanding of the role of thymic hormones in the ecology of infectious disease and cancer should illuminate the sudden death syndrome called "status thymicolymphaticus" in children and "wasting disease" in animals and should provide new avenues to cancer prevention. Insight gained from Trainin's laboratory, reported in Chapter 8, allows a hypothesis for a definitive approach to the detection of cancer susceptibility. This, together with the identification of thymic hormones, suggests a clinical survey for compounds in serum which endow lymphocyte competence for the continuous "search-and-destroy mission" of self-nonself segregation.

Finally, the importance of thymic hormones to theoretical biology cannot be overlooked. The isolation and identification of active compounds unique to the thymus will provide understanding of the complete biologic function of this organ and its interaction with other endocrines; isolation is the first step to the exact elucidation of function. The role of these compounds in antibody formation and cell-mediated immunity should reveal new concepts about the interrelationship between the antigen and the lymphocyte; this, in turn, should provide further understanding of antibody formation and possibly enzyme induction. The thymus is the spearhead of the lymphatic organ, which has as its overall purpose the maintenance of the continuity and purity of self. The fact that the total quantity of leukocytes equals that of erythrocytes provides impelling evidence of the importance of this tissue to the body. For this vigilance, the thymus operates as remote security headquarters, supply center, and maturation evoker for lymphocyte function. This continuing, nonsensory communication with the environment has been likened to that of the brain by Talmadge (1969). When leukocytes are sensitized by thymic hormones, they quickly attain the ability to identify strange molecules within their milieu and to react accordingly. The awakening of this cell potential provides a model for the initiation of recognition as a general phenomenon in biology. This concept is developed in the final chapter where consideration of the initiation of recognition is followed by a discussion of molecular imprinting to explain a variety of natural phenomona. Such concepts provide a new approach to differentiation.

This book solidified when all senior authors, excepting Dr. Potop and Dr. Milcu, gathered on August 5, 1971, following the *thymic hormones* workshop of the First International Congress for Immunology in Washington, D.C. Since our work was not well known to one another all were enthusiastic about submitting these summaries and examples of our thymic research for this book. I hereby acknowledge the fine cooperation of these authors, as well as the essential contribution of checking references by Mrs. E. J. McKinin and her staff at the Medical School Library of the University of Missouri, the critical reading by Bruce Zwilling, and the editing of the text by Mrs. Pauline Luckey.

T.D.L.

Contributors

Clara M. Ambrus, M.D., Ph.D., *Associate Professor of Pediatrics, State University of New York, and Roswell Park Memorial Institute, Buffalo, New York*

Julian L. Ambrus, M.D., Ph.D., *Director, Springville Laboratory, Roswell Park Memorial Institute, New York State Department of Health, and Professor of Internal Medicine, State University of New York, Buffalo, New York*

Benedict J. Campbell, Ph.D., *Professor of Biochemistry, University of Missouri School of Medicine, Columbia, Missouri*

Walter S. Ceglowski, Ph.D., *Associate Professor of Microbiology, The Pennsylvania State University, University Park, and Adjunct Associate Professor of Microbiology, Temple University School of Medicine, Philadelphia, Pennsylvania*

Jean Comsa, M.D., *Professor of Experimental Medicine, Saarland University School of Medicine, Homburg, Saar, Germany*

Herman Friedman, Ph.D., *Director of Clinical Microbiology and Immunology, Albert Einstein Medical Center, Philadelphia, Pennsylvania*

Terry L. Hand, M.D., *Department of Microbiology, Temple University School of Medicine, Philadelphia, Pennsylvania. Present address: Rockridge Medical Care Center, Oakland, California*

R. Robert Hook, Jr., Ph.D., *Microbiologist, Sinclair Comparative Medicine Research Farm, and Assistant Professor of Microbiology, University of Missouri Medical School, Columbia, Missouri*

Josef Kimhi, Ph.D., *Department of Biochemistry, The Weizmann Institute of Science, Rehovot, Israel*

T. Don Luckey, Ph.D., *Professor of Biochemisty, School of Medicine and Chairman of the Graduate Nutrition Area Committee, University of Missouri, Columbia, Missouri*

Stefan M. Milcu, M.D., *Professor of Endocrinology, Institute of Medicine and Pharmacy, and Director of the Institute of Endocrinology of the Academy of Medical Sciences, Bucharest, Romania*

Akira Mizutani, Ph.D., *Professor of Pharmaceutical Science, Nagoya City University, Nagoya, Japan*

Isabela Potop, C.D., *Associate Professor of Endocrinology, and Research Associate of the Institute of Endocrinology of the Academy of Medical Sciences, Bucharest, Romania*

W. Gerry Robey, Ph.D., *Research Assistant, Department of Biochemistry, University of Missouri School of Medicine, Columbia, Missouri*

Myra Small, M.D., *Department of Cell Biology, The Weizmann Institute of Science, Rehovot, Israel*

Nathan Trainin, M.D., *Department of Cell Biology, The Weizmann Institute of Science, Rehovot, Israel*

Thymic Hormones

1   Thymectomy

J. Comsa and R. R. Hook, Jr.

1.1 Introduction

Thymectomy is the surgical removal of all component parts of the thymus gland with as little damage to the remaining structures as is possible; thyroid and parathyroid glands should remain intact unless elements of these have become incorporated into the thymic structure. The multiple thymus gland may comprise as many as 14 lobes in chicks. Thus, good surgical technique involves a search for structures of thymus tissue on both sides of the neck from the jaw into the chest cavity. The time of thymectomy relative to the maturation of the thymus, endocrine organs, and lymphatic system is very important because different results can be expected by thymectomy before or following the complete maturity of the thymus and its associated functions. A search for fragments of thymus tissue at the end of an experiment usually includes histologic examination of the associated area. In the following chapters, it will be noted that guinea pigs have been of special importance for the endocrinologic studies, while mice have been of prime importance in the immunologic studies.

The result of thymectomy depends not only upon the maturation of the thymus at the time of extirpation but also upon the condition of the animal. If thymectomy led to a wasting disease or hormone deficiency, what did infection and/or stress contribute to the data? From this point of view it could be suggested that crucial experiments which have evolved from concepts presented herein should be reenacted using germ free animals. Also, certain critical experiments should be repeated in germ free animals with assurance that no stress has occurred.

This chapter will be concerned with observations pertinent to the influence of thymus insufficiency on wasting disease, changes in morphology, physiology, endocrinology, and the development of immune competence. No modern reviews are known which present a thorough study of thymectomy from a view which includes the general condition, histology, endocrinology, physiology, and immunology of the thymectomized animal. The influence of the thymus on immune responses has been studied in many species. Most of the knowledge concerning the role of the thymus in the development of immune competence came from studies on the phylogeny and ontogeny of the adaptive immune response, studies on experimentally thymectomized and/or irradiated mice and chickens, and studies of immune deficiency syndromes of man. No attempt is made here to present a review of all literature on the immune competence of thymectomized animals. Instead, this chapter presents those observations pertinent to the influence of thymus insufficiency upon the development of immune competence. Readers interested in the evolutionary development of the adaptive immune responses are referred to reviews by Fish, Pollara, and Good (1966), Hess (1968), Clem and Leslie (1969), Goldstein and Mackay (1969), and Good and Fisher (1971). The immune deficiency diseases of man are discussed in Chapter 2. *Experimental Thymectomy* by M. W. Hess (1968) presents a thorough review of the thymus as an organ essential for the development of immune competence.

1.2 Techniques and timing

The technique of thymectomy has been abundantly described in the rat (Segaloff, 1949), mouse (Dischler and Rudali, 1961), guinea pig (Comsa, 1938; Bomskov and Holscher, 1942), rabbit (Lucien and Parisot, 1910), dog (Matti, 1911), sheep (Silverstein, 1964; Silverstein, Parshall, and Uhr, 1966), and tadpole (Harms, 1952a, b). Two conditions are unanimously considered as compulsory for the development of a thymoprivic (thymus-deficient) condition: a) the thymectomy should be complete, and b) the operation should be performed in very young animals. A subtotal extirpation has no consequences on the general condition of the animals (Comsa, 1938; Gyllensten, 1953). Complete thymectomy can be confirmed by histologic section. *Xenopus* tadpoles should be operated upon in the hindleg bud stage (Harms, 1952a,b), mice (Dischler and Rudali, 1961) and rats (Jankovic, Waksman, and Aranson, 1962) within less than 24 hr of birth, rabbits within 5 days (Lucien and Parisot, 1910), dogs (Matti, 1911) and hamsters (Dameshek and Sherman, 1962) within 1 month after birth. Guinea pigs should be operated on as soon as they can be weaned and reared on the usual stock diet of oats, greens, and hay (Comsa, 1938).

Indeed, thymectomy is of no consequence in newborn guinea pigs if they are not weaned immediately after the operation. Since a too precocious weaning results in a severe dystrophy even in normal animals, this fixes the age for thymectomy in guinea pigs at 10 to 12 days after birth. Thus, thymectomized guinea pigs are animals operated upon at this age unless otherwise stated.

Gyllensten (1953) observed no consequences on the general condition of guinea pigs thymectomized at birth. However, his operation was subtotal and probably the animals were not weaned. He did not state this expressly, but he published growth curves which cannot be observed even in intact guinea pigs weaned soon after birth and reared on the diet he described.

1.3 General effects of thymectomy

Following thymectomy, a state of physiologic distress may develop which is generally lethal. Early publications of this observation are summarized in Table 1.1. An extensive account of the documentation with divergent observations was presented by Comsa (1959a). Hess (1968) provided a complete review of this subject. Wasting disease was found to be conditioned by the strain in dogs (Matti, 1911) and mice (Hess, 1968), to be sex linked in hamsters (Sherman and Dameshek, 1963), to be conditioned additionally by alimentary factors in rats (Asher and Landolt, 1934) and probably in guinea pigs (Comsa, 1959b) and by eventual infections in mice (Miller, 1961a).

Several investigators have provided good examples of wasting disease after thymectomy of various animal species (Abelous and Billard, 1896; Matti, 1911; Klose, 1914; Comsa, 1938c; Parrott and East, 1962; Miller, 1964a–c; Osoba, 1965b). On the other hand, growth, weight gain, and maturation were reported not to be altered in thymectomized animals that remained healthy (Pappenheimer, 1914a, b; Anderson, 1932). This is reviewed in detail by Miller (1961a, b). Since the wasting syndrome closely resembled the graft-*versus*-host syndrome and is associated with lymphoid atrophy and immunologic deficiences, wasting disease has often been attributed to an autoimmune process (Miller and Howard, 1964; DeVries *et al.*, 1964). However, the pathogenesis of post-thymectomy wasting disease is debatable, and experimental evidence has been obtained which supports the concept that the wasting syndrome is pre-

Table 1.1. Consequences of thymectomy on growth, wasting disease, and survival by early investigators

Reference	Year	Animal	Age (weight)	Growth	Wasting disease	Lethality
Lucien and Parisot	1910	Rabbit	Newborn	Transitorily delayed	None	None
Matti	1911	Dog	1 month	Delayed	Frequent in Danes and St. Bernards; none in fox terriers	Constant in diseased animals
Asher and Landolt	1934	Rat	(20 g)	Delayed, if reared on a poor diet	Not mentioned	Not mentioned
Rowntree et al.	1934	Rat	Newborn	Delayed	None	None
Comsa	1938	Guinea pig	10 days	Delayed	In 60% of the animals	Not strictly constant
Sandberg et al.	1940	Rat	(20 g)	Delayed	None	None
Bomskov and Holscher	1942	Guinea pig	(80 to 100 g)	Arrested	Constant	Constant
Segaloff	1949	Rat	Newborn	Normal	None	None
Harms	1952	Xenopus tadpole	Hindleg bud stage	Delayed for several years	Not fully developed	Increased[a]
Parhon and Costin	1953	Rat	(20 g)	Delayed	Not fully developed	None
Dischler and Rudali	1961	Mouse	Newborn	Not described	Not mentioned	Constant
Jankovic et al.	1962	Rat	Newborn	Not described	In 25% of the litters	Constant in diseased animals
Miller	1962b	Mouse	Newborn	Delayed	In 70% of the animals	Constant in diseased animals
Dameshek and Sherman	1963	Hamster	7 to 30 days	Not described	In 60%	Constant in diseased animals

[a]Survival was poor in control animals.

cipitated by infectious factors. Briefly, these are the experimental observations supporting this concept.

1) Germfree mice thymectomized at birth did not develop wasting disease (Wilson, Sjodin, and Bealmer, 1964; McIntire, Sell, and Miller, 1964; DeVries *et al.*, 1964).
2) Antibiotic treatment reduced the incidence of wasting disease in neonatally thymectomized rats (Azar, 1964).
3) There was no evidence of wasting disease in pathogen-free mice thymectomized at birth (Hess and Stoner, 1966; McIntire *et al.*, 1964).
4) The onset of wasting in neonatally thymectomized mice was accelerated by repeated injection of endotoxin (Salvin, Peterson, and Good, 1965).
5) Wasting disease does not occur in all thymectomized mice (Hess, Cottier, and Stoner, 1963); there is also litter effect in rats which suggests an infectious process (Jankovic *et al.*, 1962).

Wasting disease does not develop immediately after thymectomy. There is a variable interval in mice (Good *et al.*, 1962), in rats (Aisenberg, Wilkers, and Waksman, 1962), and in guinea pigs (Comsa, 1938) during which the growth rate is decreased but the animals appear otherwise normal. This transitory arrest of the growth is observed in guinea pigs, whether or not they may develop the wasting syndrome later on; it was observed also in rabbits (Lucien and Parisot, 1910), which thus far are not known to develop severe wasting disease following thymectomy. The thymus and microbial defense mechanisms are too well developed in new born lambs to allow this syndrome (Silverstein and Kraner, 1965).

The overall picture of the thymoprivic condition shows no specific clinical symptoms unless wasting occurs. In its terminal stage the animals develop typical physiologic distress characterized by severe weight loss, coarse and dirty fur, asthenia, disabled gait, anorexia, diarrhea, etc. This condition has been compared with the syndrome of graft-*versus*-host reaction, such as the runt disease of new born animals and the secondary disease of irradiated animals given injections of nonisologous cells. However, there is no evidence of a similar physiopathologic mechanism of these syndromes. It has been shown that the onset of secondary disease is somewhat delayed by previous thymectomy in irradiated mice given injections of rat bone marrow (van Putten, 1964). In fact, the thymoprivic wasting syndrome resembles any other wasted condition, such as the terminal stage of nutritional deficiency diseases.

It could be supposed that the thymoprivic condition may express an intricate hormonal unbalance. In guinea pigs simultaneous extirpation of the thymus and the thyroid results in peculiarly severe disorders. The onset of the wasting syndrome is almost immediate and most animals die within 14 to 20 days. Castration consistently prevents the wasting syndrome in thymectomized and in thymus-thyroidectomized guinea pigs as well (Comsa, 1945; 1947).

1.4 Anatomic pathology of the thymoprivic condition

In frogs thymectomized as tadpoles (Harms, 1952a, b) and in mice thymectomized at birth (Berek et al., 1967), the bones are weak and fragile. Spontaneous fractures occur frequently (Harms, 1952a). In thymectomized rats the proliferative activity of the epiphyseal cartilage is decreased (Asher and Landolt, 1934).

The skeletal muscles are atrophic in tadpoles (Harms, 1952b) and in guinea pigs (Houssay et al., 1955). Fibrosis and hyperplasia of the adipose tissue of the muscles may develop (Pora and Toma, 1960b). Myocardial lesions similar to those of the skeletal muscles have been observed (Bomskov and Holscher, 1942).

The lymphatic tissue is atrophic in thymectomized animals. The lymph nodes are shrunken in the rat (Pappenheimer, 1914; Jankovic et al., 1962), guinea pig (Comsa, 1957c), rabbit (Nakamoto, 1957a, b) and mouse (Metcalf, 1958; Miller, 1960). The lymphatic tissue of thymectomized animals does not react to interventions which induce its hypertrophy in normal animals, such as thyroxine injections (Comsa, 1959a), hemorrhage (Metcalf, 1958), adrenalectomy (Metcalf and Buffet, 1957), or skin graft (Waksman, Arnason, and Jankovic, 1962). Thyroxine injections even enhance the atrophy of lymphatic tissue in thymectomized guinea pigs. In guinea pigs the atrophy of lymphatic tissue is fully developed on the 6th day following thymectomy; this precedes by 10 to 25 days the onset of the wasting disease.

The endocrine glands show complex changes following thymectomy. The short-term and terminal conditions of these glands should be considered separately (Comsa, 1959a–d). The sensitivity of the thymectomized rat to anterior pituitary hormones is greatly modified following thymectomy; this is presented in Chapter 4. Shortly after thymectomy the endocrines show definite signs of stimulation. In the anterior pituitary this stimulation is expressed by a conspicuous increase in number and in size of the α (growth hormone) cells, the β (follicle-stimulating) cells, and the δ (thyrotropic) cells and the big chromophobes (corticotropic). The sequence of these changes is different in the rat and in the guinea pig. In thymectomized weanling rats the changes of α cells and of big chromophobes are precocious and are visible 3 days after the operation. Within numerous α cells the cytoplasm appears to be reduced to a small border under the membrane and another small border surrounding the nucleus, with several tenuous connections between both borders. The greatest part of the cell appears to be empty. This was called the "wheel cell" by Collin and "daisy bloom cell" by Dhom. This picture was interpreted by several authors to express a stimulated condition approaching exhaustion. Beta and δ cells show signs of stimulation only later (6 days after the operation). Twelve days after the operation this stimulation seems somewhat decreased. The α cells are comparatively small and dense. Some δ cells are small and stain peculiarly dark with shrunken nuclei. Big chromophobic cells are scarce. This decrease of the stimulated condition of the anterior pituitary parallels the changes of the thyroid and the adrenal (*see below*). The posterior pituitary contains numerous extracellular round homogenous drops of various sizes ("neurosecretion") stained intensely in sky-blue (Herlant's tetrachrome) staining. In thymectomized guinea pigs the β cells and the δ cells only show signs of stimulation a short time after the operation. Big chromophobes appear only 16 to 24 days after the operation. The reaction of the α cells is conspicuously late, between the 24th and 30th day. Furthermore, α cells increase in size and number only in animals which show signs of recovery (Comsa, unpublished).

The thyrotropic activity of the anterior pituitary is increased (Comsa, 1951b–d), and a significant thyrotropic activity of the urine can be detected. For this test 6 ml of urine from thymectomized guinea pigs were injected into infantile guinea pigs; within 1 day of the last injection the thyroid of these animals showed signs of stimulation. If the donor animals were thymectomized 15 days previously, the thyroid stimulation was quite strong. Urine of normal guinea pigs had no similar effect. Gyllensten (1953) could not confirm this observation, very likely because he injected only 1 ml of urine instead of 6 ml.

In thymectomized guinea pigs glandular cells of the thyroid are increased in height. Their cytoplasm and nucleus stain pale. In the center of the gland the colloid is completely resorbed from most of the follicles. Mitoses are frequent (Comsa, 1938). Similar changes occur in the thyroid of thymectomized *Xenopus* tadpoles (Harms, 1952a). Possibly the changes observed by Matti (1911) in thymectomized dogs are similar. His one photograph is difficult to interpret, and his interpretation is vague because at that time the histologic expression of the stimulated condition of the thyroid was not yet known. In the rat the histologic changes of the thyroid are not significant.

The ^{131}I uptake of the thyroid was measured in the isolated gland from thymectomized guinea pigs 2 hr after an intraperitioneal injection of 0.1 Ci of carrier-free ^{131}I. Incorporation in the thyroid was increased to about four times the normal range (Comsa, unpublished). In thymectomized rats this increase is controversial. With the technique used in guinea pigs, Comsa (unpublished) demonstrated a twofold transitory increase 6 days after thymectomy. Doniach (1957) injected 2.25 μCi of ^{131}I into thymectomized rats 24 hr after the operation and measured *in vivo* the radioactivity of the thyroid daily for 8 days. He observed no difference between thymectomized and sham-operated animals. Differences in techniques prevent direct comparison.

The protein-bound iodine content of the serum increased in thymectomized guinea pigs to 18.0 μg per 100 ml from a normal range of 4.5 to 6.0 μg. These results are in agreement with the histologic evidence of thyroid stimulation following thymectomy. The thymoprivic creatinuria gives further evidence to this supposition, since creatine excretion is suppressed by simultaneous thyroidectomy (Comsa, 1945). The increased thyrotropic activity of the urine and the increased creatine excretion are transitory; in thymectomized guinea pigs which recover during the 2nd month after the operation, these disappear gradually, as do the morphologic changes.

The adrenals are increased in size in the thymectomized guinea pig and in the rat. However, in the rat the ^{32}P uptake of the adrenal was found to be within the normal range (Shibata, 1953a).

The gonads show histologic signs of stimulation in the guinea pig (Comsa, 1938). In female rats, the onset of puberty is precocious (Anderson, 1932), but not in males (Plagge, 1940; Shibata, 1953b). The initial signs of stimulation are constantly observed in all thymectomized animals; however, this is a transitory condition. In rats it lasts more than 9 days and less than 12 days. Degenerative changes are not observed in guinea pigs which do not develop the terminal wasting condition; in those which recover, they disappear during the 2nd month after the operation.

During the terminal wasting stage in guinea pigs the endocrines show signs of exhaustion (Comsa, 1938; Bomskov and Holscher, 1942). In the anterior pituitary none of the different cell types is recognizable.

The gland appears to be composed of small chromophobic cells. The follicles of the thyroid contain a slightly basophilic, liquid-looking secretion instead of colloid, and the follicular cells are flat. The adrenals are small and they contain only traces of ascorbic acid and cholesterol. Remarkably few gonocytes can be seen in the testes. The cells of Leydig show no signs of functional conditioning. In the ovary the increasing follicles undergo atresia or cystic degeneration (Comsa, 1938). Bomskov and Holscher (1942) observed the same degenerative changes in the thyroid and in the gonads of thymectomized guinea pigs. They did not notice the initial stimulated condition of these glands, because they examined all their animals *sub finem*.

This terminal exhaustion of the endocrines is by no means specific. It occurs more or less in every case of extreme wasting, such as the terminal stage of nutritional deficiency diseases. It may be questioned whether or not the degeneration of the endocrines is a consequence of the wasted state of thymectomized guinea pigs. This question has not been examined in germfree animals which do not waste. However, in *Xenopus*, which does not develop a proper wasted condition following thymectomy, the gonads are also degenerated; they do not attain full maturity. An artificial maturation can be induced with injections of chorionic gonadotropin, but the ova thus produced are not viable when fertilized by normal sperm (Harms, 1952b).

1.5 Physiologic and endocrinologic changes in thymectomized animals

In thymectomized guinea pigs, it has been found that basal metabolism is increased (Gyllensten, 1953). In the rat the nitrogen excretion is increased; the most conspicuous feature of this nitrogen excretion is the increased creatine excretion (Comsa, 1944; Sandberg, Perla, and Holly, 1940). The phosphorus excretion is increased (Pora and Toma, 1960a). The ^{32}P uptake is decreased in the skeleton (Pora, Toma, and Oros, 1962), muscle, brain, bone marrow, and kidney of the rat (Pora and Toma, 1960a). The phosphatase activity of the bone is decreased in thymectomized guinea pigs (Fiaccavento, 1952). The effect upon calcium and phosphorus metabolism of chicks was explored by Milcu and Potop, and a compound affecting serum calcium in rabbits has been partially purified by Mizutani as reported in subsequent chapters. The high-energy phosphate content of rat muscles

(Parhon and Costin, 1953) and the glucose uptake of the diaphragm
(Pora, Toma, and Madar, 1962) are decreased. The activity of the thymic
extracts of Mizutani (Chapter 10) refutes the assumption of Hess (1968)
that defects in bone development and structure are caused by ablation
of parathyroid glands during thymectomy.

1.6 Immune competence

Before the influence of thymus insufficienty on immune competence can
be assessed, the immunologic characteristics of immunologically competent animals must be defined. Generally, it is accepted that an immunologically competent animal possesses the ability to exhibit the
following responses:

1) Production of circulating specific antibody after antigenic stimula-
    tion.
2) The capacity to reject homografts.
3) The ability to develop delayed hypersensitivity.
4) Proliferation of immunocompetent cells after antigenic stimulation.
5) The capacity for immunologic memory as assessed by the anam-
    nestic response to secondary antigenic stimulation or by the second-
    set homograft reaction.

In addition, the degree of lymphoid tissue development can be correlated with the level of immune competence; as lymphoid development
increases, the level of immune responses also increases.

The relationship of the thymus to immunocompetence has been real-
ized only recently. Since the development of immunocompetence is an
event which is dependent upon fetal and postnatal development of
primary and secondary lymphoid tissues, the effects of thymectomy vary
with the age of the animal at the time of surgery. Thymus-dependent
tissues cease further development after thymectomy but, for a time,
remain at the level attained before the thymus was removed. However,
these tissues usually degenerate with time. Metcalf (1960) and Miller
(1962a, b) pioneered the understanding of thymus function by recognizing
that mice thymectomized at birth did not attain complete immunocompetence; they developed, in fact, only a low level of immunocompetence. These studies provided an explanation for the equivocal results
obtained from other studies. Evaluation of the effects of thymectomy
in earlier studies were hindered primarily because at the time of thy-

mectomy the animals were not young enough and the experiments were of short duration. In addition, the relationship of the thymus to immunocompetence was clouded by studies in which thymectomy was incomplete. More recent studies have eliminated these earlier problems and have increased our knowledge and understanding of the relationship of the thymus to immunocompetence. It is on the basis of these studies that the influence of thymectomy on the development of immunocompetence is discussed below.

1.7 Influence of thymectomy on lymphatic tissue

A similar sequence of lymphatic tissue development is found in a variety of those animal species which have been studied thoroughly (Hammar, 1921; Knoll, 1929; Ball and Auerbach, 1960; Papermaster and Good, 1962; Good and Gabrielson, 1964; Kelley, 1963; and Block, 1964); the thymus is the first lymphoid organ to develop in most species. The mammalian thymus originates embryologically from the ventral portion of the third and fourth pharyngeal pouches (Patten, 1948) and early fetal development is epithelial. With progressive fetal growth, the thymus becomes lymphopoietic, and subsequently it becomes primarily lymphoid prior to birth. The spleen usually remains entirely erythropoietic and myelopoietic during fetal development and usually becomes lymphoid a short time after birth. The central and peripheral lymph nodes are the last lymphatic tissues to become lymphoid. The cat is an exception to this developmental sequence; lymphocytes appear in the lymph nodes before they appear in the thymus (Ackerman, 1967).

The ultimate origin of the thymocytes has been discussed passionately and at length for years (see Hammar, 1936, for an extensive review of the older references). Two theories exist which concern the origin of the lymphoid cells of the thymus, and experimental evidence supporting each viewpoint has been obtained. Ball and Auerbach (1960) have suggested that the lymphoid cells arise from the thymic epithelium, while Maximow (1901) and Hoshino et al. (1969) have obtained evidence which indicates that the first lymphocytes develop outside the thymus and later migrate to it.

In thymic grafts the thymocytes are soon destroyed by pycnosis. Thymocytes appear again on approximately the 5th day after the operation. In grafts surviving without developing vascular connections with the surrounding tissues in the anterior chamber of the eye (Gregoire, 1935) or in grafts included in a diffusion chamber (Osoba and Miller, 1963), no thymocytes will develop. These grafts remain definitely reduced to the parenchyma. Thymocytes will appear in intraocular grafts if they adhere to the surrounding tissues (Gregoire, 1935; Auerbach, 1960, 1961). These observations provide valid arguments for the immigration theory. Under adequate conditions, thymocytes will appear in explants of embryonic thymus (of mice) *in vitro*, although the explants probably contained none of these cells when explanted (Auerbach, 1960: 1961). In grafts of mouse embryonic thymus implanted on the chorioallantoic membrane of chick embryos, lymphocytes of both mouse and chick could be identified speculatively (Auerbach, 1961). This presumes a double origin of the thymocyte. Possibly this confusion would clear if embryonic and neonatal thymic grafts were considered separately.

Although the origin of the thymic lymphocytes may be debatable, Miller and Osoba (1967) established that the thymus, either directly through a cellular mechanism or indirectly through a hormonal mechanism, is responsible for the presence of the small lymphocytes in the circulating pool, lymphocytic fields of lymph nodes, and periarteriolar lymphocyte sheaths of the spleen. Thus, neonatal thymectomy performed in animals in which lymphatic tissue development is not yet complete results in the depletion of the small lymphocytes in these thymus-dependent tissues; further development of these tissues ceases with thymectomy. Although the development of thymus-dependent tissues usually stops at the level attained before the thymus was removed, such tissues degenerate with time. The diminution of the small lymphocyte population after neonatal thymectomy has been reported in the rat (Patton and Goodall, 1904; Sanders and Florey, 1940; Pappenheimer, 1914; Sloan, 1943; Reinhardt, 1945; Schooley and Kelley, 1958; and other laboratories during the past decade), guinea pigs (Patton and Goodall, 1904; Comsa, 1957c; Reinhardt and Yoffey, 1956), hamster (Sherman, Adner, and Dameshek, 1963, 1964), rabbit (Sanders and Florey, 1940; Nakamoto, 1957a, b; Good et al., 1962; Sutherland, Archer, and Good, 1964; Kellum et al., 1965), opossum (Miller et al., 1965), chicken (Warner and Szenberg, 1962; Jankovic and Isakovic, 1964; Isakovic and Jankovic, 1964; Cooper, Peterson, and Good, 1965; and Cooper et al., 1966), dog (Klose, 1914; Tilney, Beattie, and Economu, 1965), mouse (Metcalf, 1960; Miller, 1961a, b; Parrott, 1962; Good et al., 1962; Parrott and East, 1964), and man (Joske, 1958; Perla, 1960).

The striking lymphocyte deficiency which may occur after thymectomy is illustrated in the neonatally thymectomized mouse. In normal mice, the lymphocyte count and the lymphocyte to polymorphonuclear cell ratio rise progressively from birth to 8 days of age (Metcalf, 1958). Injection of either human or mouse cell-free extracts into baby mice induced lymphopoiesis; this was the first clear hint of the lymphocyte-stimulating factor of Metcalf (1956). However, in neonatally thymectomized mice there is no increase in this ratio. Total white blood cell counts of neonatally thymectomized mice are approximately one-half of those of normal mice, and this diminution is due primarily to a decrease in the small lymphocyte population (Miller, 1961a, b; 1962a, b; 1964c). This decrease has been reported to become more pronounced with increasing age, and the lymphocyte counts of mice 3 or 4 months after neonatal thymectomy have been reported to be as low as 10% of the lymphocyte counts of control animals (Miller, 1962c; 1963b). Young neonatally thymectomized mice usually have lymphoid follicles and germinal centers, but these become less active with age and are often not present in older thymectomized mice. There is no deficiency in plasma cells, which tend to accumulate in the thymus-dependent tissues of older thymectomized animals (Miller and Osoba, 1967). In addition to a decrease in the small lymphocyte population, thymectomy of neonatal mice often results in general hyperplasia of the reticuloendothelial elements, and large numbers of reticular cells, histiocytes, and macrophages replace the lymphocytes in the cortex of the lymph nodes (Miller, 1963b; Miller and Howard, 1964; Schooley et al., 1965).

Results of thymectomy in animals beyond the first few days of life, and especially in adult animals, are not as dramatic as those in neonatal animals, but the results nevertheless are functionally important. While there is usually a dramatic decrease in the lymphocyte population of neonatally thymectomized animals, the lymphocyte counts in the blood and thoracic duct lymph of animals thymectomized at 60 days of age were still 60% of the normal levels; Bieering (1960) found the lymphocyte population of the lymph nodes, spleen, and Peyer's patches did not decrease.

Intact adult mice have the capacity to regenerate their immune competence after sublethal doses of total body X-radiation. However, Cooper et al. (1967) discovered that adult mice which are thymectomized after receiving sublethal doses of total body X-radiation behave similarly to neonatally thymectomized mice; regeneration of their immune competence was postponed or inhibited. Metcalf (1965) and Miller (1965c)

reported that animals thymectomized as adults become lymphopenic and
behave much like neonatally thymectomized mice; however, lymphopenia was not significant until 3 months after thymectomy.

1.8 Effect upon antibody production

The adaptive immune response consists of a series of reactions and
interactions that eventually results in the synthesis of a unique protein
which has a high degree of specificity. This series of events has a cellular
basis; the ability to produce antibody resides in the lymphoreticular system. The small lymphocyte, in particular, has been associated with this
series of reactions and interactions. The small lymphocytes appear to
consist of at least two populations, each with perhaps a distinct function,
circulating life-span, and origin (Caffrey, Rieke, and Everett, 1962). As
far as immunologic competence is concerned, Ruhenstroth-Bauer and
Lucke-Hunle (1968) indicated that the functional properties of the two
populations of small lymphocytes are different. Since the small lymphocytes are involved in the immune response and since at least a portion of
the small lymphocyte population is either directly or indirectly under the
control of the thymus, it can be expected that thymectomized animals
would have deficiencies in their immune system.

Experimental designs used to study the influence of thymectomy on
antibody production have been so extremely different that it is difficult
to compare and evaluate results. The designs have differed so widely that
varying antibody responses have been observed; the various responses
were most likely due to the fact that different animal species, different
antigens, animals of various ages, and different response evaluation procedures had been used.

The primary antibody response to a variety of antigens, including sheep
erythrocytes, *Salmonella typhii* H. O. and Vi antigens, influenza A virus,
T_2 coliphage, and bovine serum albumin, has been examined in mice,
hamsters, rats, and rabbits which were thymectomized either at birth or
as newborns. This subject is reviewed in detail by Hess (1968). While
subnormal levels of antibody were obtained in the above studies, normal
antibody responses were obtained in thymectomized animals with tetanus
toxoid, hemocyanin, *Pneumococcus* type III capsular polysaccharide,
Salmonella flagellar antigen, ferritin, and polyoma virus (Hess *et al.*, 1963;
Fahey, Barth, and Law, 1965; Humphrey, Parrott, and East, 1964; Hess
and Stoner, 1966; Pinnas and Fitch, 1966).

The apparent differences in the results of these studies possibly can be explained by the current knowledge of the primary antibody response mechanism and interactions between lymphocytes. Several kinds of antigens elicit primary antibody responses that require the presence of two separate classes of lymphocytes; one class is derived from the bone marrow ("B" cells), and the other is derived from the thymus ("T" cells). Although the exact mechanism of the B cell–T cell interaction is unknown, it has been established that the interaction is synergistic (Claman, Chaperon, and Triplett, 1966a, b; Miller and Mitchell, 1968; Mitchell and Miller, 1968). Furthermore, it may be found that, in addition to the two types of lymphoid cells, the initiation of the immune response may require a third "accessory" cell, as is indicated by *in vitro* experiments on the immune response (Mosier *et al.*, 1970; Haskill, Byrt, and Marbrook, 1970; Shortma *et al.*, 1970; Osoba, 1970). Many antigens are dependent upon the interaction between T cells and B cells for the induction of the immune response. However, while there are other antigens which have not been demonstrated to depend upon T cells (Law *et al.*, 1964; Humphrey *et al.*, 1964; Fahey *et al.*, 1965; Taylor, 1969), recent reports question the T cell independence of these antigens (Unanue, 1970; Kruger and Gershon, 1971). Thus, the various types of primary antibody responses reported with neonatally thymectomized animals may be a result of the nature of the antigens; *i.e.*, the antibody response was related to the antigen's dependence on or independence of the thymus-derived lymphocyte. In addition, even in animals thymectomized at birth there is the possibility that a few thymus-derived cells had "seeded" other organs or the circulating pool of lymphocytes prior to thymectomy.

Unlike mammals, the chicken has a distinct separation of the thymus-dependent system and the thymus-independent system. Antibody production in neonatally thymectomized chickens was normal (Warner and Szenberg, 1962; Graetzner *et al.*, 1963; Warner and Szenberg, 1964), while bursectomy was associated with a high degree of impairment of the antibody responses (Miller and Osoba, 1967).

Conflicting reports are available concerning the ability of neonatally thymectomized mice to produce a secondary immune response. The primary response to sheep erythrocytes has been reported to be depressed, while the secondary response was nearly normal (Shewell, 1957). Other reports by Hess, Cottier, and Stoner (1963), Hess and Stoner (1966), and Basch (1966) indicate that the ability to produce an anamnestic response was more affected than was the primary response after neonatal thymectomy. John and Karlin (1971) recently reported that both thymocytes and bone marrow cells can possess immunologic memory. Under this supposition one would expect the anamnestic responses of neonatal thymectomized mice to be near normal if the animals could successfully mount a primary response.

The capability of neonatally thymectomized mice to synthesize immunoglobulins has been studied and there are conflicting reports which concern synthesis (Humphrey *et al.*, 1964; Arnason, deVaux St. Cyr, and Shaffner, 1964). However, the immunoglobulins of neonatally thymectomized mice appear to differ only quantitatively from those of normal mice; there was no qualitative differences in the immunoglobulins from normal and thymectomized mice, according to Miller and Osoba (1967). Synthesis of the IgG class of immunoglobulins appeared to be normal or slightly increased in neonatally thymectomized animals, but immunoglobulin catabolism sometimes appeared to be accelerated (Fahey, Barth, and Law, 1965).

In summary, it appears that antibody responses of neonatally thymectomized animals are influenced by the animal species, completeness of thymectomy, nature of the antigen, and immune response evaluation procedures. The primary antibody response was either normal or depressed, depending upon the system, and the anamnestic response was normal or reduced. Immunoglobulin levels are not dramatically altered by thymectomy, although there may be increased immunoglobulin anabolism and catabolism in some systems.

1.9 Effect upon cell-mediated immune response

The thymic system is responsible for the development of the small lymphocyte, which is intimately linked with the development and expression of cell-mediated immune reactions. Thus, there is considerable evidence that neonatal thymectomy impairs or inhibits the development and expression of cell-mediated immune reactions.

In animals which were thymectomized at birth, there was a marked impairment in their capacity to reject skin grafts, regardless of the magnitude in histocompatibility differences between the donor and recipient (Miller, 1961; Miller, Marshall and White, 1962; Good and Gabrielsen, 1964; Sherman *et al.*, 1964; Fisher and Fisher, 1965; Goedbloed and Vos, 1965). The grafts usually remained intact until the death of the animals, which most frequently was due to wasting disease. This impairment was evident in neonatally thymectomized chickens (Warner and Szenberg,

1962; Jankovic *et al.*, 1963; Aspinall *et al.*, 1963; Vojtiskova, Masnerova, and Viklicky, 1963; Vojtiskova and Nouza, 1965). However neonatally thymectomized puppies rejected renal homografts (Fisher *et al.*, 1965).

In mice, the severity of immunologic deficiency decreases as the time between birth and thymectomy increases. Thymectomy within the 1st week of life resulted in impairment of homograft immunity only when histocompatibility differences between the donor and recipient were minimal (Good *et al.*, 1962; Miller, 1962a, b, 1965a; Dalmasso *et al.*, 1963). A slight deficiency was detected in mice thymectomized at 35 days of age.

Generally, the ability to produce delayed hypersensitivity reactions, to develop autoallergic encephalomyelitis, to develop allergic thyroiditis, and to develop lethal hypersensitivity reactions is depressed in neonatally thymectomized animals. Neonatal thymectomy also renders animals more susceptible to tumor transplants. Cells from lymphoid organs of neonatally thymectomized animals are less efficient in inducing graft-*versus*-host reactions, and animals thymectomized as neonates are more susceptible to graft-*versus*-host reactions. For greater detail in this area refer to a review by Miller and Osoba (1967). Thus, it is evident that neonatal thymectomy results in a severe impairment of cell-mediated immune reactions in animals in which thymus-dependent lymphoid development is not well advanced at birth.

In summary, it may be concluded that if thymectomy is performed before the lymphoid tissues are well developed, there will be a severe impairment of those immune responses which depend upon thymus-derived or thymus-controlled cells either for sensitization or manifestation. The influence of neonatal thymectomy on the primary and secondary antibody responses is debatable and may to a large extent be dependent upon the animal species and the nature of the antigen. Further experimental evidence is needed to elucidate the dependency of various types of antigens on the thymus-derived and/or bone marrow-derived cells. In contrast to the influence of neonatal thymectomy on antibody responses, it is obvious that neonatal thymectomy severely reduces the population of small lymphocytes in the circulating pool, lymphocytic fields of the lymph nodes, and periarteriolar lymphocyte sheaths of the spleen. The bulk of experimental evidence also indicates that neonatal thymectomy severely impairs the cell-mediated immune responses. The majority of experiments which involved thymectomy of animals after the neonatal period or as adults apparently were of too short a duration to produce severe immunologic impairment. Longer term experiments indicate that the development of thymus-dependent tissue stops with thymectomy and that these tissues usually degenerate with time. The evidence appears to indicate that impairment of the immune responses will occur in animals thymectomized as adults if sufficient time elapses between thymectomy and response evaluation. Further experimentation is needed to elucidate this area.

2   Disorders of the Thymus Gland and Thymus Transplantation in Man

Julian L. Ambrus and Clara M. Ambrus

2.1 Normal functions of the thymus

Most of our current knowledge of the normal function and disorders of the thymus gland has been accumulated during the last decade. Much of this originated from clinical observations of "experiments of nature." Nevertheless, this knowledge has not yet made major inroads into the practice of medicine. Thymectomy and thymus transplantation are still considered experimental procedures, and hormonal thymic factor isolates have not yet reached the stage of clinical investigation. This review will briefly summarize clinical aspects of thymic disorders and discuss current studies on their treatment.

Table 2.1 summarizes some of the suggested physiologic functions of the thymus and disorders related to thymic deficiencies. In the past, the thymus was considered part of the lymphoid system and/or an endocrine gland. Yet classical endocrinologic methods of organ ablation and injection of organ extracts contributed little to the understanding of its physiologic functions. Only recently was it discovered that the thymus performs its major function on imparting immunologic competence at a definite species- and strain-specific time in embryonic or neonatal life (Miller, 1961; Archer and Pierce, 1961; Good *et al.*, 1962). Only if immunologically competent cells are destroyed by disease, radiation, antilymphocyte serum, or drugs is the thymus required for immunologic regeneration (Miller, 1962c; Cross, Leuchars, and Miller, 1964; Jeejeebhoy, 1965; Monaco, Wood, and Russell, 1965; Davis, Tyan, and Cole, 1964). In most cases of this type of injury the thymus itself is impaired and recovery depends upon the immigration of stem cells of bone marrow origin (Takada *et al.*, 1969a, b; 1970a, b; 1971a, b, c).

Table 2.1. Clinical syndromes related to thymus dysplasia

Normal functions of the thymus	Pathologic manifestations of deficiency or excess
Development of immunologic competence	Immunologic deficiency syndromes
Regeneration of immunologic competence	Autoimmune diseases
Maintenance of immunologic competence	Neoplasia related to lack of immune surveillance
Regulation of the peripheral lymphoid system	
Bone marrow-stimulating factor production	Thymoma, agammaglobulinemia with erythroid aplasia
Regulation of sex-related endocrine activity	
Hypoglycemic factor production	Hypoglycemia in leukemias
Permeability factor production	Delayed hypersensitivity reactions
Neuromuscular transmission, inhibitory factor production	Myasthenia gravis

Several authors reported that immune deficiency became evident in adult mice 6 months or later after thymectomy (Taylor, 1965; Jeejeebhoy, 1965; Metcalf, 1965; Miller, 1965c), suggesting that the available pool of immunologically competent cells becomes exhausted as lymphoid cells completed their life-span and that the thymus contributes to the maintenance of immunologic competence even in adult life. Studies with thymic extracts in various stages of purification suggest that the immune functions of the thymus are based at least in part on humoral factors (DeSomer, Denys, and Leyten, 1963; Trainin *et al.*, 1966; Takada *et al.*, 1970b; Goldstein *et al.*, 1966; Law and Agnew, 1968; Goldstein and White, 1970a,b). These factors are reviewed in more detail by Luckey and by Trainin in this book; the review includes their own studies. In addition, emigration of immunocompetent lymphocytes from the thymus into the peripheral lymphoid system may play an important immunologic role (Nossal, 1964; Harris and Ford, 1964; Davies *et al.*, 1966; Weissman, 1967).

Evidence was also presented by several investigators on the role of the thymus in regulating peripheral circulating and "sessile" lymphocyte levels (Roberts and White, 1949; Metcalf, 1956, 1960; Gowans and Knight, 1964; Parrot, Sousa, and East, 1966; Miller, 1967).

Goodman and Grubs (1970) and Goodman (1971) reviewed the evidence on interaction between thymocytes and bone marrow stem cells and suggested the existence of a thymic bone marrow-stimulating factor.

The endocrine functions of the thymus and its place in the immunologic "concert" of the body are discussed by Comsa elsewhere in this book, as is the thymic hypocalcemic factor by Mizutani. The latter may be related to parathyroid and thyroid calcitonin. Pansky, House, and Cone (1965) reported an insulin-like thymic hypoglycemic factor which may be related to the hypoglycemia seen in certain experimental and clinical leukemias. Lykke, Willoughby, and Kosche (1967) isolated a permeability-increasing factor from the thymus (TPF) related to the lymph node cell-produced permeability factor (LNPF) (Walters and Willoughby, 1965) and suggested that it may play a role in delayed hypersensitivity reactions.

Castleman and Norris (1949) reviewed the association of myasthenia gravis and pathologic changes in the thymus. A number of investigators reported neuromuscular blocking factors produced by the thymus (Adler, 1937; Torda and Wolff, 1944, 1947; Trethewie and Wright, 1944; Constant *et al.*, 1949a, b; Parkes and McKinna, 1967; Goldstein, 1968; Goldstein and Hoffman, 1968, 1969).*

2.2 Diseases of the thymus

Thymic hypoplasia and immunologic deficiencies

Table 2.2 summarizes clinical syndromes of immunologic deficiency related to thymic dysplasia; Table 2.3 summarizes immunologic deficiencies in which the thymus is apparently functional. Figure 2.1 depicts a hypothesis on the origin of the most important disorders.

The thymus is derived from the embryonic third bronchial cleft. Developmental anomalies may result in athymia alone or in combined deficiencies with other structures of related embryonic origins (parathyroid gland, aortic arch) producing the several varieties of Di George's syndrome. The bone marrow contributes stem cells in embryonic life and, possibly, in postnatal life as well, particularly after thymic injury (Takada *et al.*, 1969a, b, 1970, 1971a, b, c). Deficient stem cell production and/or delivery to the thymus may result in inadequate development of lymphoid elements of the thymus. Stem cell deficiency involving myeloid elements and stem cells which may become the precursors of the bursa-equivalent cells, as well as thymic stem cells, results in the reticular dysgenesis

---

*Foldes could not repeat some of these experiments (personal communication, 1972).

Table 2.2. Immunologic deficiency syndromes with thymic dysplasia

Syndrome	Heredity	Thymus	Immunity			Lympho-cytes	Other and occasional features	References
			Humoral	Cellular	Immune globulins			
Reticular dysgenesis		Hypo-plasia	Defic.	Defic.	Defic.	Low	Leukopenia	deVaal et al., 1959; Gitlin et al., 1964
DiGeorge syndrome (III and IV pharyngeal pouch syndrome)		Absent	Normal	Defic.	Normal	Normal and low	Lack of parathyroid, aortic arch, and cardiac anomalies	Cameron, 1965; DiGeorge et al., 1967; Dische, 1968
Swiss type agamma-globulinemia and combined types	Austosomal recessive (also a sex-linked form?)	Hypo-plasia	Severe Defic.	Absent or defic.	Defic.	Very low	Dyschondro-plasia, ulcerative colitis	Glanzman et al., 1950; Hitzig et al., 1968; Tobler et al., 1958; Rosen et al., 1966
Thymic alym-phoplasia (Gitlin)	Sex-linked recessive (males only)	Hypo-plasia	Defic.	Absent or defic.	Defic.	Low		Gitlin et al., 1963; Giedion et al., 1957; Gilbert et al., 1964

Disease	Inheritance	Thymus				Associated features	References
Nezelof's disease	Autosomal recessive	Hypoplasia	Normal or slight defic.	Defic.	Normal or slight defic.	Low		Nezelof et al., 1964
Ataxia-telangiectasia (Louis-Bar syndrome)	Autosomal recessive	Hypoplasia	Mild defic.	Defic. (some antigens)	Normal or mild defic. (low IgA)	Variable	Cerebellar ataxia, telangiectases, lymphomas, dyschondroplasia, endocrine abnormalities, neutropenia	Louis-Bar, 1941; Border et al., 1958; Peterson et al., 1964
Agammaglobulinemia with thymoma		Spindle cell tumor	Defic.	Defic.	Low	Low	Eosinopenia, red cell aplasia, diarrhea	Comings, 1965; Kirk et al., 1967; Peterson et al., 1965; Wolf et al., 1963, Fudenberg et al., 1962

Table 2.3. Immunologic deficiency syndromes without severe thymic dysplasia

Syndrome	Heredity	Thymus	Immunity		Immuno-globulins	Lympho-cytes	Other and occasional features	References
			Humoral	Cellular				
Infantile sex-linked Bruton-type agamma-globulinemia	X-linked	Normal	Defic.	Normal	Defic.	Normal	Defic. germinal centers of lymph nodes, plasma cell deficiency	Soothill, 1968; Gabrielson et al., 1969
Wiskott-Aldrich syndrome	X-linked	Normal	none to carbo-hydrate membrane antigens	Defic.	Decreased IgM	Decreased	Thrombo-cytopenia, eczema, lymphomas, defic. antigen processing by macrophages	Wiskott, 1937; Aldrich et al., 1954
Transient anti-body defic-iency of infancy	Familial	Normal	Defic.	Normal	Defic.	Normal	Plasma cell defic. spontane-ous cures	Rosen et al., 1966
Antibody deficiency with spleno-megaly	Familial	Normal	Defic.	Normal	Defic.	Normal	Plasma cell defic. spleno-megaly, lymph-adenopathy	Davis et al., 1967; Schwartz et al., 1969; Kushner et al., 1960; Troggis et al., 1961

Disorder	Genetic/Clinical notes						Clinical features	References
Antibody deficiency with elevated IgM (Type I dysgammaglobulinemia)	a) early onset x-linked form, and b) late onset form in both sexes	Normal	Defic.	Normal	Defic. IgG and IgA; normal or increased IgM	Defic. or normal	Hemolytic anemia, neutropenia, thrombocytopenia, aplastic anemia	Goldman et al., 1967; Stiehm et al., 1966
Antibody deficiency without immunoglobulin deficiency		Normal	Defic.	Normal	Normal	Normal		Blecher et al., 1968
Antibody deficiency with normal IgG levels		Normal	Defic.	Normal	IgG normal, IgA and IgM defic.	Normal		Gilbert et al., 1964
Antibody deficiency with decreased IgM levels	Familial	Normal	Defic.	Normal	IgM defic.	Normal	Eczema, steatorrhea	Stoclinga et al., 1969; Hobbs et al., 1967; Buckley et al., 1968
Isolated IgA deficiency	Some patients show abnormalities of chromosome Ig	Normal	Normal	Normal	IgA defic.	Normal	Often no infectious complications, mental retardation, thyroiditis	Rockey et al., 1964; Bachman, 1965; Ruvalcaba et al., 1969

(Cont'd)

Table 2.3. (*Continued*)

Syndrome	Heredity	Thymus	Immunity Humoral	Immunity Cellular	Immuno-globulins	Lympho-cytes	Other and occasional features	References
Antibody deficiency with nodular lymphoid hyperplasia of the intestines		Normal	Defic.	Normal	Defic.	Normal	Diarrhea, g.i. neoplasms, anemias, plasma cell defic.	Hermans *et al.*, 1966; Kirkpatrick *et al.*, 1968
Hypogammaglobulinemic sprue		Normal	Normal	Normal	Low IgA	Normal	Steatorrhea, plasma cell defic.	Crabbe *et al.*, 1967; Bull *et al.*, 1968
Immunologic deficiency with lymphocytotoxic factors	Autosomal recessive	Normal	Defic.	Defic.	Variable	Low (episodic)	Eczema	Kretchmer *et al.*, 1969
Congenital rubella syndrome		Normal	Defic.	Normal	Increased IgM; decreased IgG and IgA	Low	Plasma cell defic., no lymphoid follicles	Schimke *et al.*, 1969

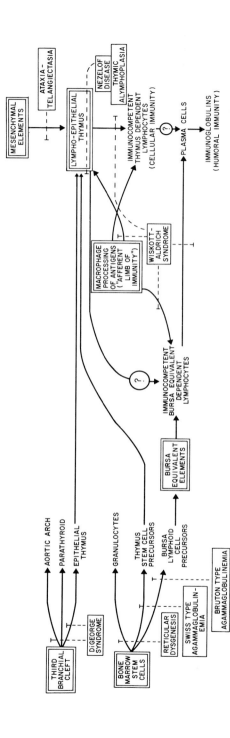

Fig. 2.1. Hypothetical origin of important immune disorders.

syndrome. These infants lack cellular and humoral immune mechanisms, as well as phagocytic cells. They usually die within a few months of birth from intercurrent infections. If the stem cell block involves only the thymic and bursa-equivalent elements, the several varieties of Swiss type agammaglobulinemia develop. Block at the bursa-equivalent stem cell level only is responsible for Bruton type agammaglobulinemia, where humoral immunity is lacking but cellular immunity is adequate.

Louis-Bar syndrome, ataxia-telangiectasia, is determined by an autosomal recessive gene. There appears to be a generalized developmental failure of mesenchymal elements which is responsible for inadequate development of the thymus, degeneration of Purkinje cells, cerebellar atrophy, abnormalities of blood vessels (including telangiectases), endocrine abnormalities (including gonadal hypoplasia), and others. Auerbach (1961) showed that organized *in vitro* development of mouse embryo thymic rudiment depends upon induction by mesenchymal elements.

In the sex-linked Wiskott-Aldrich syndrome, at an early stage, accumulation of thymus-dependent lymphocytes in peripheral lymphoid tissue, development of germinal centers, and plasma cells are all normal. With time, however, lymphocyte depletion occurs in the circulation and thymus-dependent (cortical) areas of lymph follicles. There is also impairment of humoral immunity; yet the thymus and intestinal lymphoid elements appear to be intact, and immunoglobulins are produced in response to certain antigens. The suggestion was made by Cooper *et al.* (1968) and others that this may be a disorder of the afferent limb of immunity; there may be a defect in the processing of certain antigens by macrophages, and thus there is the impairment of both cellular and selective humoral immunity in spite of apparently normal thymic and bursa-equivalent structures.

In thymic alymphoplasia and in Nezelof's disease there is inadequate development of the lymphoid elements of the thymus. The former syndrome is sex linked recessive, and the latter is autosomal recessive.

Maintenance therapy of the immunodeficiency syndromes is difficult. Periodic weekly to monthly injections of immunoglobulin preparations are helpful. Unfortunately, available preparations contain only IgG; no usable IgM or IgA preparations have been made available. For this reason, several authors prefer the use of whole human plasma. To avoid serum hepatitis, a few Australia antigen-free, clinically proven donors are recommended for plasmaphoresis. Thymus and bone marrow transplantation is discussed later.

Autoimmune diseases

Many autoimmune diseases appear to be based on reactions of the delayed hypersensitivity type (Doniach and Roitt, 1962), which in turn are dependent on thymic function as described above. In this section we will not deal with myasthenia gravis, which has both autoimmune and humoral relationships to thymic function; it will be discussed in the next section.

Burnet (1959) proposed that, in the thymus, developing lymphocyte clones are screened out and eliminated if they are potentially able to react with "self" antigens ("forbidden clones"). Failure of this screening function of the thymus results in autoimmune diseases. Howe, Goldstein, and Battisto (1970) reported that thymocytes from newborn mice can recognize antigens of isogenic spleens, as measured by blast formation and mitosis *in vitro*. This capacity is rapidly lost with increasing age.

It is widely held that autoimmunity can be induced by changed antigenicity in a group of cells because of mutation, alteration by chemicals or viruses, or introduction of a foreign antigen with determinant groupings resembling certain host antigens. For example, *Escherichia coli* 014 has cross-reacting antigens with colon tissue and may play a role in ulcerative colitis (Perlmann *et al.*, 1965). These mechanisms, however, are unlikely to explain the constant levels of autoantibodies found over a period of years in certain cases of chronic thyroiditis, atrophic gastritis, or idiopathic autoimmune adrenal failure. In systemic lupus erythematosus, the titers of antinuclear antibodies fluctuate, but they are usually present over long periods of time. The most likely explanation for persistent autoimmunity is a genetically determined mechanism. Failure of thymic and/or bursa-equivalent regulatory functions is probably involved.

Morphologic changes were found in the thymus (including enlargement and appearance of germinal centers) in a wide spectrum of autoimmune and related diseases, including thyrotoxicosis (Mackay, 1966, Gunn, Michie, and Irvine, 1964), Hashimoto's thyroiditis (Irvine and Sumerling, 1965), idiopathic Addison's disease (Irvine, Stewart, and Scarth, 1967), and systemic lupus erythematosus (Goldstein and Mackay, 1965).

In the NZB strain of mice, autoimmune hemolytic anemia is common; the F_1 hybrids of NZW mice often have a lupus erythematosus-like disease. These disorders are associated with morphologic abnormalities of the thymus, including the appearance of germinal centers (Burnet and Holmes, 1964).

Myasthenia gravis

In about 10% of the patients with myasthenia gravis, thymomas are present; conversely, 15 to 30% of the patients with thymoma suffer from myasthenia gravis. Of the patients without neoplastic thymic lesions, 70% exhibit thymic changes resembling those of autoimmune diseases and 20% have morphologically normal thymuses (Castleman and Norris, 1949). Burnet and Holmes (1964) considered the germinal centers which appear in the thymus of patients with myasthenia gravis and other autoimmune disorders as the site of "forbidden clone" production. Others thought of the germinal centers as sites of antigen-antibody reactions and as an expression, together with the appearance of significant numbers of thymic plasma cells, of autoimmune thymitis (Goldstein, 1966).

In 30% of the patients with myasthenia gravis, autoantibodies were demonstrated by the indirect fluorescent antibody-localization technique against skeletal muscle A band striations and against thymic epithelial cell cytoplasms (Strauss et al., 1965). Goldstein (1966) suggested that thymoma initiates an autoimmune response resulting in thymitis. Strauss et al. (1965) demonstrated a myoid antigen in thymomas related to muscular A band antigens. These authors suggested that in addition a humoral neuromuscular blocking substance is released from the diseased thymus (Strauss et al., 1966). Goldstein (1968) isolated a factor (termed *thymin*) from bovine thymuses which upon repeated, but not single, injections produced neuromuscular block in guinea pigs. Goldstein and Hofmann (1969) suggested that small amounts of thymin may be released from the thymus even under normal conditions.

Thymomas and the relationship of the thymus to other neoplastic diseases

Primary thymomas (benign or malignant), thymic involvement of lymphomas, leukemias, and metastatic carcinomas often produce various systemic disorders. In patients with thymomas, autoimmune myositis, myocarditis, dermatomyositis, systemic lupus erythematosus, bullous dermatitis, rheumatoid arthritis, scleroderma, and Sjogren's disease have been reported (Klein et al., 1964; Larsson, 1963; Kough and Barnes, 1964; Beutner et al., 1968; Birch et al., 1964; Lattes, 1962). Small cell carcinoma of the thymus often produces an ACTH-like substance and Cushing's syndrome (Cohn, Toll, and Castelman, 1960). The relationship of autoimmune thymitis and thymoma to the release of a thymic neuromuscular blocking agent and myasthenia gravis has been discussed above. In a number of cases with thymoma, erythroid hypoplasia develops (Hirst and Robertson, 1967). This may be due to the release of an erythropoiesis-depressing factor, to decreased production of an erythropoiesis-stimulating factor (Goodman and Grubs, 1970), or to autoimmune processes. The relationship of thymomas to immunologic deficiencies has been discussed.

Association was observed between autoimmune diseases, thymic lesions, and malignancies (Fudenberg, 1966; Damashek, 1966). Neoplastic diseases may be a consequence of loss of immunologic surveillance, which normally eliminates most mutant cell clones. In patients subjected to prolonged immunosuppression by drugs and/ or antilymphocyte sera prior and subsequent to organ transplantation, a significant incidence of neoplasms was noted (Doak et al., 1968; Balner, 1970; Starzl et al. 1968). Eilber and Morton (1970) found a correlation between the ability of cancer patients to develop dermal sensitization and delayed hypersensitivity reactions to 2,4-dinitrochlorobenzene (DNCB) and prognosis of the malignant disease. On the other hand, thymic deficiency induced by neoplastic involvement may be responsible for loss of immunologic defense against both neoplastic cells and superinfections. This may be aggravated by radiation and/or chemotherapy. Loss of cellular immunity has been demonstrated in lymphoid leukemia (Shaw et al., 1960; Cone and Uhr, 1964) and Hodgkin's disease (Casazza, Duval, and Carbone, 1966; Aisenberg, 1962, 1966; Sokal and Primilarios, 1961; Sokal and Aungst, 1969).

At the time when "status thymico-lymphaticus" was considered to be a disease entity and to be responsible for sudden deaths, particularly under anesthesia, radiation therapy of enlarged thymuses in infancy was widely practiced (Keynes, 1954). A high incidence of thymic tumors developed in this population (Simpson, Hempelmann, and Fuller, 1955; Simpson and Hempelmann, 1957; Pifer et al., 1968). Other authors (Janower and Miettinen, 1971) found an increased breast cancer rate in a similar population.

2.3 The thymus in extrathymic disorders

In addition to the autoimmune, neoplastic, and immunodeficiency diseases discussed above, changes occur in the thymus in a number of other disease states. Thymic involution is caused by increased levels of corticosteroids in stress, and thus is present in almost every serious illness.

Thymic changes include loss of thymic cortex, cystic changes of the Hassall bodies, and aggregates of spindle-shaped epithelial cells in the medulla (Goldstein and Mackay, 1967; Boyd, 1932). Plasma cells are often found in the thymus in septicemias and bacterial or antigenic penetration of the thymus (Goldstein, 1966).

2.4 Therapeutic thymectomy and thymus transplantation

Thymectomy has been tried in many clinical conditions, yet it remains a procedure that is controversial in some disorders and experimental in others. The first thymectomy for myasthenia and Grave's disease was performed by Sauerbruch in 1911 (Schumacher and Roth, 1912). Andrus and Foot reported in 1927 that thymectomy in a patient with myasthenia gravis was the first known case in which the patient survived. A reliable surgical technique was established, and the first series of thymectomies in myasthenia gravis was reported by Blalock (1944; Blalock et al., 1941; Harvey, Lilienthal, and Talbot, 1942). Of 20 cases, two with thymoma, four patients died, 13 showed objective improvement, and three showed subjective improvement. Best results were obtained in patients with a duration of myasthenia gravis of less than one year. Following these publications, several larger series were reported (Viets, 1945, 1950, 1960; Keynes, 1946, 1949, 1954; Harvey, 1948; Eaton, Clagett, and Bastron, 1942, 1950, 1953, 1955; Ferguson, Hutchinson, and Liversedge, 1955, 1962; Simpson, 1956, 1958; Schwab and Viets, 1960; Kreel et al., 1960; Kreel et al., 1967; Perlo et al., 1966). The general consensus developed that although thymectomy has a significant surgical mortality (1–8%), it results in improvement in a large number of patients (10–70%); the results were better in females than in males, better in younger patients, and better in patients with short duration of the disease. Surgery is recommended also on the basis that a significant number of the patients were found to have malignant and invasive thymomas. Failure of significant benefits in a number of patients was attributed to irreversible myopathy as shown by persistent electromyographic abnormalities and failure to respond to neostigmine. The question was also raised whether ectopic thymic tissue not removed during surgery could be involved. In thymoma cases both pre- and post-operative X-ray therapy has been advocated (Keynes 1954, 1955; Viets and Schwab, 1960; Kreel et al., 1967).

Preventive thymectomy was found to decrease the incidence of "spontaneous" (virus induced) leukemia in AKR, RIL, and C58 mice (McEndy,

Boon, and Furth, 1944; Law and Miller, 1950a), carcinogen induced leukemia in DBA mice (Law and Miller, 1950b) and X-ray induced leukemia in C56 mice (Kaplan, 1947, 1966; Kaplan, Brown, and Paul, 1953); thymus grafts restored susceptibility, but grafts in millipore chambers or thymic extracts were unsuccessful. It was thought that the thymus might provide the proper environment for the action of certain carcinogenic factors such as viruses. Based on this rationale, thymectomy was explored in human leukemias and lymphomas and generally was found to be unsuccessful (Earle, Reilly, and Dean, 1951; Dean, Earle, and Reilly, 1951; Soutter and Emerson, 1960; Gotoff, 1968; Patey, 1963).

Thymectomy has been attempted in a number of autoimmune diseases. In autoimmune hemolytic anemia of children, two apparent cures were reported following thymectomy (Wilmers and Russel, 1963; Karaklis et al., 1964). However, in adults with systemic lupus erythematosus and rheumatoid arthritis (Mackay, Goldstein, and McConchie, 1963; Mackay and Smalley, 1966; Milne et al., 1967), the results were disappointing.

Thymectomy was performed as an immunosuppressive measure in connection with organ transplantation. Insufficient data are available at this time for evaluation (Strazl et al., 1965).

Table 2.4 summarizes the literature on thymus transplantation in genetic and acquired immune deficiency states. Apart from a few cases of DiGeorge syndrome and Swiss type agammaglobulinemia, there was no evidence of permanent take of the graft. Thymic transplantation was undertaken in acquired immunologic incompetence due to neoplastic diseases (Hodgkin's disease, mycosis fungoides) in order to explore the practical value of the transplant in clinical medicine. In these diseases, immunologic impairment results partly from the disease process itself and partly from the bone marrow and lymphoid system depression due to radiation and/or chemotherapy (Sokal and Primikirios, 1961; Sokal and Aungst, 1969; Aisenberg, 1962). Aggressive treatment may eliminate the majority of neoplastic cells, but it will also destroy whatever immunologic antitumor defense may be present. In this state, thymic transplantation may restore cellular immunity and help in the elimination of the remaining tumor cells. Following regeneration of the immune system the transplanted thymus may be rejected. Embryonic thymus has been transplanted into 35 patients with Hodgkin's disease with deficient cellular immunity after intensive chemotherapy (30 have been observed for adequate periods of time) and into two patients with mycosis fungoides. Persistence of the graft was demonstrated by repeat biopsies for 22 and 224 days. A series of delayed hypersensitivity reactions was performed

Table 2.4. Transplantation in genetic and acquired immune deficiency states in man

Disease; donor; organ transplanted	No. of patients	No. of transplants	Immunologic reconstitution		Graft-vs.-host reaction	References
			Immediate	Long range		
Swiss type agamma-globulinemia						
Embryonic donors						
Thymus	11	16 ⎫	7	2	4	Allibone *et al.*, 1964; DeKoning *et al.*, 1969; Dooren *et al.*, 1968; Good *et al.*, 1969; Harboe *et al.*, 1966; Hitzig, *et al.*, 1960; Hong *et al.*, 1968; Rosen *et al.*, 1966, 1969 (unpublished).
Lymphoid tissue, liver	10	14 ⎭				
Postnatal donors						
Thymus	3	3	1	0	1	Rosen *et al.*, 1966, 1969; Bethenod *et al.*, 1966; Gitlin *et al.*, 1963
Blood	11	11	1	0	9	Allibone *et al.*, 1964; Dooren *et al.*, 1968; Hathaway *et al.*, 1965, 1966, 1967; Hitziq *et al.*, 1968; Hong *et al.*, 1968; Meuwissen, 1968; Rosen *et al.*, 1966, 1969
Bone marrow	9	9	5	2	7	DeKoning *et al.*, 1969; Dooren *et al.*, 1969; Good *et al.*, 1969; Hathaway *et al.*, 1967; Kretschmer *et al.*, 1969; Miller, 1967; O'Connell *et al.*, 1966; Rosen *et al.*, 1966: 1969

Disease / Donor					References
Compatible bone marrow	4	5	4	2	DeKoning et al., 1969; Good et al., 1969; Kretschmer et al., 1969; Rosen et al., 1969
DiGeorge syndrome Embryonic donors Thymus	2	2	2	0	August et al., 1968: 1970; Cleveland et al., 1968
Ataxia telangliectasia Embryonic donors Thymus and spleen	5	7	5	0	Goya et al., 1967: 1968
Combined defects Embryonic donors Thymus	2	5	1	0	Levy et al., 1971; Hong et al., unpublished, 1971
Hodgkin's disease Embryonic donors Thymus	30	30	21	0	Stutzman et al., 1971
Thymus and bone marrow	1	1	1	1	Kersey et al., 1971
Mycosis fungoides Embryonic donors Thymus	2	3	2	0	Stutzman et al., 1971; Ambrus et al., unpublished, 1971

periodically in these patients. In the patients with Hodgkin's disease, about one-half exhibited conversion to a positive skin test in one test or more. Before transplantation 15% of all skin tests were positive; this rose to 39% after transplantation. Reversion to pretransplant levels occurred after about 6 months. In a number of patients, low reactivity of lymphocytes to phytohemagglutinin (PHA) stimulation *in vitro* showed improvement after thymic transplantation. Of the two patients with mycosis fungoides, both showed improvement of cellular immunity after thymus transplantation. Signs of systemic disease (hepatosplenomegaly, lymphadenopathy) disappeared in one patient, and skin lesions markedly improved. This improvement was temporary. In relapse, the graft was biopsied and was found to be rejected. At this time a second thymus was implanted, but without clinical improvement (Stutzman, Mittleman, Ohkochi, and Ambrus, 1971; Ambrus, Klein, and Stutzman, unpublished; Mittleman and Ambrus, unpublished). Thymus transplantation in these conditions is obviously of only temporary benefit. Once preparations of nonantigenic thymic humoral factors become available, the hypothesis described above can be more adequately tested.

2.5 Conclusions

After many years of obscurity, the thymus has emerged as an organ of major physiologic significance in regulating the development of immunologic competence, in the regeneration of the immune system, and possibly in the maintenance of immunologic competence, particularly concerning cellular immunity. In addition, the thymus may regulate proliferation of the peripheral lymphoid system and bone marrow stem cells and may influence humoral immunity. A great deal of evidence has accumulated to suggest that many of these functions may be accomplished through humoral mediators. Isolation and identification of these substances and their eventual availability for clinical purposes may represent a major addition to our therapeutic armamentarium. In addition, the thymus may play a part in the endocrine "concert", particularly in the regulation of neuromuscular transmission, calcium and glucose metabolism, phenomena of inflammation, and sex-related endocrine activity.

Developmental anomalies and acquired disorders of the thymus are responsible for a number of immunologic deficiency diseases and may be involved in autoimmune diseases and neoplastic processes related to impairment of immune surveillance.

Myasthenia gravis is an interesting example of the complex role the thymus may play in disease states. In this condition, autoimmunity against skeletal muscle and thymic epithelial cells may play a role (thymus and muscle A bands may share antigens). Neuromuscular blocking agents released from the thymus in large quantities in thymitis, thymic neoplasms, or both may also be involved in the pathophysiology of this disease. Thymic neoplasms may initiate autoimmune processes involving muscle and may result in thymitis, which in turn may contribute to the release of neuromuscular blocking substances.

Thymectomy was investigated in a number of autoimmune diseases (particularly in myasthenia gravis) and as an auxiliary method of immune suppression in connection with organ transplantation. Further studies are needed for the evaluation of this approach. The possible therapeutic value of specific antithymic antibodies has not yet been explored in clinical investigation.

Thymus transplantation was used in a limited number of cases of immune deficiency disorders (we are aware of 23 reported cases) and in 33 patients suffering from impaired immunologic competence due to neoplastic diseases and to subsequent radiation and chemotherapy. Although a few encouraging cases were reported, this approach is still experimental. It also suffers from the general problems of organ transplantation studies, including availability of viable organs and histocompatibility factors. A major hope in this area is the eventual availability of synthetic thymic humoral factors.

The thymus may represent a favorable environment for certain carcinogenic factors, such as oncogenic viruses (at least in rodents) and ionizing radiations.

Secondary neoplastic invasion of the thymus may contribute to loss of immune competence, as for example in lymphomas. Thymic involution by increased levels of endogenous or iatrogenic corticosteroids is an important feature of almost all serious illness ("stress reaction"). This may represent a defense system for the prevention of the development of autoimmunity related to the presence of modified tissue antigens (by injury, infection, or other factors).

Acknowledgment

Original studies by the authors were supported in part by National Institutes of Health, General Clinical Center Grant 1 M01-RROO-262-2.

Addendum

In a recent paper, Vessey and Doll (1972) studied 386 patients undergoing thymectomy for myasthenia gravis at four London hospitals during the years 1942–64. These patients were followed until the end of 1967. Five of the patients died from extrathymic tumors; from the national experience 5.5 were expected to die. An additional five patients developed nonfatal extrathymic tumors during the same period. It was originally believed that prenatal or neonatal thymectomy would eliminate "immunological surveillance" and thus increase sensitivity to neoplastic processes. On the other hand, thymectomy in adult rodents was thought to have no important effect on immunologic competence. It was shown subsequently that adult thymectomy is followed by a gradual decline in immunologic competence which becomes apparent only after a period of 6–9 months, a quarter to a half of the animal's life span (Miller, 1965c; Metcalf, 1965; Taylor, 1965). Thymectomy was shown to render mice more susceptible to the carcinogenic activity of oncogenic viruses and certain chemical carcinogens (Miller *et al.*, 1963; Gaugas *et al.*, 1969). It is likely that the adult thymus influences the development of populations of immunologically competent cells which are long lived and that defects in immune capacity become apparent only after this pool has been depleted. This may cause a loss of "immunological surveillance" and an increase in the effectiveness of carcinogenic factors. The fact that this conclusion was not supported by the clinical study described above may be related to the inadequate length of the follow-up (3–25 years) of most patients.

3   Thymus Substitution and HTH, the Homeostatic Thymus Hormone

J. Comsa

After thymectomy, the thymus gland may be replaced directly by a total gland equivalent in quantity to the amount left in a sham operation, by a fragment of the thymus, or even by a few cells of the thymus from either the animal being operated upon, animals of the same species, or animals of different species. Both allogenic and xenogenic grafts are active (reviewed by Hess, 1968). In such cases the host could receive both cells and a humoral factor from the thymus graft, or the lymphocytes of the host could migrate through the thymus for a contact factor. Implants of thymus remnants or the tissue remaining in subtotal thymectomy do not hypertrophy. However, the influence of the thymus does not parallel its size. Following a brief summary of thymus replacement, this chapter provides a review of thymus substitution by a variety of extracts. Although much of the early work is controversial, it eventually led to the development of current concepts, and it introduces the work of Comsa, which culminated in the isolation of a presumably pure (purified) hormone by Bernardi and Comsa (1965a).

3.1 Thymus grafts

In *Xenopus* tadpoles, the heterotrophic autograft of extirpated thymus immediately after thymectomy completely prevented the development of the thymoprivic condition (Harms, 1952a, b). In mice thymectomized at birth, implantation of a neonatal mouse thymus prevented the development of the thymoprivic condition and restored the immunologic functions (Miller, 1962b), even when the implant was enclosed in a diffusion chamber (Osoba and Miller, 1963). The latter work has been reviewed by Miller (1964b). Barclay (1964) indicates that early criticism of the pore

size used in the early work was met by obtaining the same positive response
with millipore diffusion chambers having a pore size of 3.0, 0.45, 0.1, and
0.01 μ. Thymic grafts also restored the development of leukemia in thymectomized mice (Kaplan *et al.*, 1953; Law and Miller, 1950a; Levinthal and
Buffett, 1961). Thymus grafts in chambers placed into intraperitoneal,
subcutaneous, or kidney subcapsular areas from either newborn or adult
donors seem equally effective; both syngeneic and allogeneic thymus implants were active in either neonatally thymectomized or adult irradiated
mice (Defendi and Metcalf, 1964).

Since the adult irradiated mouse provided with bone marrow and
thymus grafts will reject the thymus following acquisition of immune competence and retain antibody-producing capabilities, it is inferred that a
short exposure to thymic hormones provides adequate activity for a long
time. This confirms previous observations that a few days of exposure of
the neonatal mouse to thymic hormones is adequate to allow maturation
of antibody-forming cells. Extirpation of the thymus at 1 to 2 days in the
newborn mouse suppresses immune competence, whereas extirpation at
the 6th day or later does not. This concept is verified by the rapid disappearance of the homeostatic thymus hormone from lymph nodes and
spleen following thymectomy as detailed in the next chapter.

3.2 Early thymus extracts with proved substitutive action

The early methods proposed for the preparation of thymus extracts which
were not tested in thymectomized animals are summarized in Table 3.1.
Preparations which are capable of suppressing the consequences of
thymectomy (substitutive) are described throughout this book and are
summarized in the final chapter.

An aqueous extract of ground thymus previously extracted with acetone and ether and precipitated by saturation with ammonium sulfate
(method of Doris Asher, 1933) proved to be substitutive in thymectomized
guinea pigs (Comsa, 1940). The same extract restored normal growth in
rats reared on a poor diet without specific deficiencies (Asher and Landolt,
1934).

A crude preparation, a suspension of ground thymus made cell-free by
centrifugation, was found to be able to restore the development of lymphatic tissue in neonatally thymectomized mice (Metcalf, 1958). This preparation accelerated the development of lymphatic tissue in normal
mice.

Goldstein, Slater, and White (1966) homogenized thymus in saline. The

Table 3.1. Techniques for the preparation of crude thymic extracts

These are listed in order of increasing lipid solubility, with omission of materials detailed in this monograph.

Reference	Technique
Thurner, 1924	Homogenate boiled in saline, filtered
Metcalf, 1958	Suspension of mash in saline, boiled, filtered
Constant et al., 1949a, b	Suspension in saline
Beauvieux, 1963a, b	Suspension of thymocytes; cells destroyed ultrasonically
Goslar, 1958	Aqueous extract from thymus of calves injected before sacrifice with large amount of distilled water; method of extraction not described
Nitschke, 1929b	Suspension in dilute acetic acid; proteins discarded by isoelectric precipitation
Rowntree et al., 1934	Extraction with NaCl (0.028 M) at 68°C; precipitate discarded; supernatant adjusted to pH 3.5
Molnar and Kovacs, 1959	Agitated with 20% trichloracetic acid, filtered, evaporated to 1 ml/g fresh thymus; adjusted to pH 6.5, and filtered
Eskelund and Plum, 1953	Extracted with ethanol; ethanol evaporated; dissolved in ether, precipitated with acetone; suspended in saline for use
Torda and Wolff, 1947	Extracted with acetone, followed by ether
Wilson and Wilson, 1955	Extracted with acetone; acetone evaporated; residue extracted with saline; lyophilized
Bomskov and Holscher, 1942	Lipid-soluble extract; method approximately described in the text
Schneider, 1957	Extracted with acetone and ether successively; both extracts reunited; solvents evaporated; residue dissolved in acetone and cooled to precipitate impurities
Schwarz et al., 1953	Aqueous extract of thymus previously extracted with ether, lyophilized
Pausky et al., 1965	Acetone extracted
Szent-György et al., 1962	Extracted with methanol; purified with chloroform; precipitated as reineckate; chromatographed

activity was purified by centrifugation and acetone precipitation. The active fraction was purified by column chromatography on a polyacrylamide gel. It contained three major proteins. Details are provided in Chapter 7. The extraction and fractionation methods of other materials will be described in separate sections of this book.

3.3 Isolation of HTH, the homeostatic thymus hormone

Bezssonoff and Comsa (1958) extract thymus with M sulphuric acid (1 ml per g of ground thymus). Less soluble impurities are discarded following neutralization with ammonium hydroxide and half saturation with ammonium sulfate. The half saturation is calculated for the added liquid only, not for the total volume of liquid plus thymus. The active fraction is salted out by full saturation with ammonium sulfate. This precipitate is dissolved in 0.03 M hydrochloric acid. More impurities are precipitated by bringing the pH to 7.0 with ethanolic ammonia and adding 20% of ethanol. The active fraction is precipitated from the supernatant by bringing the pH to 6.2 with hydrochloric acid and raising the ethanol concentration to 66%.

The purified hormone preparation of Bernardi and Comsa (1965a, b) was isolated from the extract of Bezssonoff and Comsa by successive column chromatographies. a) The thymic extract of Bezssonoff and Comsa was dissolved in distilled water (1% solution) and passed through a Sephadex G-25 column. The active material was eluted with 0.001 M phosphate buffer (pH 6.8). This process increased the activity of the extract slightly. b) The eluate was charged onto a hydroxyapatite column and eluted with phosphate buffer successively at 0.001 M, 0.5 M, and 1.0 M. The elution is surveyed by automatic record of the optical density in ultraviolet light. The eluates were desalted by Sephadex chromatography and lyophilized.

Bioassay of these eluates with the method of Comsa (1953c) shows no detectable activity in the first two fractions. The activity of the initial extract is recovered in the third fraction. This material was homogeneous by two criteria and was named HTH, for homeostatic thymus hormone. One unit was determined to be equal to 1 μg of presumably pure HTH. Its constitution is under investigation.

3.4 Physical-chemical properties of HTH

The extract of Bezssonoff and Comsa is a slightly pink, odorless, tasteless powder. It dissolves readily in water and more readily in saline. The best solvent is 0.1 M potassium phosphate buffer at pH 6.75. It is soluble in 20% ethanol at pH 7. It dissolves in 0.01 M HCl and remains dissolved in this solvent when 2 volumes of ethanol are added. It precipitates at pH 6.2, not readily from aqueous solution but massively and instantly from 60%

ethanol. It is stable to heating at 60% for 30 min. Boiling for a few seconds appears to decrease its activity. It burns without residue. It contains no phosphorus and no -SH groups. With 0.001 M potassium phosphate buffer at pH 6.8, it is eluted without any fractionation from a Sephadex G-25 or G-50 column or from a DEAE-cellulose column. It precipitates on the top of a carboxymethylcellulose or amberlite column. It is strongly adsorbed by paper and thus not susceptible to paper electrophoresis.

The presumably pure fraction of Bernardi and Comsa (*i.e.*, HTH) is a white powder. Its solubility properties are those of the total extract. Its homogeneity was demonstrated a) by ultracentrifugation and b) by bio-assay. For the bioassay test, the HTH was eluted from a hydroxyapatite column and divided arbitrarily during elution into four subfractions, which were bioassayed separately with the method of Comsa (Bernardi and Comsa, 1965a, b). The activity (expressed in units per mg) divided by the optical density of all these subfractions gave the quotient 2.97. Its size was roughly estimated by means of ultracentrifugation at more than 1800 and less than 2500. Its chemical constitution is unknown. The first attempts of hydrolysis (G. Bernardi, unpublished) yielded amino acids, sugars, and aminated sugars. Its ultraviolet absorption spectrum is shown (Fig. 3.1). The solubility properties of HTH are identical to those of the thymus extract.

3.5 Physiologic properties of HTH

This section discusses the substitutive effect in thymectomized animals. The extract of Bezssonoff and Comsa and HTH given daily in subcutaneous injections suppressed completely the consequences of thymectomy in guinea pigs. For various purposes this experiment was performed more than one-thousand times with consistent results. No treated guinea pig wasted and died. An example of these experiments (Comsa, 1965d, e, f) is summarized.

One hundred six male guinea pigs aged 12 to 16 days, weighing 136 ± 9 g, were used. The thymus was extirpated in 98 animals. They were treated as follows: a) 24 animals were given daily injections of 100 μg (8 units) of the thymic extract of Bezssonoff and Comsa per 100 g of body weight; b) 24 animals were given daily injections of 8 μg (8 units) of HTH (isolated from the same sample of extract) per 100 g of body weight; c) 50 animals received daily an injection of 1 ml of physiologic saline, the solvent of the thymic preparations; and d) eight animals were untreated.

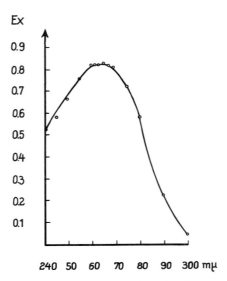

Fig. 3.1. Ultraviolet absorption spectrum of HTH. The spectrum was determined at pH 6.75 in 0.1 M potassium phosphate buffer containing 100 μg HTH/ml.

The daily weights of the 12 animals were kept for 45 days, as is summarized in Table 3.2. The weight gain of the saline-injected animals was only one-fourth that of animals given injections of total extract or HTH. HTH also protected the guinea pigs from the high mortality seen in the saline-injected control animals.

At regular intervals, four animals from each of the three groups were isolated for 24 hr in individual metabolic cages and the 24-hr creatine

Table 3.2. Weight in grams of thymectomized guinea pigs injected with thymic preparations (mean of four animals ± standard deviation)

Days after thymectomy	Total extract	HTH	Saline (controls)	No. of deaths in saline group
0	137 ± 4	133 ± 5	140 ± 4	0
5	156 ± 8	157 ± 7	141 ± 5	0
11	166 ± 3	177 ± 7	145 ± 6	1
18	189 ± 6	204 ± 5	149 ± 3	3
27	228 ± 4	232 ± 6	166 ± 7	7
35	247 ± 5	253 ± 4	172 ± 4	11
45	271 ± 6	274 ± 5	176 ± 5	3

excretion was determined (Table 3.3). Both the extract and HTH prevented the rise in urinary creatine noted in the saline-injected animals. Immediately afterward these animals were necropsied, and the following determinations were performed. a) Histologic examination of the thyroid (Helly, hematoxylin-eosin), of the testes, lymph nodes (Bouin, hematoxylin-eosin), and of the anterior pituitary revealed that administration of thymus extract of HTH to thymectomized guinea pigs completely prevented the previously described histologic changes of thyroid stimulation, the testes stimulation followed by degenerative changes, the lymph node atrophy, and the pituitary cellular changes described in my previous chapter which are uniformly noted in thymoprivic animals. Thymic extract injections also suppressed the excretion of urinary thyrotropic factor in

Table 3.3. Creatine excretion rate in thymectomized guinea pigs

The values are given as mg/100 g/24 hr and include the mean with standard deviation of four animals injected with total extract, HTH, or saline.

Days after thymec- tomy	Total extract	HTH	Saline
0	0.7 ± 0.08		
5	0.57 ± 0.17	0.49 ± 0.06	1.56 ± 0.28
11	0.69 ± 0.21	0.72 ± 0.08	2.08 ± 0.40
18	0.53 ± 0.16	0.67 ± 0.11	3.47 ± 0.15
27	0.73 ± 0.20	0.70 ± 0.18	2.99 ± 0.42
35	0.54 ± 0.14	0.56 ± 0.09	1.86 ± 0.51
45	0.60 ± 0.12	0.63 ± 0.07	1.09 ± 0.37

Table 3.4. Protein-bound serum iodine in thymectomized guinea pigs

Data are μg/100 serum with the mean and standard deviation of four animals injected with total extract, HTH, or saline.

Days after thymec- tomy	Total extract	HTH	Saline
0	5.81 ± 1.2		
5	7.90 ± 0.7	6.80 ± 0.6	9.80 ± 1.4
11	5.30 ± 1.2	5.80 ± 1.3	13.70 ± 2.1
18	4.90 ± 0.8	5.50 ± 1.0	16.30 ± 1.2
27	6.10 ± 1.1	4.70 ± 0.6	15.40 ± 1.7
35	5.20 ± 0.8	5.60 ± 0.8	11.70 ± 2.8
45	5.40 ± 0.6	5.00 ± 0.7	5.30 ± 1.6

thymectomized guinea pigs (Comsa, 1951b, c). b) The data presented in Table 3.4 show the consistent maintenance of low levels of protein-bound serum iodine (method of Lachiver and Leloup) in thymectomized animals given injections of thymus extract or HTH when compared to saline-injected control guinea pigs. c) Adrenal ascorbic acid levels determined by the method of Roe and Kuether were maintained at the control level when thymus extract or HTH was injected (Table 3.5). Saline injections did not maintain normal adrenal ascorbic acid content in thymectomized animals. d) Differential cell counts in smears of circulating blood, bone marrow, and spleen (May-Grunwald-Giemsa) (Table 3.6) indicate that the percentages of lymphocytes in blood, spleen, and bone marrow in thymectomized guinea pigs were maintained at normal levels in thymus extract and in HTH-injected animals but decreased in saline-injected animals.

These determinations were repeated at 5, 11, 18, 27, 35, and 45 days after thymectomy and performed in eight normal male guinea pigs of the same strain and age for control. Results from the intact animals are indicated as "0 days after thymectomy" in the tables.

Repeated injections of either thymic extract or HTH also restored antibody production in thymectomized guinea pigs (Comsa and Filipp, 1966). An example follows. At 5 days of age, 25 male guinea pigs were thymectomized. Following the operation, five animals received daily injections of total thymic extract, five animals received daily injections

Table 3.5. Ascorbic acid content of the adrenal glands of thymectomized guinea pigs

The data give mg ascorbate/g of fresh gland with the mean and standard deviation of four animals injected with total extract, HTH, or saline.

Days after thymec-tomy	Total extract	HTH	Saline
0	1.62 ± 0.07		
5	1.48 ± 0.10	1.53 ± 0.11	1.36 ± 0.02
11	1.55 ± 0.08	1.56 ± 0.08	0.78 ± 0.05
18	1.67 ± 0.05	1.64 ± 0.07	0.59 ± 0.03
27	1.59 ± 0.05	1.66 ± 0.05	0.61 ± 0.05
35	1.69 ± 0.10	1.65 ± 0.04	0.98 ± 0.11
45	1.63 ± 0.08	1.60 ± 0.05	1.46 ± 0.07

Table 3.6. Percentage of total lymphocytes in the blood, bone marrow, and spleens in thymectomized guinea pigs

The data give means of four animals injected with total extract, HTH, or saline. For each value, 200 nucleated cells were counted in the blood or, 1000 nucleated cells were counted in marrow and spleen.

Days after thym-ectomy	Blood			Spleen			Marrow		
	Total extract	HTH	Saline	Total extract	HTH	Saline	Total extract	HTH	Saline
0	59.0			67.0			18.2		
5	46.2	53.7	30.0	59.1	64.1	32.1	17.1	19.2	14.1
11	47.9	58.1	28.5	69.2	71.2	30.6	18.6	17.5	11.9
18	59.3	64.2	21.5	70.4	67.6	29.7	20.2	17.0	10.8
27	67.0	63.1	22.0	76.3	64.9	33.3	22.0	21.5	9.7
35	64.4	57.5	29.0	69.7	72.3	35.2	19.1	18.0	11.3
45	62.1	60.1	32.0	75.2	70.0	41.2	17.1	19.2	13.7

of the presumably pure hormone HTH, and five received daily injections of saline. Dosages were those of the previous experiment. In five animals, a sham thymectomy was performed, and five animals served as intact normal controls. The animals were weaned at 10 days of age, and the injections were continued. On days 11, 13, and 15 after the operation, and at corresponding ages in unoperated controls, an intraperitoneal injection of a commercial H antigen of *Salmonella typhosa* (10^9 cells/0.5 ml) was injected into all animals. The thymus extracts or saline injections were continued for 9 more days. Nine days after the last antigen injection the agglutinin titer of the serum of all animals was estimated in the usual way (diluted sera added with an equal volume of antigen, incubated at 37°C for 24 hr). Results are summarized in Table 3.7.

In thymectomized rats, injections of either thymic extract or HTH, 100 units per animal 24 hr daily for 7 days, restored the reaction towards an intraperitoneal eggwhite injection which had been suppressed by thymectomy (Comsa, 1965c). In this reaction, described by Selye (1950) for normal rats, the intraperitoneal injection of 2 ml of eggwhite produces an intense erythema of the face, ears, and paws. Within 1 hr the flushed area becomes cyanotic, bradycardia and hypothermia develop, and the animals usually die within 3 to 5 hr.

The toxicity of these preparations could not be determined. In intact guinea pigs, a single dose of 1 mg of the Bezssonoff-Comsa extract per 100 g of body weight had no visible consequences. Daily subcutaneous

Table 3.7. Agglutination of H antigen by diluted serum of thymectomized guinea pigs treated as shown and immunized with *Salmonella typhosa*

Parentheses denote number of animals reacting where all five were not the same.

Dilution	Normal animals	Sham-operated	Thymectomized plus injection		
			Saline	Total extract	HTH
1/20	+ + +[a]	+ + +	+ +[b](3) + + + (2)	+ + +	+ + +
1/40	+ + +	+ + +	+[c](3) + + (2)	+ + +	+ + +
1/80	+ + +	+ + +	0[d](4) 0 (1)	+ + +	+ + +
1/160	+ +	+ +	+ (1) 0 (4)	+ +	+ + + (3) + + (2)
1/320	+ +	+ +	0	+ +	+ + (3) + (2)
1/640	+ (3) 0 (2)	+	0	+	+ (3) 0 (2)
1/1280	0	0	0	0	0

[a] + + +, clot at the bottom of the tubes, supernatant limpid.
[b] + +, clot at the bottom of the tube, supernatant turbid.
[c] +, agglutination visible only under 5 × magnification.
[d] 0, suspension homogeneous.

injections of 500 μg per 100 g of body weight resulted only in an increased growth rate and after 7 to 8 months in degenerative lesions of the thryoid. Daily subcutaneous injections to mice of 100 μg of HTH showed no observable pathologic changes and no increase of the mortality rate during a period of 10 months (M. Guerin, unpublished).

The interactions between the thymic hormone and other hormones, the radioprotective potency of this hormone, and its influence on lymphocytes will be discussed below.

The extract of Goldstein and coworkers has been tested for its substitutive potency (Asanuma, Goldstein, and White, 1970) in neonatally thymectomized mice which were given injections daily of 40 μg and later 80 μg of the preparation for 63 days. The growth rate of these mice was improved when compared to that of nontreated thymectomized mice, but it was equal to about one-half the growth rate of normal mice. Mortality of the treated mice (in a wasted condition) was 34%, instead of the 70% mortality in nontreated thymectomized animals. The lymphocyte count in blood of treated mice was 3500 per mm^3 (untreated thymectomized mice had 1400/mm^3; normal mice, 7000/mm^3). Thus a substitutive effect is obvious. It is not complete, however.

The first extract of Trainin, Burger, and Kaye (1967) was tested on mice thymectomized at 20 to 40 days of age and given injections of the preparation daily from the 20th to the 50th day after thymectomy. The ^{3}H thymidine uptake of the lymph nodes of these animals was tested. It increased about twofold in thymectomized treated animals in comparison with untreated thymectomized mice. In normal mice, the thymic preparation had no obvious influence on the ^{3}H thymidine uptake (in contradistinction, the extract of Goldstein and coworkers has shown a stimulating effect in normal mice with a similar test). Small and Trainin (1967) observed that their thymic extract restored the immunologic competence of thymectomized mice. Late work from this laboratory is provided in Chapter 6.

3.6 Thymic extracts of unproved substitutive potency

The biologic effects of thymic extracts of unproven substitutive potency are summarized in Table 3.8. Most of them are controversial. All were tested in intact animals having mature thymuses; thus any resemblance to thymic hormones is probably coincidental. The thymic preparations which influence tumor growth are certainly different from the thymic hormone(s). Bomskov and Holscher (1942) failed to influence significantly the growth of thymectomized guinea pigs with their lipid extract. Their data do not support their overoptimistic summary.

Molnar and Kovacs (1953) observed a stimulating effect of their extracts (see Table 3.1) on the growth of Brown-Pearce sarcoma. Szent-Gyorgi (1962) has obtained two fractions from a methanol extract with an intricate technique, essentially by chromatography; these are promine, which accelerated the growth of implanted Ehrlich sarcoma in mice, and retine, which delayed it. The former may be compared to the extract of Maisin (1963). These materials were readily demonstrated in tissue other than thymus. Isabela Potop and coworkers (1967, 1969) made similar observations which have resulted in the isolation of compounds discussed in Chapters 5 and 11.

Table 3.8. Some biological effects of thymus preparation in intact animals. Preparations discussed elsewhere are excluded.

Reference	Preparation	Animal	Test	Result
Reviewed in Comsa, 1959d	Fresh thymus fed	Goldfish, chick, mouse, tadpole	Growth	Accelerated
Schneider, 1957	See Table 3.1, acetone soluble fraction	Xenopus tadpole	Growth	Accelerated
Gudernatsch, 1912	Dried thymus fed	*Rana temporaria* tadpole	Metamorphosis	Delayed
Abderhalden, 1926	Dried thymus fed	*Rana temporaria* tadpole	Metamorphosis	Delaying influence of thymus not specific
Krizenecky, 1926	Dried thymus fed	Chick	Growth and maturation of feathers	Accelerated
Capocaccia and Cicchini, 1955	Commercial	Rabbit	Resistance to infection fever, general condition, phagocytic index	Improved
Beauvieux, 1963 a, b	See Table 3.1	Rabbit	Lymphocyte count in blood	Improved
Molnar and Kovacs, 1953	See Table 3.1	Rabbit	Brown-Pearce tumor growth	Accelerated
Szent-Gyorgyi	See Table 3.1	Mouse	Ascites tumor growth	a) Accelerating (promin); b) inhibiting, (retin); neither is thymus specific
Nitschke, 1929 a, b	See Table 3.1	Rabbit	Calcemia phosphatemia	Decreased

Table 3.8 (*Continued*)

Reference	Preparation	Animal	Test	Result
Rowntree *et al.*, 1934	See Table 3.1	Rat	Growth development	Accelerated, cumulative effect if repeated in successive generations
Schwarz *et al.*, 1953	See Table 3.1	Rat	Calcemia phosphatemia	Increased
Eskelund and Plum, 1953	See Table 3.1	Rat	Fracture healing	Accelerated
Anderson 1932	Suspension injected	Rat	Puberty	Delayed
Goslar, 1958	See Table 3.1	Natrix	Skin casting	Accelerated
Marabini	Commercial	Rat	Influence on the cortico-tropin effect on adrenal and thymus weight	Slight inhibition
Schwarz *et al.*, 1959	Commercial	Rat	Influence of hemiadrenal-ectomy on the ascorbic acid content of the remaining adrenal	Suppressed
Diomede-Fresa *et al.*, 1959	Commercial preparation not described	Rat	Antibody production following vaccination with *Salmonella*	Increased
Pausky *et al.*, 1965	See Table 3.1	Mouse (alloxan diabetic)	Glycemia	Decreased, active fraction equals insulin (immunoassay)

A direct inhibitory action of the thymus on the growth of implanted tumors is difficult to separate from the immune function of the thymus. Thus Wistar rats rejected a transplantable mammary tumor induced in Furth rats by stilbesterol, while the tumor grew in thymectomized Wistar rats (Lazar, 1966). Mice refractory to a transplantable tumor accepted it when they were given injections at birth of an antithymus serum (Anigstein *et al.*, 1966). The immunologic explanation is certainly not exhaustive. The influence of thymic extract on tumor cells in tissue culture remains unexplained by this theory.

3.7 Secretion of thymic hormone

By definition, a hormone is a unique substance delivered from a specific tissue or gland into the circulating blood. This constitutes the difference between a hormone and a possible specific cellular constituent. Thus, the demonstration of the secretion is compulsory if a substance is to be defined as a hormone. In practice this implies two observations: in normal animals this substance must be detected both in the gland which produces it and elsewhere; and the extirpation of the gland must be followed by the disappearance of the substance from all tissues.

A preliminary attempt to demonstrate this for the homeostatic thymus hormone was made by bioassay (Comsa and Bezssonoff, 1959). It succeeded in rats and guinea pigs. A hormone-like activity could be detected in the thymus, the lymph nodes, and the spleen. No similar activity could be detected in the liver, the lung, the kidney, the testes, and the muscles. After thymectomy, the hormone-like activity disappeared from the lymph nodes and the spleen. It was concluded that a) the hormone-like activity is supported by a substance secreted by the thymus, and b) this substance is stored in organs rich in lymphocytes.

Recent results (Bernardi and Comsa, 1965b) confirmed this work under more precise conditions. Extracts were prepared with the method of Bezssonoff and Comsa from pooled thymus, pooled lymph nodes, and pooled spleens of normal rats in homogeneous age groups of 30 to 150 days with 20 or 24 animals per group. These extracts were fractionated with the method of Bernardi and Comsa, and the fraction corresponding to the homogeneous, fully substitutive fraction (HTH) isolated from veal thymus was determined by spectrophotometry at the wavelength of 270 mμ. The following quantities were found (μg per g of fresh rat organ):

Age group (days)	30	50	80	120	150
Thymus	125.2	87.0	35.0	34.0	44.0
Lymph node	77.0	51.4	29.7	0	0
Spleen	28.4	17.7	0	0	0

Similar extracts were prepared and examined from pooled lymph nodes and spleen of 1-month-old male rats at 3, 6, 9, and 12 days after thymectomy. No traces of HTH activity could be detected in these extracts. These results of bioassay estimation are confirmed by the finding of Comsa and Phillipp (in press) that the consequences of thymectomy on the thyroid and the adrenal cortex last more than 9 days and less than 12 days.

These observations demonstrate that the HTH isolated by Bernardi and Comsa (which prevented the consequences of thymectomy) is secreted by the thymus only. The appellation *thymic hormone* is thus justified. The data also suggest that the HTH may either accumulate in or be transported by the lymphocytes.

Observations in humans may give some further support to this conclusion. Extract of human thymus prepared by the Bezssonoff-Comsa method was found to be active by bioassay (Table 3.9). The activity was found to decrease in dystrophic infants. When the thymus weights decreased to about 0.02% of the total body weight, the hormone content of the thymus tended toward zero. From desiccated human urine, a fraction could be prepared by the method of Bezssonoff and Comsa which prevented the consequences of thymectomy in guinea pigs (Comsa, 1952f; see Tables 3.10 and 3.11). Examination of a 9-year-old girl who had undergone total thymectomy 1 year previously revealed that the thymus-substitutive fraction was missing in her urine. The diagnosis was of thymic hypertrophy. The extirpated thymus was splendidly complete but within normal weight limits.

Relationships similar to those in dystrophic infants are likely to be seen in calves. Thymuses from fattened calves weigh about 250 g and they contain 0.4 g of HTH per kilo of fresh weight. Thymuses of calves reared under poor conditions weighed only 50 to 80 g, and the Bezssonoff-Comsa extracts of these thymuses were found to be inactive. The above correspond roughly to the calves from beef or dual purpose cattle having high quantities of hormone in large thymuses, while calves from dairy cattle or primitive cattle have very small thymuses and reduced quantities of the hormone. By comparison, thymuses contained approximately 2 mg HTH/g in infantile guinea pigs, 0.7 mg/g in adult guinea pigs, 0.23 mg/g in weanling rabbits, and 0.125 mg/g in weanling rats.

Many authors have assumed (*see* Hammar, 1936, for older references)

Table 3.9. Hormonal activity of human thymus

Cause of death	Total body weight (kg)	Thymus weight (g/kg of total)	Activity (units) per g of thymus	Activity (units) per kg of body weight
Accidental death				
Obstetrical trauma	3.5	3.43	132.6	555.0
Obstetrical trauma	3.6	3.47	136.0	515.0
Obstetrical trauma	3.2	4.69	121.0	567.0
Obstetrical trauma	2.8	1.79	200.0	337.0
3 months, CO asphyxia	3.63	2.48	203.7	504.0
18 months, skull fracture	13.0	1.54	148.3	228.0
Infection, good nutritional condition				
3 months, pneumonia	4.4	6.14	104.3	634
13 months, pneumonia	10.0	3.0	179.0	537.0
2 months, encephalitis	4.3	2.7	156.3	434.0
6 months, pneumonia	6.5	2.2	164.6	329.2
4 days, pneumonia	2.8	3.43	108.0	129.0
16 days, pneumonia	3.4	1.9	173.0	96.7
Dystrophic condition				
15 months, pharyngitis	6.4	1.11		
1 month, antritis	3.73	1.17	92.0	102.0
13 days, pleuritis	2.80	1.17		
1 month, meningitis	2.40	1.13		
4 months, antritis	2.33	1.25		
3 months, blank p.m.	2.45	1.02	72.0	90
40 days, pneumonia	2.00	1.07		
3 months, pneumonia	2.15	0.7		
2 months, pneumonia	2.0	0.7	41.0	30.4
1 month, antritis	2.4	0.66		
1 month, antritis	2.6	0.66		
5 months, pneumonia[a]	4.5	0.49		
4 months, pneumonia	3.0	0.36	32.3	14.0
3 months, antritis	2.6	0.32		
3 months, pneumonia	4.0	0.32		

[a]The last four values were obtained from pooled samples divided by relative weight of thymus and sex.

Table 3.10. Thymus-like activity of human urine extract, normal male subjects (units/kg of body weight/24 hr)

Age	Weight (kg)	Activity
1 month	3.9	1045
3 months	5.6	1398
4 months	6.1	1107
5 months	6.2	1000
3 years	16.8	956
4 years	18.1	815
6 years	19.6	794
7 years	24.0	742
8 years	26.8	670
9 years	27.8	620
11 years	32.2	645
12 years	37.6	538
15 years	42.8	320
16 years	47.0	262
19 years	64.0	179
19 years	70.0	167
21 years	63.0	213
26 years	73.0	194
26 years	83.0	176
32 years	67.0	185
37 years	52.0	183
42 years	90.0	168

that lymphocytes may be involved in thymic secretion (possibly as vectors of the hormone). Direct evidence for this assumption is lacking, but the influence of the thymus on lymphocytes has been abundantly demonstrated.

3.8 Thymus and HTH have positive chemotaxis for lymphocytes

The chemotactic influence of the thymus on the lymphocytes is implicitly suggested in the observations mentioned above. There is definitive evidence for positive chemotaxis not only by the total thymus extract but also by HTH (Comsa and Schweissfurth, unpublished).

Thymic preparations were dissolved and mixed with two volumes of 3% agar-agar solution at 60°C. These preparations were the Bezssonoff-

Table 3.11. Thymus-like activity of human urine extract, dystrophic children

Age	Weight (kg)	Weight deficiency, corresponding to the height (%)	Activity
2 months	3.42	22	607
2 months	2.16	40	170
2 months	3.34	24	666
3 months	4.25	17	750
3 months	3.6	30	172
4 months	4.4	30	246
6 months	5.2	25	604
2 years	8.1	13	167
2 years	11.5	22	454
3 years	12.0	15	507
5 years	15.0	18	521
6 years	17.0	24	165
7 years	20.0	13	511
8 years	22.0	17	467
9 years	21.0	20	432
10 years	22.0	25	139

Comsa extract, the fraction discarded at pH 7.0 from the same extract, and the three fractions isolated from the same extract with the method of Bernardi and Comsa. These preparations were poured into Petri dishes in a layer of about 2 mm and stored at 3°C. They were cut into pieces of about 0.5 cm². These pieces were inserted in incisions of the skin of the right flank of male rats (aged 40 days) thymectomized 9 days previously. Similar pieces of pure agar-agar were inserted subcutaneously in the left flank of every animal (six rats for every preparation). Thus, every animal received: a) control agar, presumably an inactive implant (left flank); and b) preparation to be tested for its influence on lymphocytes (right flank). The implants were removed 24 hr later, and smears were made by gently rubbing their surface on microscope slides, which were then stained for differential cell counts with May-Grunwald-Giemsa stain. The following percentages of lymphocytes were found:

Implants	Control	Extract
Total extract	14.0 ± 4.4	55.2 ± 9.1
Impurity discarded carded at pH 7.0	14.0 ± 4.9	16.4 ± 3.8
Fraction I	17.8 ± 1.7	21.3 ± 3.3
Fraction II	19.0 ± 1.8	26.0 ± 2.8
Fraction III (HTH)	15.1 ± 2.9	53.5 ± 1.8

This experiment gives further support to the conclusion drawn previously from a similar experiment (Comsa, 1950): the chemotactic influence of the thymus on lymphocytes, as supposed by Gregoire (1935), is performed by the fraction which suppressed the consequences of thymectomy. This chemotactic influence of thymus extracts could be demonstrated in thymectomized animals or with thymic grafts devoid of lymphocytes (Gregoire, 1935). "It is a matter of discussion, whether or not a normal lymphocyte may enter a normal thymus" (Burnet, 1962). The parabiotic experiment of Brumby and Metcalf (1967) showed that lymphoid cells from one animal did localize in the thymic medulla of the other.

3.9 Summary

Thus far several substitutive substances in the thymus are known. The presumably pure substance of Bernardi and Comsa (HTH) has shown a peculiarly conspicuous substitutive influence. Its action can be explained (at least in an interrogative form) to a certain extent by its interaction with other hormones. Its chemotactic influence on lymphocytes is probably direct.

The substance contained in the extract of A. Goldstein and coworkers has not yet been obtained in pure form. The technique of preparation of this extract allows no speculation about its identity or nonidentity with the hormone of Bernardi and Comsa. However, the molecular weights of its major glycoproteins are 10 to 30 times greater. It is substitutive to some extent (Asanuma et al., 1970); however, it is apparently less efficient than the hormone of Bernardi and Comsa. However, Asanuma et al. (1970) tested their material in mice, whereas Comsa used guinea pigs and rats in his tests. Perhaps this difference accounts to a certain extent for the difference in the results. The action of their substance on lymphocytes is different from that of Bernardi and Comsa; however, ultimately both stimulate lymphocyte proliferation.

The action of other extracts will be presented in other chapters of this book. Most demonstrations of activity were performed in mice; the consequences of thymectomy are much less well known in the mouse than in the guinea pig.

In conclusion, several biologically active compounds have been isolated from the thymus thus far. Still more are likely to be found in the future. However, we cannot state presently how many hormones are produced in the thymus. This statement will be possible only when we know how many of the active compounds found within the thymus are actually secreted; that is, a) found in the thymus and elsewhere in the normal animal, and b) proved to disappear everywhere following thymectomy.

4   Hormonal Interactions
of the Thymus

J. Comsa

Significant observations were made in thymectomized guinea pigs. The anterior pituitary shows significant changes; the thyroid and the adrenal glands are transitorily stimulated and undergo degenerative changes in wasted animals, and the gonads give evidence of an incipient but abortive maturation. All these changes are suppressed by substitutive therapy with a thymic extract as well as with HTH. Furthermore, simultaneous extirpation of the thymus and the thyroid results in a peculiarly severe wasting syndrome; castration improves the condition of thymectomized and thyroid-thymectomized guinea pigs. These data seem to indicate that, to a certain extent, the thymoprivic syndrome may express an intricate hormonal imbalance resulting from the loss of a hormone. This justified investigations into the endocrine interactions of the thymus. The crude lipid extract of Bomskov and Kucker (1940) is a very crude extract and is likely to contain several substances with known antagonism towards thyroxine, such as cholesterol, phospholipids, carotenoids, *etc.* See Comsa (1952a) for a review. The animals used in our experiments, described below, were bred in our laboratory; guinea pigs were of the AgB strain of Bezssonoff and Comsa, and rats were of the Wistar-Commentry strain.

4.1 Thymus-thyroid interactions

The thymus and thyroid function antagonistically

Thyroxine-induced precocious metamorphosis is suppressed in *Rana temporaria* tadpoles by fresh thymus added to their food (Romeis, 1915; 1926; Sklower, 1926). Injections of a thymus homogenate suppressed the influence of simultaneously injected thyroid homogenate on respiratory metabolism in mice (Gebele, 1929). With more or less purified thymic extracts, similar observations could be made. Injection of the crude extract of Nitschke (1929a, b) into guinea pigs suppressed the influence of simultaneously injected thyroxine on respiratory metabolism (see Table 3.1). Powdered dried thymus added to the food suppressed the thyroxine influence on feather growth in chickens (Krizenecky, 1926). More purified extracts, such as that of Asher (1933), that of Bezssonoff and Comsa (1958), and HTH (Bernardi and Comsa, 1965b), were found to suppress the influence of thyroxine on creatine excretion and glucose uptake. In contradistinction, Takao (1926) observed that the influence of dried thyroid added to the food (1% of the total diet, an enormous dose) on liver glycogen was not modified in the rat by simultaneous addition of 1% of dried thymus to the food; this was probably too little. Very likely, the same error may account for Wyssmann's observation (1929) that the influence of feeding dried thyroid (160 mg daily, an enormous dose) on the working respiratory metabolism of the rat could not be counteracted with Asher's thymus extract (injected in amounts impossible to guess from his text).

The bioassay method of Comsa (1952b) for thymic preparation was based upon the above observations. A more extensive report may be of some use. The creatine test is performed on male infantile guinea pigs, previously thymectomized, thyroidectomized, and castrated. Thyroxine and thymic extract are injected simultaneously. From the 24th to the 48th hr following the injection, the animals are placed in individual metabolism cages. They are fed lettuce and oats. Creatine is determined in their urine. It is important to determine creatine separately; a determination of the so-called total creatinine, i.e., the sum of creatine and creatinine, is of no significance. An example of these determinations is summarized in Table 4.1.

The thyroxine influence on creatine excretion is considered to be suppressed if a) the average excretion rate of the four animals given injections of equal amounts of thyroxine and thymus is equal to or smaller than the excretion rate in untreated thymus–thyroidectomized castrates (0.8 ±0.07 mg/100 g of body weight per 24 hr, and b) none of these treated animals excreted 1.0 mg/100 g or more.

It can be seen that the thymus dose sufficient to suppress the influence of a thyroxine dose of 5.0 to 24.0 μg/100 g of body weight is a first-degree function of the thyroxine dose, according to the equation:

$$ax = y \qquad (1)$$

where x is the thyroxine dose and y is the corresponding dose of the thymic preparation. The first-degree law is valid for thyroxine doses

Table 4.1. Creatine excretion rate

Data give means (in mg/100 g/24 hr) with standard deviation of four animals in thymus and thyroidectomized castrated male guinea pigs injected with various amounts of thyroxine and Bezssonoff-Comsa thymic extract

Thymus (units/100 g body weight)	μg Thyroid/100 g body weight						
	5	10	15	20	24	25	26
0	2.09 ± 0.30	2.47 ± 0.30	2.78 ± 0.28	3.42 ± 0.20	3.57 ± 0.18	3.61 ± 0.24	3.82 ± 0.5
2	1.23 ± 0.28						
4	0.92 ± 0.13						
5	0.71 ± 0.09						
7		1.79 ± 0.08					
8		1.27 ± 0.09					
9		1.01 ± 0.09					
10		0.74 ± 0.04	2.56 ± 0.20				
13			2.38 ± 0.32				
14			1.17 ± 0.22				
15			0.72 ± 0.06				
17				3.12 ± 0.35			
18				1.57 ± 0.82			
19				1.11 ± 0.12			
20				0.78 ± 0.06			
22					2.04 ± 0.37		
23					1.01 ± 0.09		
24					0.94 ± 0.15		
25					0.61 ± 0.04		
26						1.44 ± 0.25	
27						1.01 ± 0.07	
30						0.72 ± 0.05	
34							3.67 ± 0.30
38							2.71 ± 0.26
							1.28 ± 0.16
40							0.74 ± 0.04

below 25 μg/100 g of guinea pig. Above this limit the efficiency of the thymic extracts decreases abruptly. The significance of this observation is discussed later.

The constant, a, is a measure of the purity of the thymic extract. In various samples of the Bezssonoff-Comsa extract, values of a from 2.6 to 18.0 were found. With various samples of the presumably pure substance, HTH, of Bernardi and Comsa the values of a were found to be between 0.97 and 1.09 (more or less equal to 1.0).

This was the basis used to define the constant a (the amount of a thymic extract able to suppress the influence of 1 μg of thyroxine) as 1 guinea pig unit of a thymic extract.

The glucose uptake is performed on the isolated rat diaphragm. The diaphragm is divided in four approximately equal parts. These are weighed and incubated for 1 hr at 37°C under 95% O_2 and 5% CO_2 in Krebs-Henseleit saline with 0.2% glucose in a Krebs apparatus gently agitated in the water bath. Sample 1 has no additions. Sample 2 has 0.1 μg of thyroxine per milliliter. Samples 3 and 4 have 0.1 μg of thyroxine per milliliter and increasing amounts of a thymic preparation.

Glucose is determined with the glucose-oxidase method at the end of the incubation. Added thyroxine increased the glucose uptake of the diaphragm by 100 to 200%; thymic extract suppressed the influence of thyroxine if 0.1 units were added to the medium. When the adequate amount was found, the determination was repeated under identical conditions four times. This method is less accurate than the creatine method, but it allows assaying of minute amounts of thymic hormone.

Both these bioassay methods were considered routine methods, suitable for assay of new samples of thymic preparations. As often as the method of extraction was modified, the first sample thus obtained was tested completely for substitutive potency in thymectomized guinea pigs and rats.

The antithyroxine action of the thymic hormone may express an acceleration of the thyroxine catabolism. This was demonstrated as follows (Comsa, 1956b). A homogenate of guinea pig liver was suspended in water (8%); 0.3 μg of thyroxine per milliliter was added and incubated at 38°C. The protein-bound iodine content of this preparation decreased gradually and reached zero within 9 to 12 hr. Addition of a Bezssonoff-Comsa extract to this preparation in amount of 3.4 units/ml resulted in an accelerated decrease of the protein-bound iodine content, which reached zero within 30 min (Comsa, 1956b). This did not occur if the liver homogenate was boiled previously. It was concluded that the thymic hormone does not denature thyroxine by itself, but it enhances the activity of a thermolabile factor contained in the liver. To a certain extent, this may explain the antagonism between thymus and thyroxine, if thyroxine catabolism occurs in the muscles (diaphragm) as well as in the liver.

Influence of the thymus on the thyroid

The consequences of thymectomy on the thyroid were described in Chapter 1. The consequences of hyperthymization are intricate. In intact guinea pigs given injections daily of 100 units/100 g of body weight of Bezssonoff-Comsa extract, there were these results. a) After 5 days a histologic picture of stimulation was found, but the serum protein-bound iodine was decreased from about 5.3 to 2.8 $\pm 0.2\,\mu$g/100 ml. The stimulation may be understood as a result of the decreased influence of circulating thyroid hormones. b) After 15 to 20 days, a picture corresponding to a resting condition was seen. The antithyrotropic influence of the thymus may account for this. c) In long-lasting experiments, degenerative changes of the thyroid were seen. The follicular cells were edematous; some contained several nuclei. Stratified epithelium appeared. In some follicles, small adenomas which seemed to disintegrate were visible (Comsa, 1957e). These aspects do not suggest consequences of a hormonal vacuum, nor do they evoke a resting condition induced by the (anti-thyrotropic) thymus; they are proper lesions and not changes corresponding to various functional states. We are bound to admit that a long-lasting hyperthymization results in degenerative lesions of the thyroid.

Influence of the thyroid on the thymus

In thyroidectomized animals, the thymus undergoes atrophic changes (Hammet, 1926). The histologic picture recalls that of senile atrophy (a similar picture can be seen in 2- to 3-year-old guinea pigs). The lobules are shrunken, particularly the cortex. Mitoses of the thymocytes are exceptional. No young Hassall corpuscles are found; all corpuscles are old, large, calcified, keratinized, and cystic. The limit between cortex and medulla is peculiarly sharp. The hormone content of the thymus, as estimated by bioassay, decreases, and so does the thymic-like activity of lymph nodes and spleen (Comsa, 1959d). The ratio of thymus:lymph node:spleen in normal animals is 10.4:2.2:1; in thyroidectomized animals, it is 10.6:2.1:1. This lack of change suggests that a) the hormone production of the thymus is decreased following thyroidectomy and b) the ratio between the thymus (the factory) and the lymph nodes and the spleen (the secondary stores) is unaffected. These facts suggest that the decrease

of the hormone production is a consequence of the decreased needs resulting from the absence of an antagonist (Comsa, 1959a).

Repeated thyroxine injections suppress these changes. The smallest
sufficient dose is 2.0 μg thyroxine per 100 g of guinea pig in 24 hr. Daily
thyroxine injections of 8.0 to 18 μg induce hypertrophy of the thymus.
Large doses, above 22 μg/100 g/24 hr, induce less hypertrophic change
with a pattern conspicuously different from that of thyroprivic atrophy;
the relative weight of the thymus is decreased, but the lobules are not
shrunken. There is no longer a visible limit between cortex and medulla.
Thymocytes decrease in number. No pycnoses are seen. Mitoses are conspicuously frequent. A great number of young Hassall corpuscles can be
seen (these are composed of three to six young, turgescent cells). The
interstices between the lobules and the interlobular veinules are crowded
with lymphocytes. Production of thymocytes is enhanced, but glandular
thymocytes decrease in number; thus the lymphocytes observed in the
veinules can be considered to be leaving the thymus. When 28 μg are
injected daily, the thymus weight decreases to slightly below normal, and
lymphocytes crowd the medulla but are nearly absent from the cortex;
this condition is called "inverse thymus."

Some emphasis should be put on the dosage of thyroxine in these guinea
pig experiments; the largest dose inducing hypertrophy was 18 μg, while
the smallest dose inducing a characteristic atrophy was 22 μg. The limit
between the smallest thyroxine dose which induces thymic atrophy (22
gamma) and the largest dose which does not (18 gamma) is of some
significance. Considering the interaction between circulating thyroxine
and circulating HTH (Table 4.1), the first-degree law of this interaction
($ax = y$) seems valid for the thyroxine doses of less than 25 gamma/100 g
body weight (Table 4.1). To suppress the effect of 25 gamma of thyroxine,
a larger dose of thymus extract is needed than that calculated with the
first-degree equation, and still more HTH is needed for doses of thyroxine greater than 25 gamma. This seems to indicate that the efficiency of
the thymus as a thyroxine antagonist decreases if the thyroxine doses
are increased beyond this limit. This observation will be reinforced in the
discussion on thyroxine-thymus-testosterone interaction. The thymus
seems to show signs of exhaustion if the efficiency of its antithyroxine
hormone decreases.

The literature concerning the influence of hyperthyrodism on the
thymus is controversial. Thyroxine injections induced hypertrophy (Glaser,
1926; mouse, 4 μg daily) or atrophy of the thymus (Schulze, 1933; mouse,
10 μg daily). Possibly the authors, who concluded that the influence of
the thyroid on the thymus was incoherent (Kliwanskaia-Kroll, 1938;

Utterstron, 1910; and others later), had arbitrarily chosen a dose range on either side of the critical point or a dose range where accessory factors such as alimentation (*see later*) are relevant.

According to our results with animals, the thymus of hyperthyroidized guinea pigs seems to tend toward exhaustion by oversolicitation. This emigration atrophy recalls those observed during deficiency diseases, but it is different in the intense proliferative activity noted in the previous paragraphs. It is conspicuously different from the atrophy induced by corticoids which begins by a wave of pycnoses (never observed following thyroxine injections).

If we accept this "oversolicitation-exhaustion" interpretation for the histological changes induced by thyroxine in large doses, the thyroprivic atrophy of the thymus could be understood as expressing a resting condition of the gland induced by a loss of a stimulant.

Influence of thyroxine in thymectomized guinea pigs

Qualitatively, thyroxine effects creatine excretion and serum cholesterol level, and ascorbic acid content of the adrenals in thymectomized animals. Still, thymectomized guinea pigs are more sensitive towards thyroxine than normal animals. The smallest thyroxine dose sufficient to induce an increased creatine excretion is $> 2 < 3 \mu g/100$ g in these animals, compared with $> 6 < 7 \mu g/100$ g in normal animals.

One conspicuous difference was noted, however. In normal guinea pigs thyroxine injections (18 $\mu g/100$ g body weight daily for 7 days) induced an increase of the blood lymphocyte count and hypertrophy of the lymph nodes. In thymectomized animals, the same injections enhanced the lymphopenia and the atrophy of the lymph nodes (Comsa, 1958b, c). The well-known lymphocytosis of hyperthyroidism (see Comsa, 1958b, for references) may express to some extent the stimulating influence of the thyroid on the thymus.

Influence of the thymus extract in thyroidectomized animals

In intact guinea pigs injected with thymic extract in large amounts a) the general appearance was unaffected; b) the growth rate was increased, but gigantism was not induced (the growth stops sooner); c) a resting condition of the adrenal cortex was found (Comsa and Leroux, 1956); d) the consequences on the thyroid were intricate (*see previous section*); e) the anterior pituitary showed significant changes (*see previous chapter*); and f) the lymphocyte count increased in the blood, the bone marrow, and the spleen.

In thyroidectomized animals, the consequences of the hyperthymic state were different from normal animals (Comsa, 1957e); a) their general condition was affected, they were apathetic, placid and dirty; b) their growth rate was significantly slower; c) the protein-bound iodine content of the serum decreased to traces (0.7 μg/100 ml); d) the pituitary showed no histologic difference from that of untreated thyroprivic animals; and e) the adrenal cortex was found to be in a resting state, as in hyperthymic or thyroidectomized animals (Comsa and Leroux, 1955; 1956). Since the lymphocyte count was increased, lymphocytosis is unaffected by thyroidectomy in the presence of large amounts of thymic extract, whereas the lymphocytosis induced by thyroxine is suppressed by thymectomy.

The thymus seems to be a permitting factor for the action of the thyroid on lymphocyte proliferation. Since the thymic hormone seems to be of primordial importance for the functions of lymphatic tissue, this is easily understood.

Thus, the thymus-thyroid interaction seems to be intricate. As noted previously, the antagonism between circulating thyroxine and circulating thymic hormone was demonstrated. Important factors considered were the range of thyroxine doses used for testing and the ratio between thyroxine and thymus doses.

The thymus seems to be a permitting factor for the action of the thyroid on growth, as it was demonstrated to be for the action of pituitary growth hormone (reviewed by Comsa, 1952c, e). Nowinsky's observations (1930: 1933) may be understood in these terms. Nowinsky tested thyroxine and Asher's thymic extract on young rats fed poor food without any specific deficiency. He observed that the (deficient) growth of these animals was stimulated by repeated injections of small amounts of thyroxine (5 μg/day) and inhibited by large amounts (500 μg/day). Asher's extract, given simultaneously, enhanced both these effects. Possibly 5 μg of thyroxine were just about substitutive for the thyroid of his rats, which were probably thyroid-deficient (this is known in many nutritional deficiencies, see Comsa, 1952b).

4.2 Thymus-gonad interactions

The thymus is involuted in adults. This was discovered by Friedleben in 1854. Its histologic picture is comparable to that seen in thyroidectomized animals. It may express a resting condition. Its HTH content decreases in guinea pigs to about 30% and in rats to about 34% of that of the infantile thymus. The influence of the thymus on the organism decreases with aging. Thymectomy is followed by a transitory increased creatine excretion; so is castration (Table 4.1). In guinea pigs, thymiprivic creatinuria decreased, while castration creatinuria increased with aging (Comsa, 1947).

The thymus is hyperplastic in castrates (Calzolari, 1898). Its histologic picture shows nothing peculiar; it resembles that of an infantile thymus. Its hormone content is increased, whereas the thymus-like activity of the lymph nodes and the spleen is decreased. The ratio of thymus/lymph nodes/spleen in normal animals is 10.4:2.2:1, in castrates it is 48:2.4:1, and in thyroidectomized castrates it is 10:2.4:1 (Comsa, 1959a, d). The interference of the thyroid in the thymus-gonad interaction is indicated here; there is further evidence for this interaction. In thyroidectomized castrated rabbits (Marine, Manley, and Bauman, 1924) and guinea pigs (Comsa, 1947) the thymus involuted as it did following thyroidectomy alone, and creatine excretion was not increased (Comsa, 1947).

Atrophy of the thymus could be induced in infantile rats by injection of a gonadotropic pituitary preparation, but not in castrates (Arvin and Allen, 1928) or in animals given estradiol (Selye, Harlow, and Collip, 1936; and others) or testosterone (Selye and Masson, 1939).

The above outlines an interaction between thymus and gonads with interference of the thyroid. Further observations on the influence of sexual hormones revealed some more details of this interaction (Comsa, 1953a). When given in more or less physiologic amounts (in the experiments quoted above the dosage was massive) to castrated guinea pigs, estradiol (0.5 to 0.7 μg/100 g) induced a wave of pycnoses, elicited as well in thyroidectomized castrates. Testosterone (100 μg/100 g) elicited an emigration atrophy similar to that induced by thyroxine; previous thyroidectomy suppressed this effect. One could postulate a direct influence of estradiol on the thymus and an influence of testosterone conditioned by the thyroid. Further investigations might confirm this supposition.

Interaction between circulating homeostatic thymic hormone, thyroxine, and sexual hormones

The following information was obtained with the creatine excretion test. Indeed, creatine excretion is influenced by all hormones considered: a) thyroxine enhances it; b) thymic extract given in large amounts increases it; c) estradiol administration reproduces the creatinuria of estrus (Butcher and Persike, 1938; Comsa, 1947; and others later); and d) testosterone inhibits creatinuria, reproducing the situation in adult males which excrete creatinine only (Jailer, 1941; and others later). The next information needed is the smallest dose of a sexual hormone sufficient to elicit the effect on creatine excretion and whether this minimal dose (called below "the threshold dose") will be modified by injections of thyroxine, homeostatic thymic hormone, or both.

For obvious reasons, these experiments must be performed in thymus-thyroidectomized castrates. The general conditions of these experiments are those of the bioassay of thymic preparations. Under these conditions, young guinea pig thymus-thyroidectomized castrates excrete 0.8 ± 0.07 mg of creatine per 100 g body weight in 24 hr.

Thymus-thyroxine-estradiol interactions

The threshold dose of estradiol was defined as the smallest dose of this hormone which induced, within 24 hr after injection in four animals out of four, a creatine excretion amounting at least to 1.8 mg/100 g body weight. This threshold dose is increased by thyroxine or thymic extract, given 24 hr prior to the estradiol injection (Tables 4.2 and 4.3).

In both experiments, the estradiol threshold dose increased in a second-degree function of the thyroxine or of the thymic extract dose. The following empirical equations could be proposed:

Influence of thyroxine:

$$\text{In males:} \quad 0.04x^2 - .005x \times 0.05 = y \tag{2}$$

$$\text{In females:} \quad 0.016x^2 - 0.01x + 0.004 = y \tag{3}$$

where x is the thyroxine dose and y the corresponding estradiol threshold dose.

Influence of the thymus:

$$\text{In males:} \quad 0.06x^2 - 0.01x + 0.005 = y \tag{4}$$

$$\text{In females:} \quad 0.022x^2 - 0.02x + 0.004 = y \tag{5}$$

where x is the thymic extract dose and y is the corresponding estradiol threshold dose.

Table 4.2. Effect of thyroxine upon estradiol threshold

Variation of the threshold dose of estradiol (μg of benzoate/100 g body weight) in thymus and thyroidectomized castrated guinea pigs injected with thyroxine.

Thyroxine	Estradiol threshold dose	
(μg/10 g)	Males	Females
1	0.05	0.04
1.0	0.07	0.05
2.0	0.18	0.07
3.0	0.35	0.15
4.0	0.65	0.25
5.0	1.0	0.44
6.0	1.40	
7.0	2.00	0.85
8.0	2.60	1.10
9.0	3.50	1.50

Table 4.3. Effects of thymus extract upon estradiol threshold

Variations of the estradiol threshold dose in thymus and thyroidectomized castrated guinea pigs injected with Bezssonoff-Comsa thymus extract.

Thymus dose (units/100 g body weight)	Estradiol threshold dose (μg benzoate/100 g body weight)	
	Males	Females
0	0.05	0.04
1.0	0.10	0.05
2.0	0.27	0.12
3.0	0.55	0.23
4.0	0.95	0.34
5.0	1.50	0.50
6.0	2.10	0.70
8.0		1.20
10.0		1.70
12.0		3.0

The threshold dose of estradiol is increased in animals of both sexes by previous injections of thyroxine and thymic extract. Both these substances appear to antagonize estradiol. The influence of thyroxine and thymic extract are mutually suppressed to a large extent when injected simultaneously (Table 4.4). The numeric laws of these interactions are different in thymus-thyroidectomized castrated males and females. A sexual difference not related to the presence of the gonads is thus revealed, as reviewed by Comsa (1963).

When both thyroxine and thymic extract are injected simultaneously (Table 4.4), the estradiol threshold increases to a level similar to that determined in castrated guinea pigs and is not influenced by further parallel increase of thyroxine and thymus doses until the dose of 23 μg of thyroxine. This limit is significant. It is very close to the smallest thyroxine dose which induced exhaustion atrophy of the thymus (22 μg/ 100 g body weight) and to the dose corresponding to the upper limit of the first-degree law of thymus-thyroid interaction (25 μg/100 g body weight).

Table 4.4. Effect of thymus extract and thyroxine upon estradiol threshold

Variation of the estradiol threshold dose (μg of benzoate/100 g body weight) in thymus and thyroidectomized castrates injected with thyroxine and thymic extract (one unit of thymic extract per μg of thyroxine).

Thyroxine (μg/100 g body weight)	Estradiol threshold dose	
	Males	Females
0	0.05	0.04
2.0	0.10	
4.0	0.16	0.10
6.0	0.20	0.12
8.0	0.22	0.12
15.0	0.21	0.12
21.0	0.21	0.13
23.0	0.24	0.22
25.0	0.33	0.58
26.0	0.63	1.60

Thymus-thyroxine-testosterone interactions

The threshold dose of testosterone is defined as the smallest dose (in micrograms of testosterone propionate per 100 g body weight) which stops creatine excretion for 24 hr from the 24th hr after the injection in all four animals injected with this dose. This threshold dose in young guinea pigs is 9 μg/100 g body weight in males and 54 μg/100 body weight in females.

Injections of Bezssonoff-Comsa thymic extract alone in doses as high as 50 units per 100 g body weight did not modify this threshold dose. Thyroxine, injected alone, induced an increase of the threshold dose (see Table 4.5).

The increase of the testosterone threshold dose is a second degree-function of the thyroxine dose. The equations are:

$$\text{In males:} \quad 0.09x^2 + 17x + 9 = y \tag{6}$$

$$\text{In females:} \quad 2.54x^2 + 1.3x + 50 = y \tag{7}$$

Table 4.5. Effect of thyroxine upon testosterone threshold

Variations of the testosterone threshold dose (μg propionate/100 g body weight) in thymus and thyroidectomized castrated guinea pigs injected with thyroxine.

Thyroxine (μg/100 g)	Testosterone threshold dose	
	Males	Females
0	9	54
3	55	
5	100	130
8		220
10	185	320
12	225	430
15	285	640
20	385	1100
22	425	1450
25	470	1750
30	600	

where x is the thyroxine dose and y is the corresponding testosterone threshold dose.

Thymic extract antagonized this influence of thyroxine, as shown in the following experiment.

Thymus-thyroidectomized castrated guinea pigs, male and female, were injected with various amounts of thyroxine and Bezssonoff-Comsa thymic extract. The threshold testosterone dose corresponding to each dose of thymic extract was determined (Tables 4.6 and 4.7). For each dose of thyroxine, the threshold dose of testosterone decreased as increased amounts of thymic extract were injected. Note that 25 μg of thyroxine allowed no response from any dose of thymic extract. This again marks the limit of the "unphysiologic dose" of thyroxine between 20 and 25 μg/100 g body weight. The thyroxine influence was suppressed when (in males) 1.6 units and (in females) 2.0 units of thymic extract were injected per μg of thyroxine given.

The numeric laws found for these interactions are:

$$\text{In males:} \quad 0.09x^2 + 17x - 12z + 9 = y \tag{8}$$

$$\text{In females:} \quad 2.5x^2 + 1.5x - 17z + 50 = y \tag{9}$$

where x is the thyroxine dose, z the thymic extract dose, and y the corresponding testosterone threshold dose.

Table 4.6 Effect of thymus extract and thyroxine upon the testosterone threshold in males

Variations of the testosterone threshold dose (μg propionate/100 g) in thymus and thyroidectomized castrated male guinea pigs injected with various amounts of thyroxine and Bezssonoff-Comsa thymic extract.

Thyroxine (μg/100 g)	Thymus dose (units/μg thyroxine)						
	0	0.2	0.5	0.8	1.0	1.2	1.6
0	9						
3	55						
5	100	80	65	53	38	30	9
10	185	160	120	100	62	44	9
15	285	250	210	170	120	85	9
20	385				150		9
26	500		520	480	500	490	510

Table 4.7. Effect of thymus extract and thyroxine upon the testosterone threshold in females

Variations of the testosterone threshold dose in thymus and thyroidectomized castrated female guinea pigs injected with various amounts of thyroxine and Bezssonoff-Comsa thymic extract.

Thyroxine (μg/100g)	Thymus doses (units/μg of thyroxine)			
	0	0.6	1.2	2.0
0	52		80	
8	220	140	130	52
10	320	210	180	50
12	430		290	51
15	640	400	570	50
20	1100		1720	52
25	1750	1780		1750

Thus we can conclude that there is no direct antagonism of synergism demonstrated between thymic hormone and testosterone. These substances are synergists insofar as both of them antagonize thyroxine.

Investigations with thymectomized guinea pigs gave further evidence of this synergism between thymus and testosterone. Castration or thymectomy is followed by a transitory increase of the thyrotropic activity of the urine and by a transitory stimulation of the thyroid (as shown by histologic examination). Creatine excretion is transitorily increased in thymectomized or castrated guinea pigs. It is definitely increased in thymectomized castrates. Serum cholesterol level is decreased in thymectomized castrates. Simultaneous thyroidectomy suppressed thyrotropic activity of the urine and restored normal serum cholesterol and creatine level. Thus these changes are correlated to the stimulation of the thyroid.

In an illuminating experiment, Comsa (1954) divided 16 male thymectomized castrated guinea pigs into two groups. Group 1 received daily injections of 13 units/100 g body weight of thymic extract, and group 2 received daily injections of 250 μg testosterone propionate/100 g body weight (see Comsa, 1953b, for justification of this dosage). The experiment was pursued for 7 days. On the 8th day, no thyrotropic activity could be detected in the urine; the serum cholesterol level increased to the normal range and creatinuria decreased to 0.8 $\pm$0.07 mg/100 g body weight/24 hr in the thymic extract group and to zero in the testosterone group. Thus, the syndrome which developed following the loss of thymus *and* gonads could be suppressed by substitution of thymus *or* gonads (Comsa, 1954).

4.3 Thymus–adrenal cortex interrelationships

Influence of the thymus on the adrenal cortex

Pertinent concepts of the influence of the thymus on the adrenal cortex are summarized. Following thymectomy, the adrenal cortex of guinea pigs was found to be in a stimulated condition (*see* Chapter 3 and Table 3.5). This could be suppressed by repeated injections of thymic extract (Comsa, 1957d) or HTH. Simultaneous castration was found to suppress the thymiprivic stimulation of the adrenal in guinea pigs (Comsa, 1957b). Castration by itself has peculiarly intricate consequences on the adrenal cortex. Within the 1st month following the operation, a resting condition resulted. The ascorbic acid content of the gland is increased (Comsa, 1957d, e), corticosteroid metabolite excretion in urine is decreased in guinea pigs (Zondek and Burstein, 1952), and corticosteroid content of the plasma is decreased in rats (Telegdy and Endroczy, 1959), whereas in long-lasting experiments (1 year in mice by Houssay *et al.* (1955) and 2 or more years in guinea pigs by Parkes, (1945)) an extreme stimulation of the adrenal was observed in castrates. The gonoducts were found to be fully conditioned by the androgens secreted by these adrenals, and adrenal tumors developed in some guinea pigs (adenomata) and in about one-half of the mice (malignant). Thus it is improper to consider a definite steady state of the adrenal in castrates. Very likely, the changes remain evolutive until the death of the animals. However, in our experiments, relatively short-term consequences were considered (1 to 2 months), and within this interval the adrenals of castrates were proved to be in a resting condition.

The consequences of hyperthymization in guinea pigs were exactly opposite to those of thymectomy. The adrenal cortex was shrunken, and its ascorbic acid content was significantly increased. Total extract was used in these experiments (Comsa and Leroux, 1955).

Neither thymectomy nor castration, nor both these operations, nor hyperthymization was of any consequences in thyroidectomized guinea pigs. By itself, thyroidectomy is followed by atrophy of the adrenal cortex (reviewed by Comsa, 1952a, b). Thus, whichever of the interventions enumerated above were performed in addition, the thyroid appears as a permissive factor in this intricate interaction.

Influence of the adrenal cortex on the thymus

Thymectomy is of no consequence on the mortality rate of adrenalecto-mized rats (Selye, 1952). Adrenalectomized and thymectomized dogs were active when compared with adrenalectomized animals (Adler, 1938).

Following adrenalectomy, the thymus increased in size (Boinet, 1895, in Jaffe, 1924a, b). This increase is peculiarly important in castrates, although it does not develop in thyroidectomized rabbits (Marine, Manley, and Bauman, 1924). Chiodi (1939) did not observe thymic hypertrophy in adrenalectomized castrated rats.

In long experiments, the thymus of adrenalectomized rats was found to be hyperplastic and peculiarly rich in lymphocytes (Jaffe, 1924a, b). Jaffe gave no saline to his adrenalectomized rats. He did not notice significant mortality. Thus one may question whether or not his adrenalectomies were complete; in some strains of rats, the accessory adrenocortical tissue is very abundant and may suffice to insure survival. In short-term experiments, no evidence of thymic hypertrophy was found in adrenalectomized rats (Comsa, 1959c). The gland was hyperemic and edematous. The histologic picture was that of involution by emigration presented previously.

Hormonal activity of the thymus was found to be decreased in adrenalectomized rats (Comsa, 1959c). Normal activity could be restored by substitutive therapy.

A significant experiment is outlined: 30 male rats of 130 ± 8 g were adrenalectomized. During the following 7 days, 10 animals received no treatment, 10 animals received 200 μg of cortisone daily in subcutaneous injections, and 10 animals received 200 μg of desoxycorticosterone daily. These doses are minimal for survival. Rats of this strain die without exception within less than 15 days following adrenalectomy. The relative thymus weight was (in percentage of the total body weight) in normal rats, 0.25 ± 0.03; in untreated adrenalectomized rats, 0.33 ± 0.05; in the cortisone group, 0.32 ± 0.04; in the desoxycorticosterone group, 0.54 ± 0.06.

The thymuses of each group were pooled, extracted, and assayed. The hormonal activity found was (in units per gram of fresh organ) in normal rats, 62.5; in untreated adrenalectomized rats, 33.0; in the cortisone group, 39.4; and in the desoxycorticosterone group, 79.0.

The histologic picture was similar in the untreated group and in the cortisone group. In the desoxycorticosterone group, the thymus was almost normal; possibly the lymphocytes were increased in number.

It is generally admitted that injections of any corticosteroid result in thymus atrophy. This was observed with total extracts (Ingle, 1938), cortisone or corticosterone (Wells and Kendall, 1940), dehydrocorticosterone, and desoxycorticosterone (Dougherty, 1952; Litwac, 1970). In all these experiments, several milligrams were injected into normal animals. Most of the workers estimated thymic atrophy just by weighing. Those who made histologic examinations unanimously described the corticoid-induced thymic atrophy as a result of quite generalized pycnosis of lymphocytes. In contradistinction, using cortisone and desoxycorticosterone in substitutive amounts, there was no increase of the pycnosis rate and one can observe conspicuous differences between the effect of cortisone and desoxycorticosterone. Furthermore, adrenalectomized rats treated with desoxycorticosterone had a somewhat enlarged thymus. Thus, the observation of thymolytic effects of corticoids within the physiologic range may be questioned.

Interaction between thymic hormone and desoxycorticosterone

Thymic hormone was found to inhibit glucose uptake of the isolated rat diaphragm. So was desoxycorticosterone. This action of desoxycorticosterone is not specific. It is common to most steroids (*see* for references, Verzar and Wenner, 1949). Desoxycorticosterone was chosen because it was the only corticosteroid available which dissolved in water for accurate dosage. In a typical experiment, rat diaphragms were divided in four approximately equal parts and incubated for 1 hr in Krebs saline to which was added 0.2% glucose and gassed with 97% O_2 and 5% CO_2 in a water bath under agitation.

One part of the diaphragm was incubated with pure glucose in saline. In three other vessels, thymic preparations were added either alone (0.1, 0.5, or 1.0 μg/ml) or at one of the above concentrations together with 6, 12, or 18 μg desoxycorticosterone/ml. Glucose was determined with the glucose-oxidase-peroxidase-orthodianisidine reagent.

Under these conditions HTH added to the medium inhibited glucose uptake (as shown by the percent of control). Glucose uptake of four parts of the same diaphragm was 100% with no HTH, 82 $\pm$ 6.3% with 0.1 μg/ml HTH, 46.3 $\pm$ 4.5% with 0.5 μg/ml HTH, and 39 $\pm$ 1.4% with 1.0 μg/ml HTH. When thymic preparations and desoxycorticosterone (6, 12, or 18 μg) were added to the medium, glucose uptake was still more inhibited (Table 4.8). One microgram of thymic hormone together with 12 μg of desoxycorticosterone completely inhibited the glucose uptake in two of four diaphragms; when administered with 18 μg of desoxycorticosterone, all four preparations were completely inhibited.

Conclusions from these experiments may be stated. The thymus seems to exert a moderating influence on the adrenal cortex. The adrenal cortex seems to stimulate the function of the thymus under physiologic conditions. This influence is supported by the corticoids such as desoxy-

Table 4.8. Influence of thymic preparations and desoxycorticosterone on glucose uptake of isolated rat diaphragm

The data give the percentage of the uptake rate of the same diaphragms incubated in pure Krebs-saline with 2% glucose.

Thymus preparation	Concentration (μg/ml)	%Glucose uptake in presence of these desoxycorticosterone levels			
		0	6 μg/ml	12 μg/ml	18 μg/ml
		100	79.9 $\pm$ 17	56.3 $\pm$ 14	38.0 $\pm$ 13
T[a]	0.1	100	76.3 $\pm$ 11	51.8 $\pm$ 6	34.8 $\pm$ 5
P[b]	0.1	100	67.9 $\pm$ 19	42.5 $\pm$ 17	28.5 $\pm$ 7
T	0.5	100	61.1 $\pm$ 5	36.2 $\pm$ 4	20.9 $\pm$ 3
P	0.5	100	47.6 $\pm$ 10	22.2 $\pm$ 6	13.5 $\pm$ 3
T	1.0	100	48.1 $\pm$ 5	27.8 $\pm$ 3	18.5 $\pm$ 3
P	1.0	100	33.1 $\pm$ 2	7.9[c]	0

[a]T, total extract.
[b]P, presumably pure hormone.
[c]Mean not valid (in two of the four samples, the glucose uptake was zero).

corticosterone, which enhance inflammatory reactions. Under physiologic conditions no influence of cortisone on the thymus was detectable. At least to one corticosteroid (desoxycorticosterone) the thymic hormone appeared to be synergistic. This was demonstrated with a test common to all steroids. It is a matter of speculation whether such would be the case for all steroids.

4.4 Thymus-insulin interactions

The glucose uptake of rat diaphragm is a valid test of insulin action (*see* Weill-Malherbe, 1955, for references). The general conditions in this experiment are those used for testing the thymus-desoxycorticosterone interaction. When added to the medium, insulin, 23 units per ml, measurably stimulates the glucose uptake. A sharp threshold of this action can be delineated; no measurable effect was obtained with 1 or 2 μg; glucose uptake was increased 50% by 3 μg and 100% by 4 μg. Thus, 3 μg/ml can be considered to be the threshold dose of insulin in this test.

Addition of total thymic extract to the medium gave a significant increase in the insulin threshold dose:

Extract concentration	Insulin threshold
2×10^{-7}	4 μg
5×10^{-7}	6 μg
8×10^{-7}	10 μg
1.2×10^{-6}	20 μg
1.5×10^{-6}	40 μg

Thus the thymic extract appears to antagonize insulin.

The variations of the insulin threshold in relationship to thymus concentration follow a continuous exponential curve (*see* Comsa, 1963, for mathematical analysis of this law).

4.5 The thymus-pituitary axis

Thymus-anterior pituitary interactions have been alluded to in previous chapters.

Influence of the anterior pituitary on the thymus

The thymus involutes after hypophysectomy (Benedict, Putnam, and Teel, 1930). The histologic picture is that of the age involution. Injections of crude anterior pituitary extracts were followed either by hypertrophy (Caridroit, 1924) or by atrophy of the thymus (Schokaert, 1930). With fractionated pituitary preparations, it could be seen that growth hormone induced hypertrophy of the thymus (Benedict, Putnam, and Teel, 1930). Corticotropin induced atrophy (Crede and Moon, 1940), as did gonado-tropin (Arvin and Allen, 1928), but not in castrates (Evans and Simpson, 1934).

The hormone content of the thymus is decreased in hypophysectomized rats (Comsa, 1959b). It increases in hypophysectomized rats injected with growth hormone or corticotropin, whereas thyrotropin or hypophyseal gonadotropin shows no influence. This was shown in an experiment in which 100 hypophysectomized male rats of 130 to 150 g were divided into five groups: a) 20 animals received daily injections of 0.5 ml of phys-iologic saline; b) 20 animals received 2 units of corticotropin daily; c) 20 animals received 2 units of growth hormone daily; d) 20 animals received 0.1 units of thyrotropin daily; and e) 20 animals received daily injection of 2 units of an ambivalent gonadotropic pituitary preparation. After 7 days, the animals were killed with chloroform, and the thymuses were divided in four pools of five glands in each experimental group.

Extracts were prepared (Bezssonoff and Comsa, 1958) and bioassayed using the throxine glucose uptake test. The units of hormone were (per gram of fresh organ): in saline-treated rats, 34.0 ± 6 units; in growth-hormone treated rats, 59.0 ± 6 units; in corticotropin-treated rats, 50 ± 7 units; in thyrotropin-treated rats, 30 ± 4 units; in gonadotropin-treated rats, 26.3 ± 3 units; and in normal control rats, 63 ± 8 units.

Thus the secretion of the thymus is stimulated, although not exactly conditioned, by the anterior pituitary through the growth hormone and the corticotropin. This confirms the mineralocorticoid stimulation previously noted.

Following injections of cytotoxic antipituitary antibodies, Pierpaoli and Sorkin (1968, 1969) observed in mice a wasting syndrome resembling the consequences of thymectomy. They could reproduce this syndrome with injections of antigrowth hormone serum. They concluded that suppression of the growth hormone resulted in a loss of the secretion of the thymus, which in turn induced the wasted condition. However, their mice probably did not lose only their thymic hormone but certainly their pituitary growth hormone as well. These observations call for further research which could be of capital interest.

Influence of the thymus on the anterior pituitary

As previously mentioned, HTH was found to suppress the changes in the anterior pituitary induced by thymectomy. Overdosage of HTH, about three times the substitutive dose in guinea pigs, results in: a) almost complete disappearance of α cells; and b) a peculiar picture of the δ cells. These cells appear to be decreased in size and stained peculiarly dark (Herlant's tetrachrome). The nucleus is shrunken, and c) there is an increase in the number of big chromophobes. In rats under the same condition, α cells were still detectable, but they looked shrunken; δ cells changed as in guinea pigs, many δ cells looked empty, and the cytoplasm was reduced to narrow borders at the periphery and around the nucleus and some tenuous expansions between these borders. These cells recall the "wheel-cells" of Collin or the "daisy-flower cells" of Dhom.

Interactions between circulating homeostatic thymic hormone and circulating anterior pituitary hormones

1) Circulating thymus-growth hormone interaction
   (Comsa, 1958, 1965).

An experiment showing the interaction between circulating HTH and growth hormone is informative. Male rats of the Wistar-Commentry strain were hypophysectomized at 40 days of age, and 5 days later the rats of one group were thymectomized. Beginning the day of thymectomy, all animals received various amounts of a commercial growth hormone daily by intraperitoneal injection, four animals receiving each dose. Their weight increase was compared to that of the preperiod, 5 days from hypophysectomy to the first injection. The results are summarized in Table 4.9. It can be seen that the growth rate of the thymectomized and hypophysectomized rats receiving growth hormone decreased when compared with that of only hypophysectomized animals receiving corresponding doses of growth hormone.

In a second experiment, 90 thymectomized and hypophysectomized rats received daily subcutaneous injections of either the total thymic extract or HTH singly or in combination with 2.0 units daily of the growth hormone preparation used in the first experiment. General conditions were those of the first experiment. The results are summarized in Table 4.10. These results allow several conclusions. a) Thymic preparations, given alone, have no influence on the growth of thymectomized and hypophysectomized rats. b) These preparations enhance the influence of a growth hormone preparation. Conclusions from these experiments are that in the absence of the thymus the influence of the anterior pituitary is decreased, but still significant, and in the absence of the pituitary the influence of the thymus on the growth is lost. This seems to indicate that the thymus stimulates growth only insofar as it is an adjuvant to the pituitary growth hormone.

Table 4.9. Influence of growth hormone on growth of rats

Mean weight increase (g) in 15 days $\pm$ standard deviation.

Daily dose (units per animal)	Hypophysectomized	Thymectomized and hypophysectomized
0	-12.8 ± 3.0	-12.0 ± 1.0
0.5	4.5 ± 1.0	0
1.0	15.0 ± 3.8	6.5 ± 2.2
2.0	30.0 ± 5.1	11.5 ± 2.0
3.0	41.0 ± 7.2	12.0 ± 3.0
4.0	56.0 ± 5.0	17.0 ± 3.0

Table 4.10. Influence of thymic preparations on growth of thymectomized and hypophysectomized rats

Weight increase (g) in 15 days following thymus injections.

Daily dose (units per animal)	Single administration		Together with 2 units of hypophyseal growth hormone	
	T^a	HTH	T	HTH
0 (preperiod) 5	−12.0 ±		11.5 ± 2.0	
10	−8.0 ± 0.8	−8.7 ± 2.5	30.0 ± 4.0	36.0 ± 4.0
	−0	−6.1 ± 1.8	45.0 ± 7.0	54.0 ± 3.0
20	−0.5 ± 0.2	−3.0 ± 2.1	58.0 ± 60	68.0 ± 5.3
35	−3.0 ± 0.5	−2.6 ± 1.6	69.0 ± 6.4	74.0 ± 6.1
50	−1.5 ± 0.6	−2.1 ± 0.9	80.0 ± 4.8	78.0 ± 3.0

[a]T, Bezssonoff-Comsa extract.

2) Thymus-corticotropin interactions (Comsa, 1959a, c; 1965f)

One experiment designed to show thymus-corticotropin interaction involved 32 hypophysectomized and 24 thymectomized, hypophysectomized male rats given various amounts of a commercial corticotropin preparation. Hypophysectomy was performed 11 days before the corticotropin injections and thymectomy 5 days after hypophysectomy.

Two hours after the corticotropin injection, the ascorbic acid content of both adrenals was determined in all rats (method of Roe and Kuether). The results, summarized Table 4.11A, indicate that ascorbic acid content decreased in the adrenals of thymectomized and hypophysectomized rats following corticotropin injections in doses; ascorbic acid was not changed in the hypophysectomized rats. Following injection of 0.3 units of corticotropin, ascorbic acid content desceased in the adrenals of thymectomized and hypophysectomized rats by as much as 53.6% (when compared with untreated animals), whereas it remained in the limits of the standard deviation of only untreated hypophysectomized rats injected with the same dose. Thymectomy seemed to increase sensitivity toward corticotropin in hypophysectomized rats.

In the second experiment, thymectomized and hypophysectomized rats were injected daily with various amount of thymus preparations from the 6th to the 11th day following hypophysectomy. Immediately

Table 4.11A. Effect of corticotropin upon adrenal ascorbic acid content

Ascorbic acid content of the adrenal glands of rats (% of fresh organ) 2 hr after a corticotropin injection (means of 4 animals ± standard deviation).

Corticotropin dose (units per animal)	Hypophysectomized	Thymectomized and hypophysectomized
0	3.90 ± 0.1	3.68 ± 0.07
0.2	3.88 ± 0.06	2.07 ± 0.04
0.3	3.79 ± 0.03	1.71 ± 0.02
0.4	2.70 ± 0.01	1.57 ± ns
0.6	2.08 ± 0.02	1.52 ± ns
0.8	1.63 ± 0.02	1.31 ± ns
1.0	1.43 ± 0.02	
1.5	1.30 ± ns[a]	

[a] ns, not significant.

Table 4.11B. Effect of thymus extracts upon adrenal ascorbic acid content.

Ascorbic acid content of the adrenals in thymectomized and hypophysectomized rats injected with Bezssonoff-Comsa extract (T) or presumably pure thymic hormone (HTH) 2 hr after corticotropin injection of 0.3 units per animal.

Thymus dose (units per animal)	T	HTH
0	1.71 ± 0.02	1.71 ± 0.02
30	2.00 ± ns[a]	1.86 ± 0.07
60	2.31 ± 0.27	2.38 ± 0.07
90	3.36 ± 0.15	3.15 ± 0.08
120	3.70 ± 0.08	3.81 ± ns

[a] ns, not significant.

after the last thymus injection, a uniform injection of 0.3 units of corticotropin was given to all animals, and the ascorbic acid content of the adrenals was determined as in the first experiment. The results of this experiment (Table 4.11 B) show that the increased sensitivity of thymectomized-hypophysectomized rats towards corticotropin was suppressed by previous injections of either the total thymic extract or HTH. This seems to indicate that the homeostatic thymus hormone antagonized corticotropin.

3) Thymus-gonadotropin interactions (Comsa, 1959a, d; 1965f) Two experiments illustrate thymus-gonadotropin interactions. In the first experiment, various amounts of an ambivalent pituitary-gonadotropic preparation were injected four times, at intervals of 12 hr, to 48 hypophysectomized female rats of 100 g body weight. Hypophysectomy was performed 15 days before the gonadotropin injections, and one-half of the animals were thymectomized 5 days after hypophysectomy. The ovaries of all animals were weighed to 0.1 mg 12 hr after the last gonadotropin injection.

Obviously, thymectomized-hypophysectomized rats were more sensitive towards gonadotropin than hypophysectomized animals (Table 4.12A). Following four injections of 0.2 units of gonadotropin, the ovaries of thymectomized-hypophysectomized animals increased 335%, whereas those of hypophysectomized animals increased only 44.6%.

In a second experiment, thymectomized-hypophysectomized female rats (conditions of experiment 1) where injected daily from the 11th to the 15th day after hypophysectomy with various amounts of total thymic extract (T) or of HTH. On the 14th and the 15th days, they uniformly received four injections of gonadotropin, and the ovaries were examined as in the first experiment (Table 4.12B). The increased sensitivity of thymectomized-hypophysectomized rats towards gonadotropin seems to be suppressed by previous injections of the total thymic extract, and of HTH as well. In other words, the homeostatic thymic hormone seems to antagonize gonadotropin.

Table 4.12A. Effect of gonadotropin upon ovary size

Weight of both ovaries (mg) in rats injected four times within 48 hr with ambivalent hypophyseal ambivalent gonadotropin (means of four rats ± standard deviation).

Gonadotropin dose (units per animal)	Hypophysectomized	Thymectomized and hypophysectomized
0	9.2 ± 0.6	9.0 ± 0.3
4 × 0.2	13.3 ± 1.0	39.2 ± 0.8
4 × 0.5	26.7 ± 1.2	50.7 ± 0.3
4 × 0.7	44.6 ± 1.5	64.1 ± 0.3
4 × 1.0	58.0 ± 0.4	68.2 ± ns[a]
4 × 2.0	61.0 ± ns	76.2 ± ns

[a] ns, not significant.

Table 4.12B. Effect of thymus extracts upon ovary weight

Weight of both ovaries (mg) in thymectomized and hypophysectomized rats injected during 7 days with thymic preparations (T, Bezssonoff-Comsa, HTH, presumably pure hormone)
and four times within 48 hr with 0.3 units of hypophyseal
gonadotropin (See text for details.)

Thymus dose (units per animal)	Animals injected with	
	T	HTH
0	39.2 ± 0.8	39.2 ± 0.8
15	35.7 ± 1.6	33.1 ± 1.2
22	21.8 ± 1.0	22.5 ± 1.4
30	16.3 ± 0.9	17.6 ± 1.6
50	12.1 ± 0.7	11.8 ± 0.8

4) Thymus-thyrotropin interactions

An experiment is presented to show thymus-thyrotropin interactions
(Comsa, 1965a, e). Infantile normal male guinea pigs, 10 to 12 days of age,
weighing 130 to 140 g, were divided into three groups: a) 24 animals
received daily injection for 7 days of 0.5 ml of physiologic saline; b) 24
animals received daily injection for 7 days of 100 units of total thymic
preparation; and c) 24 animals received 100 units of HTH daily for 7
days. On the 6th to 7th day, they received various amounts of a commercial preparation of hypophyseal thyrotropin. Twenty-four hours after
the last thyrotropin injection, the thyroids were weighed and subjected
to histologic examination (Helly, hematoxylin-eosin). The degree of
activation was expressed according to Junkmann and Schoeller (*see*
Comsa, 1951d, for references). The results (Table 4.13) indicate that
previous and simultaneous injections of total thymic extract or HTH
inhibited the influence of thyropin on the thyroid of infantile guinea pigs.

The interaction between thymus and thyroid is probably different.
Thyroxine injections are followed by lymphocytosis, but not in thymectomized guines pigs (Comsa, 1958b, c) (Table 4.14). Thus, the thyroxine influence on lymphoid tissue appears to be thymus-mediated.

Summary of thymus-pituitary interactions

All these experiments reveal an intricate interaction between the thymus
and the pituitary. Possibly under normal conditions the thymus is one
of the regulators of the influence of the pituitary on the organism.
The consequences of thymectomy are easy to understand in these

Table 4.13. Weight and activity index of thyroids in infantile guinea pigs injected with thyreotropin

See text for techniques. The data give percentages of body weight, mean ± standard deviation and Junkmann-Schoeller estimation of activity.

Thyreotropin doses, international units	Saline Weight	Saline Activity[a]	Additional Injections Total extract Weight	Additional Injections Total extract Activity[a]	HTH hormone Weight	HTH hormone Activity[a]
0[a]	0.13 ± ns[b]	0.02 ±	0.13	0.02 ±	0.13	0.02 ±
2 × 0.05	0.22 ± ns	+ +				
2 × 0.10	0.23 ± ns	+ + +	0.15 ± ns	0	0.14 ± ns	0
2 × 0.20	0.31 ± 0.04	+ + + +	0.19 ± 0.01	±0.2+	0.17 ± ns	±
2 × 0.30	0.35 ± 0.05	+ + + +	0.22 ± 0.02	+0.2+ +	0.20 ± ns	+
2 × 0.40	0.39 ± 0.01	+ + + +	0.25 ± 0.05	+ + +	0.26 ± ns	+ + +
2 × 0.50	0.44 ± 0.02	+ + + +	0.32 ± 0.01	+ + + +	0.31 ± 0.03	+ + + +

[a]Activity is evaluated by the following:
0, a resting condition. Follicles wide, epithelium flat, colloid dense and acidophilic.
±, in the center of the gland, small follicles, high epithelium.
+, picture of (±) extended over the whole gland.
+ +, in the center of the gland, follicles, empty of colloid. epithelium high.
+ + +, picture of (+ +) extended to the whole gland, some mitoses.
+ + + +, extreme stimulation. in some follicles stratified epithelium, mitoses frequent.
[b]ns, not significant.

Table 4.14. Lymphocyte count in blood, bone marrow and spleen of guinea pigs

Animals	Blood		Marrow		Spleen	
	0^a	$+^b$	0	+	0	+
Normal^c	43 $\pm$ 3	66.5 $\pm$ 8	13.9 $\pm$ 4	25.0 $\pm$ 6	47.5 $\pm$ 7	49 $\pm$ 3
Days thymecto-mized^d before						
6	30	30	14.5	10.0	34.7	24.1
12	30	29	12.2	8.0	33.1	24.2
18	30	29	11.5	6.5	33.1	23.1
24	30	28	12.0	7.5	32.7	22.8
30	30	25	12.6	7.5	35.1	20.8

^{a}0, No injection.

^{b}+, Thyroxine (16 μg/100 g body weight/24 hr for 6 days).

^{c}Normal animals, mean of 10 $\pm$ standard deviation.

^{d}Thymectomized, mean of 3 animals.

terms. In thymectomized guinea pigs: a) the influence of growth hormone is decreased as the growth rate is decreased; b) the influences of corticotropin, gonadotropin, and thyrotropin are increased as the effectors of these hormones show signs of stimulation; and c) a counter regulation may be induced later, since these effects of thymectomy are transitory.

It would be of interest to investigate the endocrines of other animals, such as mice or hamsters, known to be affected severely following thymectomy. This implies examinations at various intervals after thymectomy, principally at short term before the onset of wasting syndrome. Examinations in wasted animals only would not suffice, since it is known that every wasting disease induces degenerative changes of the endocrines (*see* Chapter 1). The slight consequences of thymectomy in the rat are possibly correlated with the peculiarly small hormone content of its thymus, whereas the hormone content of the guinea pig thymus is by far the highest of all species investigated.

The indirect thymus-anterior pituitary interaction

As mentioned previously, thymectomy is followed by an increase of the thyrotropic activity of the urine in guinea pigs; so is castration or thyroidectomy (reviewed by Comsa, 1951d). Simultaneous extirpation of all three glands had no similar consequences (Comsa, 1951b; 1954); in thymus-thyroidectomized castrates, no thyrotropic activity of the urine could be detected. Thus an imbalance between the influences of thymus, thyroid, and testes seemed to result in an increased thyrotropic activity of the pituitary. Perhaps this could be suppressed by putting the three terms of balance equal to zero. This supposition was verified by the following experiment. In thymus-thyroidectomized castrates the injection of thyroxine (13 μg/100 g of body weight), or total thymic extract (13 units/100 g of body weight), or testosterone (250 μg/100 g of body weight) (*see* Comsa, 1953a, for explanation of the dosage) was followed within 24 hr by an increase of the thyrotropic activity of the urine (corresponding to degree $+++$ of Junkmann and Schoeller; Table 4.13), but simultaneous injection of all three of these hormonally balanced preparations had no such effect. This is an example of the stimulation of the anterior pituitary by an induced imbalance between several of its effectors. Most likely more of these examples could be found if one looked for them.

4.6 Summary of hormonal interactions

The hormonal interactions of the thymus may provide an explanation for its influence on lymphocyte production. The thymic hormone antagonizes the corticotropic influence of the anterior pituitary, and thus it may inhibit the lympholytic effect of corticotropin (mediated by the adrenal cortex). It is a synergist of the growth hormone which enhances the proliferative activity of the lymphoid tissue and which antagonizes the lympholytic effect of massive corticoid injections (Selye, 1952). In adrenalectomized mice, thymectomy is not followed by lymphopenia (Metcalf and Buffet, 1957). Thus the influence of the thymus upon the lymphoid tissue may be mediated, at least partly, by the anterior pituitary and the adrenal. However, a direct influence of the thymus on lymphocytes is demonstrated by the observation of the chemotactic influence of the thymus on lymphocytes (Comsa, 1950) and of the stimulation of ^{3}H-thymidine uptake of incubated lymphocytes by thymic preparations (Goldstein, Slater, and White, 1966).

The interaction between thymus and thyroid is probably different. Thyroxine injections are followed by lymphocytosis, but not in thymectomized guinea pigs (Comsa, 1958b) (Table 4.14). Thus the thyroxine influence on lymphoid tissue appears to be mediated by the thymus.

It is a matter of discussion whether or not hormonal interactions of the thymus may play a role in its influence on leukemogenesis. The development of leukemia in mice is truly inhibited by thymectomy (Law and Miller, 1950a, b, c; Kaplan, Brown, and Paul, 1953) or by thyroidectomy (Nagareda and Kaplan, 1959). It is accelerated by adrenalectomy and by castration (Law, 1947). However, the thymus of leukemic mice is abnormal during the latent period of the disease (Smith and Kaplan, 1961). It would be audacious to suppose that this thymus exerts its influence on leukemia only by means of its normal secretion. An indirect influence of the thymus on lymphoid tissues by means of its intricate hormonal interaction is thus revealed. The present state of documentation does not permit one to differentiate this influence from the direct one.

To a certain extent the consequences of thymectomy upon immunologic reactions may result from the thymiprivic imbalance between the pituitary hormones. The balance between inflammatory (growth hormone, mineralocorticoids) and anti-inflammatory influences (corticotropin, glucocorticoids) appeared to influence antibody production (Hoene, Rindani, and Heuser, 1954). The hormonal influences on the egg-white shock in the rat provide some circumstantial evidence for this supposition. Thus, egg-white shock is particularly severe in adrenalectomized rats (Selye, 1950); it is suppressed following thymectomy. Simultaneous removal of the thymus and the adrenal enhances the egg-white shock, as does adrenalectomy alone. Thymic hormone injection restores the normal sensitivity of thymectomized rats, but it has no enhancing influence on the egg-white shock in thymectomized and adrenalectomized rats (Comsa, 1965c).

Concerning the influence of the thymus on the lymphocytes and on immunologic reactions, Miller (1962b, c) presumed that the thymus provides an environment for the lymphocytes where these cells can fulfill their potential, such as proliferation, antibody production, and malignant degeneration. According to Osoba and Miller, (1964) this environment still exerts its influence across a millipore membrane (by means of one or several specific substances delivered to the organism). Thus, the "environment" may be understood as a specific position of the hormonal balance, conditioned by the presence of the thymic hormone and, at least partially, by its interference with the influence of other hormones.

The hormonal interactions of the thymus could provide a complete explanation of all aspects of the influence of the thymus. For example, the stimulated condition of the adrenal cortex following thymectomy may account for the thymiprivic lymphopenia and for the thymiprivic deficiency of immunologic reactions. This supposition tends to define the thymiprivic condition as a form of the general adaptation syndrome peculiarly aggravated by the loss of a mechanism, *i.e.*, the thymus which contributes normally to moderate the stimulation of the adrenal. The thymus has been proven to influence other forms of stress (*e.g.*, the radiation syndrome in guinea pigs, which was improved by injections of thymic extract; Comsa and Gros, 1956). However, this explanation is probably oversimplified. The knowledge of the hormonal interactions of the thymus does not prohibit the presumption of a direct influence of the thymus in cellular physiology. It would be a matter of further research to separate those two roles of the thymus, but it would be misleading to investigate the role of the thymus in cellular physiology without taking into account its hormonal interactions.

4.7 Thymus effects in radiation sickness

The nearly complete involution of the thymus in irradiated animals is well known. Summarized here are descriptions given in reviews (Bloom, 1948; Comsa, 1964; Lacassagne and Gricouroff, 1941).

The consequences of heavy ionizing irradiation on the thymus are brutal. Two hours after the irradiation almost all lymphocytes are pycnotic. The nuclei disintegrate, and the chromatin is agglutinated to homogeneous round drops of various size which are reabsorbed within 3 to 5 days. The regeneration begins between the 5th and the 10th day after irradiation, but it is completed very slowly. In guinea pigs the limit between cortex and medulla is not clearly discerned 60 days after irradiation. Lymphocytes are scarce in the cortex, in spite of the greatly increased mitosis rate (Comsa, 1956c).

This deleterious influence of irradiation is generally explained by the peculiar sensitivity of thymic lymphocytes toward irradiation. However, this explanation is not complete.

The thymus involutes in rats after an irradiation of the hind legs, the thymus being shielded with lead. In adrenalectomized animals, direct irradiation of the thymus only is followed by involution, and the histologic picture of this involution differs conspicuously from that observed in normal rats (Leblond and Segal, 1942). This recalls normal senile involution. The thymus does not involute following a LD 50 lethal irradiation in thyroidectomized guinea pigs receiving substitutive doses of thyroxine (Comsa, 1964). Thus, to a certain extent, the thymic involution in irradiated animals seems to result from disorders induced in other endocrine glands.

The antithyroxine efficiency of the thymus was found to be decreased in irradiated guinea pigs when tested in the usual way. The dose of Bezssonoff-Comsa thymus extract sufficient to suppress the influence of 10 μg of thyroxine in irradiated thymus-thyroidectomized castrates was found to be a first-degree function of the X-ray dose administered in a single total body irradiation, after 24 hr at 200 r it was found equal to 70 units; at 250 r it was found equal to 100 units; at 300 r it was found equal to 130 units; at 350 r it was found equal to 155 units; and at 400 r it was found equal to 200 units.

Later this consequence of irradiation decreased in a second-degree function of time. The normal reactivity (10 μg of thyroxine correspond to 10 units of thymic extract) was restored 20 days after the irradiation. Thus, the efficiency of thymic extract is significantly decreased in irradiated guinea pigs. It could be imagined that the persistence of the involution of the thymus (of the "exhaustion" pattern) may result to some extent from the oversolicitation of the thymus. This suggested that repeated injections of a thymic extract may be beneficial to irradiated guinea pigs.

Three experiments were performed to investigate this supposition (Comsa and Gros, 1956).

1) Forty male guinea pigs of 140 to 150 g received one single total X-ray irradiation with 300 r (the LD 50 in our strain); 20 of the animals received daily injections of 100 units per 100 g of Bezssonoff-Comsa thymic extract. Within 50 days, 18 of these animals survived, whereas only 6 nontreated animals survived.

2) Forty guinea pigs of 140 to 150 g were irradiated with 1000 r (LD 100 in our strain); 20 received daily injections of 100 units of the Bezssonoff-Comsa extract used in experiment 1. All treated and nontreated animals died within 7 to 9 days following irradiation (Comsa, 1964).

3) One hundred twenty guinea pigs were irradiated under the condition of experiment 1; 44 were injected with thymic extract. At various intervals from 1 to 60 days after the irradiation, four animals of every group were autopsied. Histologic examination of the thyroid, pituitary, thymus, and gonads was made. Smears of bone marrow, spleen, and lymph nodes were examined. The functional condition of the adrenal cortex was estimated

by determination of the ascorbic acid content of the gland. (For details, see Comsa and Gros, 1956.)

It could be concluded that thymic extract injections did not prevent the initial lesions of the examined organs, but that they accelerated significantly their restoration. The increased thyrotropic activity of the urine was suppressed (Comsa 1952d, f). The thymus, adrenals, gonads, thyroid, hematopoietic organs, and thyroid were found to be normal 15 days after the irradiation in thymus-injected guinea pigs.

The consequences of irradiation were still conspicuous in nontreated animals 60 days after the irradiation (Comsa, 1956a, c; Comsa and Gros, 1956).

From these observations two conclusions were drawn. The thymic extract had a demonstrable radioprotective influence within the limits of the potentially lethal X-ray dose, but it is inefficient after an LD 100 lethal irradiation. The radioprotective action of the thymus is different from that of synthetic radioprotective drugs (*see* for references, Comsa, 1964). None of these drugs has any radioprotective action when administered after irradiation. Thus far, two other substances are known to protect against irradiation under the same conditions: hypohyseal growth hormone (Selye, Selgado, and Procopio, 1952) and desoxycorticosterone (Ellinger, 1947). It can be recalled that thymic hormone was found to be synergistic to both these substances.

Furthermore, ionizing irradiation is considered as a stressor. It elicits a peculiar form of general adaptation syndrome characterized by simultaneous development of signs of the resistance stage and of the exhaustion stage of this syndrome (Comsa, 1964). Since the thymic hormone is known to antagonize corticotropin, it can be imagined that in these experiments it acted as an antistressor.

Since thymic extract was unable to influence the consequences of an LD 100 irradiation (Comsa, 1964), it seems doubtful that it could influence the specific, primary consequences of irradiation when these reach the limit where the resistence of the organism approaches zero. Thymus therapy may be beneficial insofar as it suppresses the hormonal imbalance resulting from the irradiation.

It has been observed that the thymic nucleic acids of irradiated mice (expected to become leukemic) show a chromatographic pattern different from that of a normal mouse thymus several months before the onset of leukemia (Smith and Kaplan, 1961). It would be of major interest to know if this change also occurs in a normal thymus grafted in an irradiated, thymectomized mouse.

4.8 The thymus in nutritional disorders

Influence of fasting on the thymus

Fasting is followed by a severe involution of the thymus; the thymus decreases by about 70% of its normal weight when the total body weight is decreased in fasting pigeons by 30%. Chronic underfeeding also results in a nearly total involution of the thymus; in rabbits the thymus decreased by 94% when the total body weight was decreased by 40% (Jonson, 1909). Hammar (1936) described the hunger involution as characteristic; no pycnoses are seen, mitoses almost cease, lymphocytes decrease in number within the thymus, the small interlobular veins are crowded with lymphocytes, and no young Hassal corpuscles are seen. Thus, the hunger involution seems to result from an increased emigration of the lymphocytes similar to the involution caused by thyroxine injections in unphysiologic amounts. In contradistinction to thyroxine-induced involution, mitoses are not increased and no new Hassal corpuscles are differentiated in hunger involution. In other words, the thymus in starvation shows no histologic evidence of stimulation. However, the two involutions may be related to each other; Courrier (1925) has demonstrated that the thymus of thyroid-injected rabbits may hypertrophy if the animals are allowed to compensate for their increased energetic needs by increasing their food intake, whereas it involutes under the influence of identical doses of thyroxine in animals kept on limited food intake.

Specific nutritional deficiencies affect the thymus in a similar way. The thymus was found involuted to nearly unrecognizable rudiments in protein deficiency (Salkind, 1915) and in experimental beriberi (Funk and Douglas, 1913), scurvy (Lopez-Lomba, 1923a, b), avitaminosis A (Sampson and Korenchevsky, 1932), B_1 (Deane and Shaw, 1947), B_2 (1947), B_6 (1947), choline (Gyorgy and Goldblatt, 1940; Klein, Goldstein, and White, 1966) or pantothenic acid deficiency (McQueeney et al., 1947). In most of these publications, the weight loss is only indicated. The histologic examinations which were made suggested that the involution resulted from underfeeding.

Influence of the thymus on the evolution of deficiency diseases

Deficiency diseases were found to be peculiarly severe in thymectomized animals. The latent phase was shortened, the weight loss was precocious, and the animals died sooner. This was observed in "polished rice disease" (Caridroit, 1924) and in McCollum rickets (Hirota, 1938). Thymectomized rats constantly developed severe rickets when reared in the dark with a diet of skim milk and bread; under these conditions, normal rats incidentally developed slight rickets (Asher and Landolt, 1934).

Several authors have observed that addition of fresh thymus to a deficient diet allows increased survival of rats. Possibly in these experiments the thymus feeding supplemented a deficient ration. This is likely, since Hirota (1938) failed to increase the survival rate of rats reared on a McCollum diet or on polished rice with injections of Asher's thymus extract.

Influence of the thymus in underfed animals without specific deficiencies

When fed a poor diet with which normal rats survived indefinitely, thymectomized rats died in a cachectic condition in 20 to 40 days (Asher and Landolt, 1934). Asher and coworkers tested their extract as follows (Asher, 1933; Asher and Landolt, 1934; Asher and Scheinfinkel, 1929; Glazmann, 1923; Ratti, 1940): weanling rats were fed skim milk and bread or lean horsemeat. They developed no signs of specific deficiency disease, but they did not grow and their general condition was poor. Daily injections of a thymic extract allowed normal growth in these animals.

Asher and coworkers used this observation as an assay of their extract following the different steps of preparation. They concluded that under optimal conditions the thymus is not necessary, but that it becomes relevant under unfavorable conditions.

A similar observation was shown with guinea pigs (Comsa, 1959d). The deficient condition was obtained by early weaning. The survival rate and growth rate were significantly improved by daily injections of a Bezssonoff-Comsa extract using the daily dose of 100 units per 100 g of body weight. As reported in Chapter 1, thymectomy was of no consequence in newborn guinea pigs when they were not weaned at the time of operation.

Thus it is seen that thymic extract therapy improved the condition of animals fed poor diets (diets low in several nutrients but completely deficient in none). It failed to influence the development of specific deficiency diseases (the complete deficiency of one single essential nutrient).

All deficiency diseases are known to induce a hypertrophy of the adrenals (Lopez-Lomba, 1923a, b). Possibly these diseases represent the general adaptation syndrome, as well as specific disorders resulting from the lack of specific nutrients. Under conditions leading to malnutrition, the role played by the general adaptation syndrome in the disease becomes relevant, whereas it is overwhelmed in specific deficiencies. Thus we again find the supposition suggested by the irradiation experiments. The thymus may influence all these syndromes insofar as it acts as an antistressor, *i.e.*, as a corticotropin antagonist.

4.9 Pathogenesis of thymoprivic conditions

An understanding of why some animals waste and die following thymectomy while others do not may be approached from any of several viewpoints developed above.

1) The endocrine consequences of thymectomy are numerous. Conspicuous changes of the endocrines were found in thymectomized animals whenever this was studied. Some of these changes, such as the stimulation of the thyroid, the adrenal, and the gonads, are transitory; these changes may result from a feedback effect on the respective cells of the anterior pituitary. Some other changes, for instance, the stimulated condition of the pituitary alpha cells in the rat, last indefinitely. Still it should be emphasized that none of these changes is known to be lethal. The thymoprivic hyperthroidism, for instance, does not reach a toxic range, and there are no signs of toxic excess of corticoids in thymectomized animals. The stimulated condition of growth hormone from α cells does not result in gigantism; it just seems to compensate for the loss of the synergistic thymus effect. In other words, the endocrine consequences of thymectomy may provide the partial explanation of the thymoprivic wasting; the fast-reacting rat pituitary may provide an efficient counter-regulation, whereas the sluggish pituitary of the guinea pig does not (but this explanation is not exhaustive).

2) The decrease of antibody production may explain the thymoprivic wasting. The constant and definite survival of thymectomized germ-free mice is considerable, but it would be a dangerous oversimplification to conclude that in germfree mice thymectomy is of no consequence. Such conclusions are often drawn from such conspicuous facts and may lead at length to a conclusion which is difficult to substantiate. Here the incomplete description of the thymoprivic condition must be underlined. Nothing is known about the endocrine consequences of thymectomy in mice; an investigation of these consequences in germfree

and classic mice would be of capital interest. We recall the conspicuous consequences of thymectomy on the endocrines of the resistant rat.

Moreover an interspecific comparison of consequences of thymectomy does not entirely support the explanation of thymoprivic wasting as merely a decreased resistance to infection. The infection-resistant rat does not waste after thymectomy, nor does the infection-sensitive rabbit. A parallel can be found in guinea pigs, rabbits, and mice, which shows that animals which seem to need the thymic hormone the most (considering their peculiar hormonal status) produce the most of it. This is plausible, but it is not an explanation.

3) Nutritional problems should be considered. According to Asher there are optimal alimentary conditions where the thymus is unnecessary for normal growth and survival. The thymus is an emergency gland, according to Asher, necessary only to meet abnormal conditions such as malnutrition. Here again we must warn against the tendency to equate survival with an entirely normal state. I believe that the interactions between thymus and nutritional influences deserve further investigation. Asher has just shown the way. We might recall that general malnutrition, as well as specific deficiencies, results in conspicuous changes in the endocrines and an extreme decay of immunologic functions.

The proper function of the thymus in cellular physiology can be approached from present standards in a speculative way only. This attempt may be of interest for future research.

The thymus interacts with several other endocrine glands, in fact with all hormones investigated thus far. In infantile animals, the presence of the thymus seems compulsory for hormonal homeostasis. Following thymectomy, a compensatory mechanism seems to develop in the rat which apparently survives thymectomy. It is characterized by the intense stimulation of the growth hormone-producing cells of the anterior pituitary (the synergist of the thymus). In guinea pigs this reaction is sluggish, and it develops only in animals which show signs of recovery. This seems to suggest an alternative; either a compensatory mechanism develops quickly, or the animal marks its inability to compensate and the approach of death.

Hormones may react by enhancing the production of cellular enzymes. This idea approaches classic clarity in the case of insulin, but more and more hormones were investigated in this direction. Speculatively, it can be imagined that the thymus may act in this point of cellular physiology, enhancing some other hormones, such as growth hormone, and interfering with others such as thyroxine or corticotropin. However, the first step to illustrate this respect of the function of the thymus is still to be demonstrated. Here the different aspects of the function of the thymus may find a common denominator. Enzymes are proteins, and so are antibodies. Furthermore, the action of the thymus on overall growth (synergistic to growth hormone) and on lymphatic tissue may suggest its involvement in coordination of protein synthesis (for complete review, consult Litwac, 1970). From our present knowledge, this is purely speculative, but it suggests that further research is needed. Thus our knowledge of the endocrine function of the thymus is far from classic clarity; however, the very existence of this function of the thymus was categorically negated not so long ago. The function is clear; still, our knowledge is not. The endocrine function of the thymus has been known since 1940, but it has not been generally admitted.

5   Biologic Activity of Thymic Protein Extracts

S. M. Milcu and I. Potop

5.1 Introduction

Evidence accumulated in the past two decades from experimental and clinical observations has created renewed interest in the thymus for a widening circle of biologists, chemists, and physicians. "The golden age of thymology has started" (Miller, 1967), arrived at by investigations resorting to thymectomy, transplants, and extracts. As reviewed in the first chapters of this book, the bulk of this information shows the participation of the thymus in immunology and endocrinology.

The involvement of the thymus in immunogenesis implies its interference with neoplastic mechanisms, thereby furnishing a valid explanation for the inhibitory action of thymus extracts on tumor growth. Research confirmed the involvement of the thymus in body growth and metabolism. One of the questions with which we have been particularly concerned since 1943 (Milcu and Pitis, 1943a, b; Milcu and Simionescu, 1953: 1960; Milcu *et al.*, 1954) is that of the histophysiology of the thymus and its interrelation with the endocrine system; this led to studies on the pharmacodynamics of proteins from the thymus (Potop, 1963; Potop and Juvina, 1967; Milcu and Potop, 1971).

Among the saline-soluble thymus extracts is that of Asher (1933), which is seemingly a polypeptide. In 1935, Maisin and Pourbaix (cited by Masin, 1963) demonstrated the presence of two compounds in the thymus and other organs which have an antagonistic action on tumor growth; these were a water-soluble activating compound and an inhibitory substance soluble in chloroform and ether. Their effects were tested in mice with tar-induced cancer. Comsa and Bezssnoff (1958) isolated from calf thymus and human urine an extract of protein nature with a similar chemical character and biologic action. Bernardi and Comsa (1965a, b) isolated an active compound in a presumably pure state by column chromatography, as reported in Chapter 3. Apart from its replacing activity in thymectomized animals, this compound influences metabolic processes and establishes correlations between the thymus and endocrine glands, thus supporting the concept of the thymus being an endocrine gland (see Chapter 4). Pelletier, Huron, and Delaunay (1960) prepared an extract of polypeptide nature which acts on bacterial respiration. The nucleic acid extracts isolated by Dufour and Rochette (1961) from thymus had a protective, albeit unspecific, action in tumor transplantation and in cold stress. Szent-Györgyi and coworkers Hegyeli and McLaughlin (1962) studied the components of the thymus and their relations with growth, fertility, muscular activity and cancer. They separated two substances with antagonistic action on tumor growth, retine and promine, and a third factor which exhibits sexual maturation by retarding the onset of gametogenesis. In most animal tissues and some vegetable tissues and in urine there is a balance between retine and promine, which have similar physical and chemical properties. According to Szent-Györgyi, retine is apparently a general constituent of the tissues rather than a thymus hormone. Chemically it is likely that retine is a methylglyoxal derivative (Szent-Györgyi, 1966; Szent-Györgyi, Együd, and McLaughlin, 1967). A lymphocyte-stimulating factor (LSH) which is a pure protein with a molecular weight of 17,000 ± 5,000 (Hand, Caster, and Luckey, 1967), a lymphocyte-maturation factor of molecular weight 79,800 which is a pure protein, isolated by Robey, Campbell, and Luckey (1972), an active steroid isolated from thymus by our laboratory, and purified extracts of others are detailed in separate chapters.

5.2 Protein extraction procedures for TP, a thymic peptide preparation

In investigations initiated in 1949, we used an extract prepared from calf thymus according to the method of Ioana Milcu, the polypeptide nature of which we have established. Subsequent research demonstrated that this extract, which we called thymus polypeptide (TP), plays a direct or indirect role in growth, alters certain metabolic processes, inhibits the growth rate of tumors either transplanted or induced by some chemical carcinogens, and modifies blood leukocyte ratios and/or number and immune reactions of the body. The activity of these extracts was tested *in vivo* in thymectomized mammals and in intact chick embryos and *in vitro* tumor cell cultures.

Thymus polypeptide (TP) fraction

A thymic polypeptide fraction (TP) was isolated by Ioana Milcu's original method (Milcu and Simionescu, 1953). Fresh calf thymus was minced and exhaustively extracted with acetone at room temperature and dried. The lipid-free powder was subjected to alkaline hydrolysis, *i.e.*, 1000 ml of 0.1 N NaoH was added to 100g of thymus powder, boiled 20 min, cooled, and filtered. The filtrate was adjusted with 0.1 N HCl to pH 4.5 to 5. After complete precipitation, the filtrate was made alkaline with N NaOH to pH 10; then it was boiled, cooled, and again filtered. The filtrate was neutralized with N HCl to pH 7. The clear extract was placed into vials and tyndallized. This is TP. The concentration was 856 mg per 100 ml.

Using the same procedure, similar protein fractions were obtained from calf, horse, and human embryo thymus.

Electrophoretic analysis with Tiselius apparatus (Fig. 5.1) showed the extract to contain a single fraction. Chemical analysis indicated TP contained amino acids and polypeptides but no proteins according to biuret color and trichloroacetic acid (TCA) reactions. Paper chromatography of the extract demonstrated 13 spots indicative of 11 free amino acids or groups of amino acids: cystine, the arginine, histidine and lysine group, aspartic acid, glycine, glutamic acid, threonine, alanine, proline, thyrosine, the methionine and valine group, and the leucine and isoleucine group. The total nitrogen content of the TP extract (1 g of fresh thymus equivalent per 1 ml contains 44 mg/ml) ranged between 114 and 119 mg N per 100 ml; 31% was polypeptide nitrogen, and 69% was amino acid

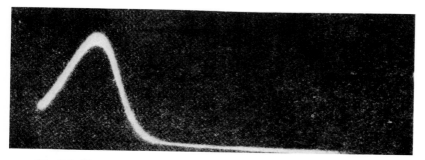

Fig. 5.1. Electrophoretic analysis of extract TP made with the Tisselius apparatus. (Veronal buffer; pH 8.6.)

nitrogen (Milcu, Potop, and Mreana, 1963). TP is stable, retaining its biological characteristics for a long period; heating to boiling fails to alter the metabolic activity of the fraction (Potop, Boeru, and Mreana, 1966).

TPE from horse embryo thymus

A polypeptide extract derived from horse embryo thymus collected during the 7th month of gestation was prepared by a method analogous to that used for TP (Potop, Biener, and Mreana, 1965) and is called TPE for thymus peptide embryo.

Analysis of the final extract of TPE demonstrated a concentration of protein-derived material of 16.5 mg per 100 ml, evaluated according to the Lowry method. Paper chromatography of TPE revealed the presence of 13 free amino acids (Fig. 5.2). When compared with TP, the extract derived from embryo thymus contained qualitatively the same set of free amino acids, but in reduced quantities (Fig. 5.2).

Extracts of human thymus

Our method was also used for preparing an extract of human thymus obtained from a stillborn child. This extract had an antiproliferative activity on tumor cell cultures. A striking fact in our experiments was the variability of the antitumor activity of the extracts when related to factors such as age, nutrition, and physiologic conditions of the cultures. These polypeptide extracts showed no toxic effects during long-term administration with increasing doses. Analyses of this extract are in progress.

5.3 Action of thymic extracts on metabolism

The action of TP was first investigated in metabolism related to normal growth. Evidence found in the literature stresses the role played by the thymus in some metabolic processes involved in growth. Although this was reviewed in previous chapters, certain aspects will be emphasized here.

Lucien, Parissot, and Richard (1927) showed in various animal species that thymectomy causes a delayed maturation of the skeleton, a reduction in volume, weight, and length of the bones, and a reduction in Ca deposition in the bony tissue. Thymus administration gave diametrically opposed effects. C. I. Parhon also showed the influence of the thymus on water and Ca and K metabolism (Parhon, Cahane, and Marza, 1927;

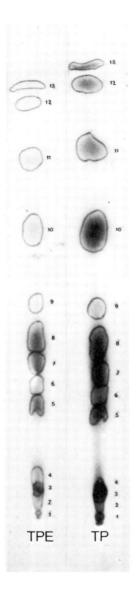

TPE TP

Fig. 5.2. Paper chromatography of free amino acids from the thymus extract prepared from embryonic thymus (TPE). Unidimensional chromatography, Whatmann paper No. 1; solvents: butanol + acetic acid + water (40:15:5); two migrations at 20°C; developed with ninhydrine, 0.2 g/100 ml in alcohol.

Parhon and Cahane, 1939) and attempted to establish a correlation between the hydrating and the hypercalcemic actions of the thymus.

By studying the effect of the thymus on growth and P and Ca metabolism, Milcu *et al.* (1951a, b) showed that administration of TP causes significant changes both in intact rabbits and in rabbits previously subjected to X-ray irradiation of the thymus. In the final stage of growth, the weight of the animals was increased by the thymus extract and was reduced by thymus irradiation (Fig. 5.3). Thymus extract administration unevenly increased Ca and P levels in all the bones, most notably in the long bones. The results warrant the conclusion that TP exerts a stimulating effect on growth and on Ca and P deposition in bone tissue. These findings were confirmed by studies based on ^{32}P and ^{45}Ca incorporation performed by Toma (1961). Pora, Toma, and Oros (1962) demonstrated the positive influence of the thymus in ossification. In contrast to the effects obtained in mammals, TP proved to inhibit maturation of chick embryo (Potop *et al.*, 1960). However, it is of significance that Ca and P accumulation in chick embryo tibia is stimulated by the administration of TP (Fig. 5.4).

The action of the thymus on serum Ca and inorganic P was shown by Potop, Boeru, and Mreana (1966) in immature thymectomized rabbits treated with TP in short- and long-term experiments. Removal of the thymus resulted in decreased serum Ca and increased inorganic P level. TP has a totally opposite effect than that of thymectomy; it elevated serum

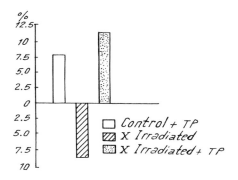

Fig. 5.3. Percentage of change in weight of X-irradiated rabbits and rabbits treated with TP extract. Zero on the ordinate represents the values for normal, nonirradiated, and untreated (controls); three groups of 5 animals each. The bars were calculated from the mean values in the individual groups. Rabbits in the final growth period, weight: approximately 1750 g. Increase in mean weight of controls: 141 g; decrease in mean weight of X-irradiated animals: 155 g; mean increase of weight in the TP-treated group: 190 g.

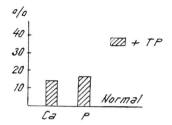

Fig. 5.4. Percentage of change in tibia Ca and P concentration of TP-treated embryo. Zero on the ordinate represents the values for control embryos. The bars were calculated from the mean values of the groups. Two groups of 45 embryos each. (a) Control: Ca, 2.31 ± 0.08; P, 1.22 ± 0.04; (b) TP-treated: Ca, 2.91 ± 0.13; P, 1.61 ± 0.06; Ca and P are calculated in g/100 g moist tissue. Ca, control embryos: treated embryos, $p < 0.003$; P, control: treated, $p < 0.001$. The control:TP-treated ratio is significant. The statistical evaluation used the following formulas:

$$\sigma_1 = \frac{\Sigma d_1^2}{n(n-1)}; \qquad \sigma_2 = \frac{\Sigma d_2^2}{n(n-1)}; \qquad r = \sqrt{\sigma_1^2 + \sigma_2^2} \qquad (1)$$

R_1 = mean control values; R_2 = mean values in TP-treated embryos. (2)

When $R_1 - R_2 \geq 2r$, the difference is significant (sig.); when $R_1 - R_2 \geq 2r$, the difference is unsignificant (unsig.).

Ca levels and decreased serum inorganic P concentration (Table 5.1). An extract derived from skeletal muscle under the same conditions had no effect on P metabolism but influenced Ca metabolism, a fact indicating that TP has a specificity for P metabolism. Potop, Felix, and Ciocirdia (1959) demonstrated that extracts from another lymphatic organ, the spleen, have no influence on P metabolism. The homeostatic action of TP on serum Ca and inorganic P levels following thymectomy should be stressed. Pora and Toma (1960a) found the ^{32}P elimination rate to be increased in thymectomized animals; this was alleviated by thymus extract administration.

Investigations made on plasma iron, liver catalase, and hemoglobin levels in thymectomized rats and in rats given TP (Potop, 1963) showed the influence of the thymus on these parameters. Thymectomy induced a significant decrease in plasma iron (Fig. 5.5) with a decrease in liver catalase (Fig. 5.6), whereas administration of fraction TP enhanced liver catalase activity and elevated hemoglobin levels. The action of thymus on liver catalase activity proved to be specific. TP again exhibited a replacement effect in thymectomized rats.

In previous work (Potop and Boeru, 1951), it was shown that adminis-

Table 5.1. Calcium and inorganic phosphate concentration in serum[a] of thymectomized rabbits before and after injection of thymus and control extract (MP); short-term experiment (2 hr)

Determination	Control animals	Thymectomized	Thymectomized + TP	Thymectomized + MP	Control animals	Sham thymectomized
Calcium in serum (mg Ca/100 ml)	12.4 ± 0.21 (70)	10.0 ± 0.16 (70) sig.	11.1 ± 0.21 (15) sig.	12.17 ± 0.05 (10) sig.	11.3 ± 0.06 (15)	11.6 ± 0.42 (15) unsig.
Inorganic phosphate in serum (mg P/100 ml)	8.30 ± 0.12 (70)	10.0 ± 0.23 (70) sig.	7.3 ± 0.24 (15) sig.	9.4 ± 0.10 (10) unsig.	7.53 ± 0.18 (15)	7.40 ± 0.05 (15) unsig.

[a]Values are given as means with the numbers of observation in parentheses. In this table, the statistical interpretation was calculated from the following formulas: $\sigma_1 = \dfrac{d_1^2}{n(n-1)}$; $\sigma_2 = \dfrac{d_2^2}{n(n-1)}$; $\tau = \sqrt{\sigma_1 + \sigma_2}$. $\overline{R}_1$ and $\overline{R}_2$ are the means of controls and treated animals, When $\overline{R}_1 - \overline{R}_2 \geqq 2\tau$, the difference is significant (sig.).

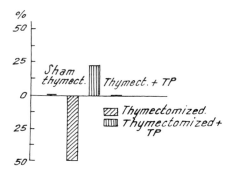

Fig. 5.5. Percentage of change of plasma iron in thymectomized and TP-treated rats. Zero on the ordinate represents normal control values. Four groups of 20 animals each. a) Controls: 304 ± 4; b) thymectomized ($-T$) animals, 251 ± 10 ($p < 0.001$); c) sham-thymectomized animals, 300 ± 9 ($p > 0.32$); d) thymectomized and treated with TP, 373 ± 4 ($p < 0.001$). ($-T/-T + TP$). Plasma iron is given as $\mu g/100$ ml plasma.

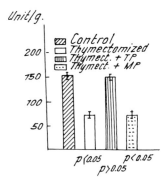

Fig. 5.6. Changes in liver catalase activity in thymectomized and TP-treated rats. Four groups of 20 animals each. a) Control, $153 + 2.31$; b) thymectomized, 50 ± 2.50 ($p < 0.001$); c) thymectomized + TP, 150 ± 2.80 ($-T/-T + TP$)$p > 0.001$; d) thymectomized + MP, 50 ± 20 ($-T/-T + MP$)$p > 0.32$.

tration of TP and X-ray irradiation of the thymus have opposite effects on hematopoiesis and leukocytopoiesis. Thus, TP elicites an increase in blood lymphocytes and erythrocytes, while thymectomy causes them to decrease.

The correlation between Fe and hemoglobin levels has frequently been reported in the literature. Several authors feel that Fe *per se* could well be an activating factor of hemoglobin synthesis, exerting a kind of erythropoietic pressure, and that a direct erythropoiesis/Fe relationship could be established (Paoletti, 1955). Two decades ago it was recognized that hemoglobin synthesis implicates some complex enzymatic systems, and a correlation was set up between Fe absorption and hemoglobin levels. Our studies indicated a stimulating role for the thymus in these processes. The concurrent elevation of Fe and liver catalase after TP administration in thymectomized rats in which this action was reduced substantiates the hypothesis that Fe acts on reconstruction of hemoprotein enzymes, which play an essential part in hematopoiesis, and at the same time points to the stimulating role of the thymus in these processes.

There is general awareness that the thymus is the organ with the highest concentration of nucleic acids characterized by a very active RNA and DNA metabolism (Ogier, Bastide, and Dastigue, 1966). Some of the first workers in this field suggested a role for the thymus in the protein synthesis and considered it a nucleoprotein store. Parhon *et al.* (1950) demonstrated that administration of a thymic protein extract stimulates liver DNA synthesis. More recently, Beauvieux (1963a, b) showed that supplying thymus cells to thymus-deprived animals enhances growth and osteo-genesis and the building up of the tissues and injury repair, probably because of their content in DNA and histones which represent basic anabolic materials.

In a series of investigations, Milcu and Potop (1966: 1970) reported a significant reduction in liver RNA and DNA in rats subjected to experimental thymectomy (Table 5.2). In contradiction, administration of extract TP both in the intact and thymectomized rat caused a rise in liver nucleic acids. It was demonstrated that TP acted with specificity when compared with the control extract prepared by the same method from skeletal muscle (Fig. 5.7).

Table 5.2. Variations in RNA and DNA concentrations in the liver of thym-ectomized rats treated with thymus fraction TP and control extract from skeletal muscle (MP) (in mg/100 g of tissue)

Groups	No. of animals	RNA	p	DNA	p
Control	50	972 ± 17		359 ± 12	
Sham thymectomy	15	980 ± 23	>0.05	336 ± 21	≥ 0.05
Thymectomized	20	758 ± 25	<0.05	317 ± 21	<0.05
Thymectomized + MP	15	753 ± 33	>0.05	306 ± 9	>0.05
Thymectomized + TP	15	815 ± 22	<0.05	333 ± 20	<0.05
Normal + TP	20	1640 ± 17	<0.05		

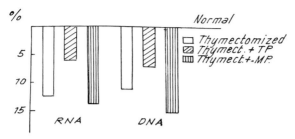

Fig. 5.7. ±Percentage changes of liver DNA and RNA in thymectomized rats and rats treated with TP and with a control muscle extract (MP). Zero on the ordinate represents normal control values. Four groups of animals. Number of animals and results are given in Table 5.2. RNA and DNA levels are given as mg/100 g fresh tissue.

Potop, Felix, and Ciocirdia (1959) showed that thymectomy induces a drop in liver nucleoproteins and a parallel reduction in ^{32}P incorporation, while administration of TP increases nucleoprotein levels conjointly with ^{32}P incorporation (Fig. 5.8). These results obtained with tests using radioactive phosphorus suggest thymus stimulation of the synthesis and metabolism of nucleic acids.

Investigations on protein metabolism revealed an action of TP in thymectomized immature rabbits (Milcu *et al.*, 1963). While thymectomy caused a rise in serum globulin concentration, administration of fraction TP induced a decrease in these compounds. TP administration modified the electrophoretic serum protein pattern. The most significant changes were noted in alpha and beta globulins, a fact also reported by other workers. Especially interesting is the fact that the protein fraction design-

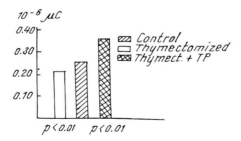

Fig. 5.8. Changes in ^{32}P incorporation into nucleoproteins of thymectomized and TP-treated animals. Three groups of 15 rats each. a) Control, 0.250 ± 0.04; b) thymectomized, 0.180 ± 0.02 (N/−T) $p = 0.13$; c) treated with TP, 0.340 ± 0.01 (N/+TP) $p < 0.001$. Activity is given as $10^{-6} \mu C$.

ated by us as β_3 (located between β_2 and γ globulins) is absent from the electrophoretic pattern in thymectomized rabbits (Fig. 5.9).

Radioisotopes have provided insight into glucose metabolism and glycogen synthesis. As early as 1950 the presence of glycogen in the thymus was reported along with its fluctuations during growth and post-irradiation regeneration. Pora, Toma, and Madar (1962) observed glycogen synthesis and muscle contraction to be decreased following thymectomy; they also noted that administration of thymus protein extract restored the normal contracting ability of the muscle after being strained or poisoned with lactic and monoiodoacetic acids. Gaburro and Volpato (1966) noted the influence of thymectomy on carbohydrate metabolism; decreased glycogen levels in liver and striated muscle paralleled the depression of respiratory activity. They also noted a decreased insulin,

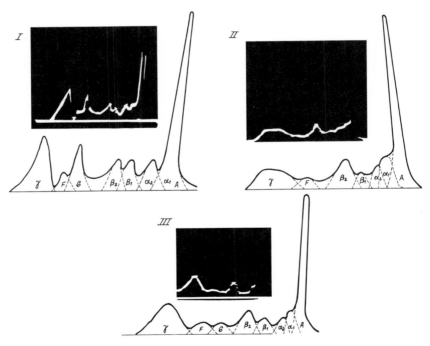

Fig. 5.9. Changes in the electrophoretic pattern (Tiselius apparatus) in thymecto-mized animals. Experiments were performed in young male rabbits, weight about 500 g. Groups: a) normal animals (I); b) thymectomized animals 4 days after surgical removal of the thymus (II); c) as b) treated with TP.

glucagon, and adrenalin sensitivity which paralleled an increased response to the hypoglycemic action of tolbutamide. These biochemical changes point to the existence of thymus endocrine gland interactions. The authors also claim that the thymus exerts an action on carbohydrate metabolism resembling that of insulin and that thymectomy induces beta cell hyperplasia, probably compensatory, in the pancreatic isles.

Luca, Santangelo, and Cotadini (1966) noted post-thymectomy changes in some enzymatic activities of the Krebs cycle, increased glucose-6-phosphate, AMP and ADP concentrations, and decreased levels in ATP. Our results demonstrated metabolic changes in the thymectomized animal, illustrated by a low concentration of glycogen, glucose-6-phosphatase, ATP, and lactic acid (Figs. 5.10 and 5.11). These findings are in keeping with those of the above authors. The decreased glycogen synthesis following thymectomy bears out the hypothesis advanced by Bentiglio in 1939 (cited by Rusescu et al., 1964), according to which the thymus stimulates a glycogen-generating action synergistic to that of insulin in rat striated muscle. The mechanism whereby liver glycogen is reduced after thymectomy is not known. The low insulin sensitivity caused by thymectomy and the reduced glucose consumption by muscle may be taken as indicating a thymus-Langerhans isle synergism.

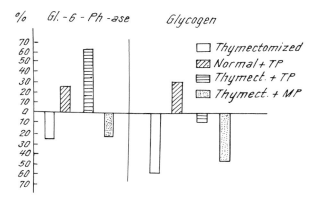

Fig. 5.10. Percentage of change of glucose-6-phosphatase and of liver glycogen following thymectomy and TP administration. Zero on the ordinate represents the values for normal controls. The number of animals is given in parentheses. Glucose-6-phosphatase: a) control, 7.79 ± 0.36 (11); b) thymectomized, 5.85 ± 0.26 (11) $p < 0.01$; c) thymectomized + TP, 12.61 ± 0.16 (6) $p < 0.01$; d) normal + TP, 9.73 ± 0.34 (6) $p < 0.01$. Glucose-6-phosphatase is given as mg P/g moist tissue/15 min. Glycogen: a) controls, 1297 ± 128 (12); b) thymectomized, 525 ± 126 (10); c) thymectomized + TP, 1180 ± 108 (6); d) normal + TP, 1688 ± 135 (7). Glycogen is given as mg/100 moist tissue.

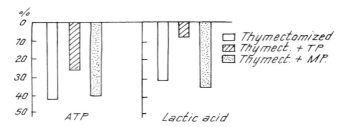

Fig. 5.11. Percentage of change of liver ATP and liver lactic acid in thymectomized and TP-treated animals. Zero on the ordinate represents the values of normal rats (controls); the number of animals is given in parentheses. ATP: a) control, 8.30 $\pm$ 0.70 (7); b) thymectomized, 4.76 $\pm$ 0.60 (4) $p < 0.001$; c) thymectomized + TP, 5.99 $\pm$ 0.70 (4) $p < 0.003$; thymectomized + MP, 4.98 $\pm$ 0.58 (6) $p < 0.003$. ATP is given in mg P/100 g moist tissue. Lactic acid: a) control, 27.50 $\pm$ 2.4 (12); b) thymectomized, 19.40 $\pm$ 2.5 (11) $p < 0.05$; c) thymectomized + TP, 24.8 $\pm$ 3.2 (12) (N/ $-$ T + TP) $p > 0.32$. Lactic acid is given as mg/100 g moist tissue.

In our experience, the reduced glucose-6-phosphatase following thymectomy is coincident with a reduction in both liver glycogen synthesis and blood sugar levels. The depressed activity of the enzyme responsible for glucose-6-phosphate cleavage is parallel with the increase in glucose-6-phosphate found by Luca *et al.* (1966). The decreased glycogen levels suggest an inhibition of the metabolic pathways of glucose-6-phosphate. The reduced glucose-6-phosphatase concomitant with a decline in ATP production in the liver and the decreased lactic acid level constitute relevant facts in support of the view held by Luca that metabolic pathways of glucose-6-phosphatase are blocked in thymectomized animals.

Both in thymectomized and in intact animals, administration of TP brings about an elevation in glycogen levels (Fig. 5.10) which parallels the rise towards normal values in ATP and lactic acid (Fig. 5.11). Modifications observed after administration of TP suggest the action of this material on carbohydrate metabolism as well as its thymus replacing action; its specificity is shown by the inactivity of the muscle peptides (MP).

There are conflicting views regarding the action of the thymus on muscular function and metabolism at this level. Studies made by Parhon *et al.* demonstrated the specific stimulating effect of the thymus on respiration of muscle tissue (Parhon and Apostol, 1954) and the decrease in the various forms of acid-soluble phosphorus in thymectomized rats (Parhon and Costin, 1953). Following thymectomy, Pora *et al.*, 1961 found signs of muscular atrophy associated with a reduced ergogram and chronaxy,

whereas after administration of the thymus protein extract there was a
significant rise (300%) in chronaxy.

Studies carried out by Potop *et al.* (1966) and Milcu, Potop, and Mreana
(1963) on ATP in striated muscle (biceps femori) following thymus
removal or administration of extract TP revealed alterations of ATP
metabolism. Fraction TP induced an increase in ATP towards normal
values in immature thymectomized rabbits (Fig. 5.12). The specificity of
the effect demonstrated by fraction TP was evidenced by the fact that
control muscle extracts gave no meaningful increase. The decrease in ATP
is accompanied by elaboration of P. These decreased ATP levels induced
by thymectomy and their increase upon TP administration illustrate the
replacing effect of TP and support the hypothesis that the thymus plays
a role in energy metabolism of muscle tissue. Toma and Roman (1969)
noted that TP, prepared in our laboratory, changed the contractions in
the isolated frog heart when given in pharmacologic dosage and that it
had a far lower toxicity than commercially available extracts.

The increase in ATP concentration induced by administration of
thymus extract was explained by some authors (Hohorat, Reim, and
Barthel 1962) either as an enhanced ATP synthesis or as a reduced ATP
turnover rate and enhanced storage. Pora and Toma (1960a) studied the
role of the thymus in ^{32}P in various organs with the viewpoint that consumption of inorganic P in energy processes may represent an indirect
index of the metabolic rate. It was noted that the ^{32}P incorporation rate

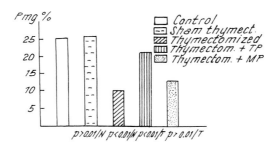

Fig. 5.12. Variations in muscle (biceps femori) ATP concentration in thymectomized
and TP-treated rabbits. Prepubescent rabbits weighing 400 to 500 g were used. Some of the
animals were thymectomized and killed 4 days after operation. Control animals (untreated):
the animals were killed 24 hr after a single intraperitoneal TP injection. The number of
animals is given in parentheses; 135 animals divided into 5 groups: a) controls, 23.2 ± 1.17
(50); b) thymectomized (−T), 11.10 ± 0.85 (40) (R_1 − R_2 > 2τ, sig); c) sham-thymectomized, 25.80 ± 0.72 (20) (control/sham thymectomized is sig.); d) thymectomized + TP,
23.3 ± 2.32 (15) (−T/−T+TP is sig.); e) thymectomized + MP, 13.2 ± 3.80 (10) (−T/
−T + MP is unsig.). ATP is given in mg P/100 g moist muscle tissue.

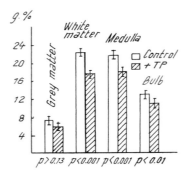

Fig. 5.13. Changes in the total lipid content of some segments of brain tissue in TP-treated rabbits. Two groups of 10 animals each. a) controls, grey matter, 7.77 ± 0.53; white matter, 22.70 ± 0.83; medulla, 21.70 ± 0.68; medulla oblongata, 13.90 ± 0.72. b) TP-treated; grey matter, 6.50 ± 0.82; white matter, 17.80 ± 0.80; medulla, 18.40 ± 0.59; medulla oblongata, 11.30 ± 0.58. The total lipids are given as g/100 g moist tissue.

into the striated muscle was much lower in thymectomized than in control animals. This fact may account for the extensive atony caused by thymectomy. Szent-Györgyi (1957) related the lymphatic system as a whole to the thymus, establishing correlations with neuromuscular activity. There is a likelihood of myotonia and muscular dystrophy being conditioned by the functional activity of the thymic-lymphatic system.

TP also affects lipid metabolism. Parhon *et al.* (1950) demonstrated a decrease of total lipids and cholesterol in brain, liver, and muscles of senescent guinea pigs following administration of the thymus extract; this was taken as an index of rejuvenation. Reversed effects were obtained in the muscular tissue of thymectomized rats. Milcu and Potop (1955) found that TP administration decreased the total lipid concentration of rabbit brain tissue (Fig. 5.13). This action partially compensated for the increased water content. TP induced hydration of cerebral structures when compared with untreated rabbits; thymectomy consistently induced a decreased water content (Fig. 5.14).

5.4 Action of thymic extracts on tumor growth

The following section presents a short survey of the most relevant data to illustrate the action of thymus extracts upon tumor growth. Antitumor activity of the extracts was tested both *in vivo* in animals and chick embryo and *in vitro* in tumor cell cultures.

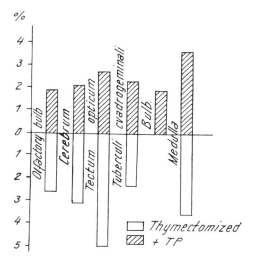

Fig. 5.14. Changes in water content of some segments of brain tissue of thymecto-mized and TP-treated rabbits. Zero on the ordinate represents the values for normal controls. Thirty rabbits (1200 g) divided into 3 groups: controls, thymectomized, and TP-treated (during 30 days, 1 ml per animal daily, corresponding to 0.5 g fresh gland). Examination of various brain segments:

	Control	Thymectomized	TP-treated
Olfactive bulb	83.90 ± 0.36	81.67 ± 0.62	85.57 ± 0.60
Encephalon	78.98 ± 0.81	76.47 ± 0.44	80.66 ± 0.51
Optical layers	77.44 ± 0.61	73.43 ± 0.75	79.54 ± 0.30
Quadrigeminal tubercles	77.62 ± 0.46	75.30 ± 0.70	79.89 ± 0.30
Medulla oblongata	72.60 ± 0.60	—	74.19 ± 0.84
Medulla	66.95 ± 0.84	64.45 ± 0.37	69.44 ± 0.54

The water content is calculated in terms of 100 g of fresh tissue.

In the early decades of this century, Hanson (cited by Davies, 1969a), Ficchera (1933), and Leriche (1948) drew attention to the role of the thymus in neoplastic processes. Then Parhon et al. (1952), Milcu and Lupulescu (1952a, b), and Milcu and Potop (1971) demonstrated the effect of thymus extracts upon the development of tumors induced by methyl-cholanthrene and dimethylaminobenzene. In further investigation with rats bearing methylcholanthrene-induced tumors, it was shown that the neoplastic incidence was lowest in rats given thymus extract. This was best seen in the group of rats treated with thymic extract prior to trans-plantation or methylcholanthrene injection (Fig. 5.15); it was less evident in rats given thymic extract after transplantation. Administration of TP

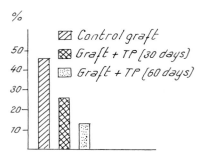

Fig. 5.15. Incidence of methylcholanthrene-induced tumors in animals treated during 30 and 60 days with TP. Three groups of 50 animals each: control group, group treated with TP 30 days prior to carcinogen administration and for a further 30 days (total period of TP-treatment: 60 days); group treated with TP during 30 days after tumor induction (total TP treatment, 30 days).

extract modified the character of the transplanted methylcholanthrene-induced tumor; the volume and weight were consistently lower in TP treated animals than in untreated controls. It should be emphasized that in animals given TP prior to or following the transplant, the tumors involuted within the first 2 weeks; after a long-term treatment (60 to 90 days), some of them regressed, while others became ulcerative with elimination of the proliferative process.

Administration of extract TP also modified the structure of the tumor. Rats given methylcholanthrene or grafted methylcholanthrene-induced tumors developed myeloblastic or polymorphous sarcomata. In a comparable series of animals the tumors were, for the most part, termed by Parhon *et al.* (1955a, b) as "mesenchymoma." These tumors were thought to be less malignant than the polymorphous, myeloblastic, or giant cell sarcomata observed in the untreated animals. The histologic appearance of the tumor was different in treated than in untreated animals. In animals treated with thymus extract, the tumor was found to contain collagen fibers and connective bands forming a connective stroma. In TP-treated animals, the thymus presented a high lymphocyte content; this indicates its functional capacity and the subsequent adverse affect on tumor growth.

Of all the organs examined, the thymus exhibited the most characteristic changes in the presence of the tumor; the reduction in the size of the thymus may be interpreted as atrophy of the gland. It was of particular interest to ascertain which of the two portions of the thymus was responsible for inhibition of tumor growth. Milcu *et al.* (1954) suggested the thymus is an organ composed of two distinct parts, one structural and one functional. Morphologic examination showed that the two parts act differently in tumor-bearing animals; the cortical zone presents a highly active proliferative process of its lymphoid elements which occasionally expanded into the medullary zone; the medullary zone undergoes a regression culminating in the total disappearance of its constitutive elements. The process of thymus cortex hypertrophy is consistent with the increased lymphocyte count observed by Potop and Boeru (1951). Parhon *et al.* (1955b) noted changes in the spleen and particularly in the bone marrow, where a hyperplastic process of white blood cells was present, a fact also reported by earlier authors.

The antineoplastic effect of TP was demonstrated during the process of malignant tumor induction by dimethylaminoazobenzene (DAB) (Potop *et al.*, 1960; Potop, Lupulescu, and Biener, 1961). Morphologically, the liver of sacrificed animals given DAB or a carcinogenic synthetic diet demonstrated hyperplasia and disorganization of the liver cords caused by bile canaliculi hyperplasia. The central lobular veins were dilated, and the

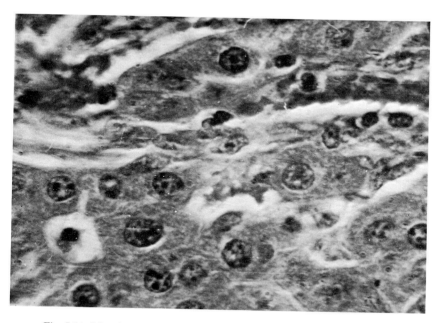

Fig. 5.16. Morphologic examination of the liver in normal untreated rat (V. Gieson, × ob.im.).

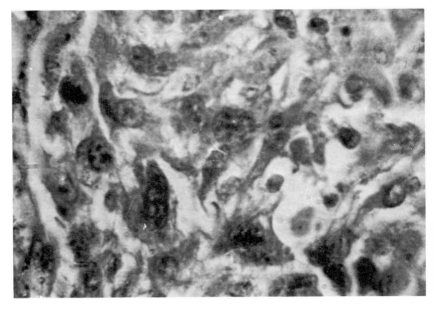

Fig. 5.17. Morphologic examination of the liver in the rat with DAB and a synthetic carcinogenic diet (V. Gieson × ob.im.).

Kiernan space was packed with cells. The nucleus was hypertrophied and frequently gigantic, due to an atypical mitosis (Figs. 5.16 and 5.17). This was a cholangioma with a hepatoma.

In animals receiving TP as well as DAB, a decreased nuclear polymorphism and hypertrophy of liver cords were noted. An arrest occurred in the development of the cholangioma and the hepatoma. Also the cellular infiltration of Kiernan's space was less extensive. The liver cords were formed of cells with an effaced contour, and degenerative changes of the nucleus indicated kariolysis and pycnosis. Hemorrhages were also noted (Fig. 5.18). From the histologic viewpoint, TP administration gave a protective action against the neoplastic process. Some authors found an increased incidence of hepatoma following thymectomy, a fact which confirms indirectly our findings.

TP extract also acts on the development of tumors in chick embryo (Potop *et al.*, 1962) by decreasing tumorigenesis and reducing tumor weight when measured by the 19th day of incubation (Figs. 5.19 and 5.20). The pathologic examination of the embryo bearing an implanted Ehrlich

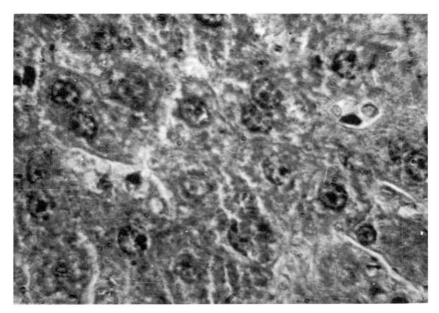

Fig. 5.18. Morphologic examination of the liver in rats given DAB, synthetic carcinogenic diet, and TP extract (V. Gieson × im.ob.).

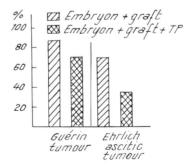

Fig. 5.19. Influence of TP extract on tumor genesis in chick embryos bearing Ehrlich ascites carcinoma and Guerin carcinoma. Four groups of 30 embryos each; two groups of embryos treated with TP extract (8 injections corresponding with 0.40 g fresh thymus). Two groups with Guerin carcinoma: a) untreated embryos, 83.1%; b) treated with TP, 64.8%. Two groups of Ehrlich ascites carcinoma; a) untreated embryo, 68.8%; b) TP-treated embryo, 34.0%.

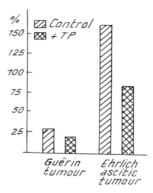

Fig. 5.20. Tumor weight variations in the chick embryo under the effect of TP extract. Four groups of 30 embryos each; two groups of embryos given 8 TP injections, corresponding to 0.40 g fresh thymus. Mean tumor weight in Guerin carcinoma-bearing embryos; a) untreated embryo, + 26.2 mg (range, 5 to 52 mg), b) treated embryo, 21.7 (range, 5 to 60 mg). Mean of tumor weight in embryo with Ehrlich ascites carcinoma: c) untreated embryos, 157.2 mg (range, 5 to 480 mg); d) TP-treated embryo, 84.0 mg (range, 5 to 164 mg).

tumor demonstrated the development of an invading carcinoma which originated in the chorioallantois. In the embryo implanted and treated with TP, a significant reduction of the expanding areas of the tumor, predominantly in the collagenic tissue on the hemorrhagic surfaces, was 'noted. There were relatively fewer atypical mitoses and giant nuclei, and capillaries in the neoplasia were also more sparse. The direct or indirect inhibitory action of fraction TP on tumor growth in the chick embryo is thus exhibited.

The antineoplastic effect of embryo thymus extract (TPE) was tested on the development of Ehrlich ascites carcinoma in mice (Potop, Biener, and Mreana, 1965). The results (Table 5.3) show that TPE administration

Table 5.3. Weight variations in mice transplants following administration of embryonic thymus extract (TPE) for 10 and 20 days

Group	Weight gain (g) after 10 days	p	Weight gain (g) after 20 days	p
Transplant	6.7 ± 0.60		25.3 ± 1.63	
Transplant + TPE	4.30 ± 0.30	<0.05	13.3 ± 2.10	<0.05

for 10 and 20 days after transplanting the tumor caused a reduction in the weight and size of the tumor when compared with untreated controls. The mean survival at 20 days was 60% in mice which were given extract TPE for 20 days, and 20% in nontreated controls. This shows the inhibitory action of TPE on Ehrlich ascites carcinoma in mice. Apparently the potency of this extract is higher than that of extract TP.

Thymectomy of the adult animal increased the development of methylcholanthrene-induced tumors (Parhon et al., 1956). Removal of the thymus in the adult animal caused some changes in tumor histology compared with tumors in intact animals. For instance, it was seen that the structure of the tumor was characterized by the presence of morphocellular sarcomata with giant cells, numerous nuclei, and frequent atypical karyokineses.

Experiments performed in newborn rats subjected to thymectomy 72 hr after birth and in which Walker carcinosarcoma was transplanted showed that thymectomy stimulates tumor growth (Boeru and Potop, 1971). Our pathologic examination demonstrated that in intact controls the tumors exhibit either necrobiosis and fibrosclerosis or proliferative areas (Fig. 5.21). In thymectomized animals, the pathologic examination revealed an active proliferation pattern with neoformed vessels and frequent mitoses (Fig. 5.22). These data agree with those available in the literature. A more significant development of the Jensen sarcoma was noted in thymectomized newborn rats as compared with controls (Perri et al., 1963). The former exhibited a shorter latency of tumor growth than did controls (Allison and Taylor, 1967). Neonatal thymectomy reduced latency and increased the incidence of skin tumors induced by 3,4-benzopyrene in mice (Miller, Grant, and Roe, 1963). The sensitizing role of neonatal thymectomy in the production of polyoma-virus neoplasia, mammary tumors, and methylcholanthrene-induced tumors was demonstrated, and immunologic deficiences of these tumor-susceptible animals were stressed. Our investigation shows that extracts TP and TPE have an inhibitory effect on tumor growth, while thymectomy has a stimulating effect on neoplastic growth.

5.5 Action of TP on tumor metabolism

From work initiated in 1952, Parhon et al. (1954 and 1958) demonstrated the influence of protein thymic extracts on nucleic acid levels in the liver and tumor tissue in rats with methylcholanthrene-induced tumors. Con-

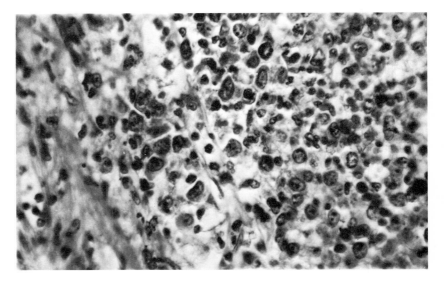

Fig. 5.21. Pathologic examination of Guerin tumor transplants in intact rats 30 days following transplantation. Implantation of tumor grafts in a 12-day-old rat; the animal was sacrificed 30 days later.

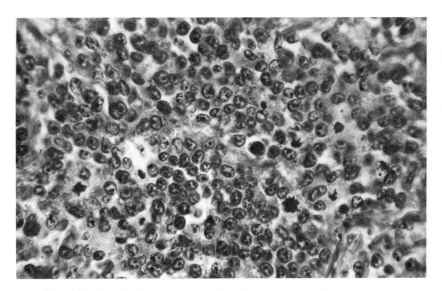

Fig. 5.22. Pathologic examination of a Guerin tumor in the thymectomized rat. Thymectomy was performed 72 hr after birth. Implantation and sacrifice of the animals was made under the same conditions as in unthymectomized controls (*see* Fig. 5.21).

siderable data have accumulated (Milcu and Potop, 1966; Parhon *et al.*, 1958a, b; Parhon, Potop, and Niculescu-Zinca, 1957; Potop *et al.*, 1961) on the influence of thymic protein extracts upon carcinogenic agent-induced changes in nucleic acid synthesis and metabolism. The presence of the tumor elevates liver RNA and DNA (Fig. 5.23), as does also methyl-cholanthrene administration (Fig. 5.24). In animals given simultaneously methylcholanthrene and thymic extract, the increase in nucleic acid concentration was moderate, particularly in animals with necrotized tumors. The slightly increased nucleic acid level could be a consequence of the relative shrinkage of the cytoplasm and of a higher nuclear content in the liver of the host, as shown in our histologic studies.

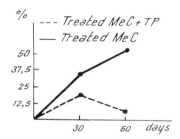

Fig. 5.23. Changes in nucleic acid concentration in the liver of rats with methyl-cholanthrene-induced tumor after 30 to 60 days TP administration. Groups of 15 animals each. Liver nucleic acid content is expressed as mg P/100 g fresh tissue. Control, 148 mg (135 to 156 mg); treated with methylcholanthrene and treated during 30 days with TP, 174 mg (168 to 177); treated with methylcholanthrene and treated 60 days with TP, 157 (150 to 163 mg).

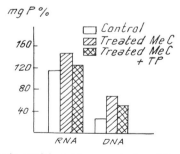

Fig. 5.24. Changes in nucleic acid concentration following methylcholanthrene administration after 30 and 60 days. Three groups of 15 animals each. The liver nucleic acid content is expressed as mg P/100 g fresh tissue. Controls, 148 mg (135 to 156 mg); 30 days methylcholanthrene administration, 200 mg (198 to 212 mg), 60 days administration of the carcinogen agent, 225 mg (208 to 233 mg).

Thymus extract inhibits tumor growth, resulting either in necrosis or in a complete regression of the tumor and biochemically in alterations of nucleic acid metabolism. These alterations, which prove the oncolytic action of the thymus, depended on the length of extract administration and of the stage of the tumor growth (Fig. 5.25). Liver ribonuclease activity (Fig. 5.26) decreased with the rise in DNA content and increased toward the control value upon administration of thymus extract in rats bearing tumors (Potop, 1959).

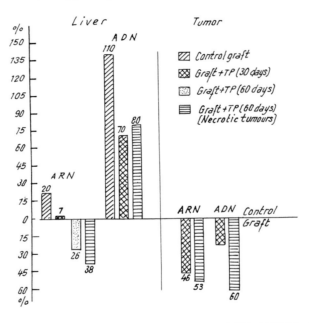

Fig. 5.25. Percentage of variations in RNA (ARN) and DNA (ADN) in the liver and tumor of rats bearing methylcholanthrene-induced tumor and treated with TP. Group of 30 animals each. Values are expressed as % of control.

Liver
1) Controls: RNA, 117 mg (110 to 123 mg); DNA, 30 mg (25 to 33 mg) P/100 g fresh tissue.
2) Rats with methylcholanthrene-induced tumors: RNA, 140 mg (136 to 152 mg); DNA, 63 mg (62 to 72 mg).
3) Rats bearing methylcholanthrene-induced tumors, treated with TP for 30 days: RNA, 120 mg (118 to 126 mg); DNA, 51 mg (44.8 to 52.5 mg).
4) Rats bearing methylcholanthrene-induced tumors, treated with TP for 60 days: RNA, 79 mg (76 to 82 mg); DNA, 54 mg (46 to 58 mg).

Tumor
1) Controls: RNA, 109 mg (91 to 152 mg); DNA, 77 mg (58 to 104 mg).
2) Group treated with TP (30 days): RNA, 59 (48 to 67); DNA, 61 (52 to 64).
3) Group treated with TP (60 days): RNA, 52 mg (40 to 58); DNA, 31 mg (25 to 36).

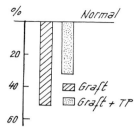

Fig. 5.26. Variations of hepatic ribonuclease activity in tumor-bearing rat after TP administration. Three groups of 12 rats each. Two groups had methylcholanthrene-induced tumors. Ribonuclease activity is expressed as mg P/100 g moist liver tissue. a) Normal controls, 7.80 ± 0.08; b) control graft, 3.50 ± 0.02 $p < 0.001$; c) graft + TP (30 days), 4.80 ± 0.06 $p < 0.001$. Values are expressed as % of control.

In a recent work on animals bearing methylcholanthrene-induced tumors (Milcu and Potop, 1966), chemical assays and ^{32}P incorporation determinations demonstrated that TP decreased RNA and DNA both in the tumor and liver. At the same time, there was a decreased incorporation of ^{32}P into these compounds (Table 5.4). The increased incorporation rate of ^{32}P noted in our experiments on tumor-bearing animals confirmed the data of other authors (Neogy and Bose, 1963; Mandel, 1963) emphasizing the essential alterations in nucleic acid and protein metabolism in cancer.

TP administration decreased tumor growth and nucleic acid metabolism, and impaired nucleic acid synthesis and protein synthesis. TP decreased nucleic acid metabolism in DAB-induced hepatoma toward values obtained for normal liver during a period of 120 days (Fig. 5.27) (Potop et al., 1960; Potop, Lupulescu, and Biener, 1961).

The influence of the thymus on protein metabolism in experimental cancer was studied following reports of large changes in proteins relative to nucleic acid and energy metabolism (Bickis and Henderson, 1966). Amino acid estimations in liver and tumor revealed both quantitative and qualitative variations of these compounds following thymus extract administration. Administration of TP decreased protein metabolism in the liver of chick embryos bearing Guerin tumors (Potop et al., 1962) as assessed by 35S-methionine uptake (Fig. 5.28).

Electrophoresis of blood protein fractions in chick embryo showed that TP influenced neither the low albumin levels nor the elevated globulin in tumor-bearing embryos (Table 5.5). Examination of lymphoid organs was not made. Tumor grafts transplanted in chick embryo induced an essential decrease in the activity of some enzymes: liver mitochondria

Table 5.4. Effect of TP on RNA and DNA concentration and incorporation of ^{32}P in liver and tumor of rats

Group	No. of animals	RNA (mg%)	p	DNA (mg%)	p	No. of animals	RNA P/g/S[1]	p	DNA[a] P/g/S	p
		Liver					Liver (^{32}P)			
Control animals	50	872 ± 18		354 ± 9		20	41 ± 0.2		14 ± 0.3	
Animals with methyl-cholanthrene-induced tumor graft	100	1129 ± 22	0.05	670 ± 20	<0.05	20	58 ± 0.9	<0.05	21 ± 0.2	<0.05
Animals with graft + TP	100	882 ± 30	0.05	407 ± 21	<0.05	20	46 ± 16	<0.05	17 ± 1.4	<0.05

Group	RNA (mg%)	p	DNA (mg%)	p	RNA[+] DNA[a] P/g/S[a]	p
	Tumor				Tumor (^{32}P)	
Control animals						
Animals with methyl-cholanthrene-induced tumor graft	780 ± 9		670 ± 20		54 ± 17	
Animals with graft + TP	577 ± 21	<0.05	430 ± 18	0.05	46 ± 3	<0.05

^{a}P/g/S = counts per gm tissue per second.

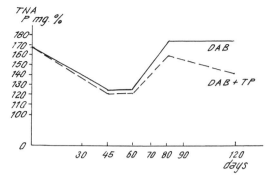

Fig. 5.27. Fluctuations of nucleic acid levels in DAB-induced hepatoma under the influence of fraction TP. Eight groups of 20 rats each: a) controls with DAB and synthetic carcinogen diet (according to LeBreton, 1953, Ann. Nutr. Aliment. 363: 404); b) group with DAB, synthetic carcinogen diet, treated with TP during 120 days (1 ml extract/100 g body weight, 1 ml corresponding to 1 g fresh gland.) The amount of total nucleic acid is given in mg P/100 g fresh tissue. After 45 days: a) control group, 120.8 ± 4.8; b) TP-treated group, 125 ± 5.47. After 60 days: c) control group, 120.8 ± 4.8; d) TP-treated group, 124.0 ± 3.87. After 80 days: e) control group, 174.7 ± 6.0; f) TP-treated group, 160.0 ± 6.9. After 120 days: g) control group, 176 ± 2.23; h) TP-treated group, 141.6 ± 8. The changes are statistically significant only after 80 ($p < 0.05$) and 120 ($p < 0.001$) experimental days. TNA = total nucleic acid.

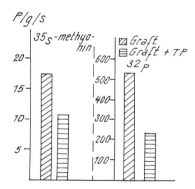

Fig. 5.28. Changes in ^{35}S-methionine and ^{32}P incorporation into tumor tissue of Guerin tumor-bearing embryo, under the effect of TP administration. The results are given as the number of counts per gram per second. Four chick embryo (Rhode Island) groups of 25 embryos each. a) controls (nontreated with TP): Guerin tumor-bearing embryo given ^{35}S-methionin, 17.9 ± 2.42; b) Guerin tumor-bearing embryo given ^{35}S-methionine, treated with TP, 10.9 ± 1.42 ($R_1 - R_2 > 2\gamma$ is sig.); c) controls, Guerin tumor-bearing embryos given $H_2Na^{32}PO_4$ (nontreated with TP), 532.5 ± 98.1; d) Guerin tumor-bearing embryos given $H_2Na^{32}PO_4$, treated with TP, 236.1 ± 24.1 ($R_1 - R_2 \geq 2\tau$ is sig.).

Table 5.5. Changes in the electrophoretic pattern of serum of embryos bearing Guerin tumors under the influence of thymus fraction TP

Electrophoretic fraction	Control embryo	Untreated tumor-bearing embryo	Tumor-bearing embryo, treated with TP
Prealbumin and albumin (mobility 1)	45.5 ± 1.60	40.1 ± 1.70 sig.[a]	40.5 ± 2.39 unsig.
α and β-globulins (mobility 2 corresponding to α and β globulins)	25.3 ± 1.25	30.0 ± 1.70 sig.	31.1 ± 2.00 unsig.
γ globulins (mobility 3 corresponding to globulins)	25.5 ± 1.11	29.9 ± 1.20 sig.	28.5 ± 0.61 unsig.

[a]Statistical interpretation was done as in Table 5.1.

ATPase and hepatocyte glucose-6-phosphatase and transaminase (Potop et al., 1961; 1962). Administration of TP increases the activity of glucose-6-phosphatase and reduced that of ATPase. Table 5.6 summarizes the results obtained with glucose-6-phosphatase and fructose 1,6-diphosphatase after treatment of mice carrying Ehrlich ascites carcinoma with TPE (Potop, Biener, and Mreana, 1965).

TP increases toward normal levels the iron and liver catalase activity in rats with Walker tumors (Potop and Juvina, 1966). A correlation has been suggested to exist in liver catalase, erythrocyte count, and hemoglobin content in the blood of the tumor recipient (Masson et al., 1960). Unlike normal organ homogenates, tumor homogenates were found to cause a decline in these variables (Ralph et al., 1960). The fraction responsible for this is apparently located in the tumor microsomial fraction. Parhon et al. (1955a) demonstrated that thymus protein extract increased liver catalase and O_2 consumption concurrently with increased erythrocyte concentration and erythrocyte count in tumor-bearing animals.

The activity of polypeptide fraction TP was tested on tumor cell cultures derived from a cancer of the buccal epithelium (KB). TP exerted a specific or nonspecific inhibitory action on tumor cell growth (Milcu et al., 1965: 1966); concomitantly, using control extracts prepared from lymph nodes and muscles by the same method, the effects produced were null, mild, or inconstant (Tables 5.7 and 5.8). Three types of results were found

Table 5.6. Changes in enzymatic activity of glucose-6-phosphatase and fructose-1,6-diphosphatase in mice bearing Ehrlich ascites carcinoma treated with embryonic horse thymus extract (TPE)

Groups	Glucose-6-phosphatase (P/g/15 min)[a]	p	Fructose-1,6-diphosphatase (P/g/20 min)	p
Control animals	7.32 ± 0.31 (25)[b]		3.80 ± 0.047 (25)	
Animals with transplants	5.84 ± 0.20 (25)	<0.05	2.52 ± 0.16 (25)	<0.05
Animals with transplants + TPE	7.40 ± 0.12 (25)	<0.04	2.70 ± 0.10 (25)	<0.05

[a]P/g/15 min = phosphorus released per gm tissue per 15 minutes.
[b]The number of animals is given in parentheses.

with TP: significant results where the inhibitory effects rose in proportion with the dose, results in which the effects were mildly inhibitory, and results in which the effects were null or paradoxically reversed in terms of the increasing dosage. Histologic studies of the cells revealed ordinary patterns of proliferative inhibition or, with high extract concentrations, of degenerative lesions. The KB line, which is characterized in cultures by cellular and nuclear polymorphism and by differentiated mitoses, demonstrated the most definite effects. In cultures treated with thymus extract in high concentrations, nuclear monstrosities were a very rare finding. Numerous cells were hyperchromophilic, and the nuclei had an angular or protruding outline. The population density was reduced, and several cells were fusiform or stellate. Morphologically, degenerative lesions and necroses were only visible when high concentrations of the extract were administered (Fig. 5.29, a, b, c); these could be caused by a toxic effect.

These results demonstrate that cell cultures are sensitively dependent upon the action of TP. Hence, significant results were obtained on KB lines when using higher dilutions. A lower sensitivity was exhibited by a culture from a spontaneous mammary adenocarcinoma in a A_2G mouse. Administration of protein extract prepared from human thymus proved to have a moderate antineoplastic activity, as tested on KB tumor cell cultures. In cultures treated with thymus extract, a concomitant reduction of the cell population and of protein levels was noted only with large doses of extract (0.2 ml). Thus, thymus in newborn children contains active

Table 5.7. Inhibitory action of thymus fraction TP compared with that of control extracts prepared from skeletal muscle and lymph nodes on proliferation of some tumor cell cultures *in vitro*

Culture used	Extract	Parameter investigated	Control culture	Concentration of extracts used		
				10^{-2}	10^{-1}	$1.5\ 10^{-1}$
KB[a]	TP	Protein assay	15.9 ± 0.002	10.2 ± 0.20^b	5.2 ± 0.01^b	
				11.6 ± 0.50^b	9.2 ± 0.03^b	
KB	TP	No. of cells	235.0 ± 6.5	173.0 ± 6.5^b	73.0 ± 2.6^b	51.7 ± 7.9^b
KB	Protein muscle	Protein assay	10.8 ± 0.19	14.2 ± 0.43	12.6 ± 0.34	10.7 ± 0.32
KB	Protein ganglion	Protein assay	13.7 ± 0.002	24.8 ± 1.20	15.6 ± 1.10	13.6 ± 0.80
Human thyroid cancer	TP	Protein assay	10.8 ± 0.19	11.2 ± 0.19	8.9 ± 0.26^b	8.5 ± 0.16^b
Human thyroid cancer	TP	No. of cells	96.0 ± 5.12	50.3 ± 12^b	34.0 ± 0.34^b	24.7 ± 2.7^b
Mammary tumor	TP	Protein assay	11.2 ± 0.21	10.8 ± 0.007	10.0 ± 0.30	9.6 ± 0.38^b
Mammary tumor	TP	No. of cells	102.0 ± 1.2	106.8 ± 1.9	102.2 ± 2.8	85.5 ± 1.9^b

[a]KB, buccal epithelium.
[b]Statistically significant inhibition, $p < 0.05$.

Table 5.8. Results of experiments made with protein extracts from thymus, lymph nodes, and muscles

Type of extract	Assay	Null or paradoxical effect	Mild effect	Effect in proportion with the dose	Net results/ No. of experiments
TP Lymph node extract	Cell count		1	6	7/7
Muscle extract		3	3	1	4/7
TP Lymph node extract	Protein assay	1		11	11/12
		1	1	1	2/3
Muscle extract		6		0	0/6

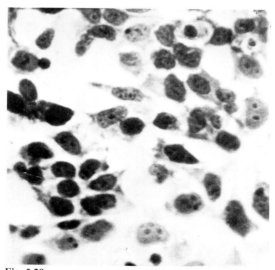

Fig. 5.29a

Fig. 5.29. The morphologic examination of the cells in KB cultures, either treated or not with thymic extract TP. a, Untreated; b, treated with a dose of 0.1 ml. c, treated with a dose of 0.2 ml.

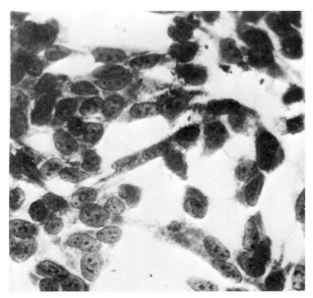

Fig. 5.29b

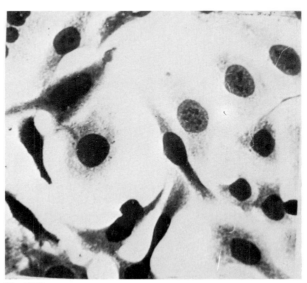

Fig. 5.29c

principles of protein nature which show inhibitory action on growth of KB cell cultures *in vitro* (unpublished observation with the assistance of our coworkers R. Petrescu, E. Ghinea, and G. Mreana).

5.6 Action of TP on immune reactions

It is known that the thymus plays an essential part in immunity; both cellular and humoral theories are postulated. The possible cellular mechanism has been extensively debated. Also there is evidence that a noncellular factor of the thymus confers immunologic competence on cells of the lymphopoietic system (Taylor, 1963; Parrott and East, 1964; Miller and Osoba, 1967). These are briefly reviewed in the first chapters.

The reactivity of TP was investigated by us (unpublished observations with N. Olenici and G. Mreana) on immune reactivity in immature chinchilla rabbits given increasing doses of *Salmonella paratyphi* AH antigen. Serum titrations were made with the somatic antigen. One of the groups had been pretreated with TP. TP was administered subsequently for 30 days. Agglutinin titers in animals given thymus extract proved to be higher compared with untreated animals. The differences were more evident with H antigen than with O antigen. Actually, antigenicity was more significant with flagellar than with somatic antigens.

A remarkable fact was that an elevated titer was maintained in TP-treated animals over a period of approximately 2 months following cessation of the TP treatment. On the other hand, it was noted (Babes *et al.*, 1970) that administration of thymus extract to hamsters immunized with flu antigen induced an earlier development of antiflu antibodies, and the titers were higher and more persistent than in controls. Thymus extract injected during 21 to 28 days produced more antibody formation than did short-term administration (7 days). Finally, it was found that administration of TP stimulated antibody formation more than did muscle peptides extracted by the same procedure (Fig. 5.30).

The stimulating effect of the thymic extract on antiviral and antibacterial antibody formation was also investigated by other authors using similar experimental designs (Comsa and Fillipe, 1966; Li *et al.*, 1963).

The results obtained thus far demonstrate that TP stimulated antibody formation in rabbits injected with *Salmonella typhi* H antigen and in hamsters immunized with antiflu antigen.

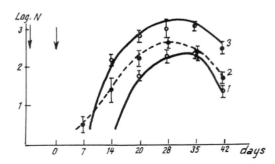

Fig. 5.30. Changes in flu antibodies following TP treatment. Ordinate gives the log of the dilution of active titer. 1, flu antigen; 2, flu antigen plus muscle extract; 3, flu antigen plus TP.

5.7 Thymus-endocrine correlations

Earlier experimental work demonstrated a thymus/parathyroid gland antagonism. Administration of a thymus extract caused a rise in blood calcium with a shift of calcium from the osseous tissue. At puberty, the period when the thymus involutes, parathyroid glands undergo a structural change. Following thymectomy, Parhon (1959) found a hyperfunction of the parathyroid glands assessed according to histocytologic criteria.

When Milcu and Pitis (1943a, b) administered pineal extract in longterm experiments, they found an increase in thymus weight, more accentuated in males, and structural changes of the thymus with a proportionate shrinkage of the medullary zone, expansion of the cortical zone, lymphoid cell hyperplasia in both zones of the gland, and reduction of the epithelial cells. It should be stressed that the structural changes of the thymus are similar to some forms of involution. The stimulating action of pineal extract on lymphoid cells is similar to that of the infantile and prepuberal thymus. These data allowed the advancement of a hypothesis on the thymotropic action exerted by the pineal gland on thymus. In males, inhibition of testicular activity promotes thymic hypertrophy as a part of this phenomenon.

Milcu and Simionescu (1953: 1960) investigated the relationship between the thymus and the adrenals based on the compensating hypertrophy of the adrenals and the role of the central nervous system in this process. In intact animals, compensatory hypertrophy was accentuated by TP administration; after thymectomy, the hypertrophy was reduced when TP was given.

The effects of thymectomy on increasing total blood nucleoproteins were demonstrated in immature rabbits (Milcu *et al.*, 1960). The increase in nucleoprotein levels following cortisone administration (Milcu *et al.*, 1960) was also modified in the absence of the thymus. The results obtained showed a significant effect of cortisone-induced involution of the thymus to be the rise in blood nucleoproteins, although the role of mobilization of these compounds from the thymus by cortisone is not yet understood. Metabolic modifications produced after cortisone administration in thymectomized animals was also demonstrated by others from this laboratory (Stanescu, Florea, and Dinulescu, 1961).

5.8 Conclusions

Data from the literature and our laboratory support the idea that the thymus gland and thymus extracts directly or indirectly affect growth, immunity, oncogenesis, and metabolism. Although exact mechanisms are not known, the effect upon tumor regression *in vivo* may be due to a stimulation of the immune response.

A thymus extract exhibiting manifold actions was obtained by us from the calf (TP), horse embryo (TPE), and the newborn child. Electrophoresis with the Tiselius apparatus and chemical determinations proved the extract isolated from calf to be constituents of a single polypeptide fraction.

Investigations with thymus extracts (TP and TPE) and thymectomy provided evidence which allowed the following conclusions: a) in animals or chick embryo TP stimulates Ca and P deposition in bone tissue and alters serum Ca and P concentration in opposition to thymectomy; b) iron metabolism, lymphocytosis, and erythropoiesis are all stimulated by TP; c) the thymus extract stimulates the synthesis and metabolism of nucleic acid and proteins; d) the thymus stimulates glycogen synthesis, enhances glucose-6-phosphatase and fructose 1,6-diphosphatase activity, and increases ATP levels in hepatic tissue; e) thymectomy and administration of TP result in opposing metabolic changes; f) TP has a replacing action in thymectomized animals which operates on the parameters investigated; g) similar extracts from muscle, spleen, or lymph nodes were inactive; h) as a rule, the action of TP and TPE seemed to be specific; i) TP has an antiproliferative action in KB tumor cell cultures *in vitro*; j) the thymic extracts administered result in a shift towards normal values of the metabolic processes of the host affected by the presence of the tumor, notably in nucleic acid metabolism; and k) there is a good correlation between results obtained *in vivo* and those obtained *in vitro* in tumor cell cultures. These extracts of polypeptide nature are inhibitory to tumors induced either by methylcholanthrene or dimethylaminoazo-benzene when assessed *in vivo* in animals and chick embryos bearing Guerin and Ehrlich ascites carcinoma. A decline in the incidence and volume of the tumor and a reduction in malignancy of tumors are obtained by treatment with TP.

It may be concluded that the thymus contains active factors of poly-peptide nature which influence metabolism, neoplastic growth, immune reactivity, blood lymphocyte and erythrocyte levels and establish morpho-functional correlations with the endocrine glands.

The activity of the polypeptide extracts (TP and TPE) is dose-depen-dent and exhibits a replacing ability in thymectomized animals. These extracts also possess a certain degree of specificity. Taken as a whole, these data seem to indicate the production by the thymus of a hormone-like compound.

6 Characteristics of a Thymic Humoral Factor Involved in the Development of Cell-Mediated Immune Competence

Nathan Trainin, Myra Small, and Yosef Kimhi

6.1 Introduction

Immunologic responses appear to be divisible into two categories, those which are cell-mediated and those which involve circulating antibodies. In fowl, the lymphoid cells responsible for cell-mediated immunity have been found to be under the control of the thymus, while the cells capable of synthesizing antibody molecules have been shown to be dependent upon the bursa of Fabricius. In mammals, thymic function is essential in the establishment of cell-mediated responses, whereas most antibody-synthesizing cells to most antigens appear to be independent of thymic control. Knowledge of the role of the thymus in the development of mammalian immune responses derives from experiments in which the thymus was removed either prior to complete development of the lymphoid system or later in life with concomitant irradiation of the existing lymphoid system. Both of these procedures resulted in decreased numbers of circulating lymphocytes in the blood, depletion of paracortical areas of the lymphoid tissues, and a marked decrease in the small lymphocyte population of the thoracic lymph duct (Miller, 1961a; Parrott, Sousa, and East, 1966; Miller and Mitchell, 1967; Miller, Mitchell, and Weiss, 1967). The long-lived recirculating small lymphocyte pool appears to be most affected by removal of the thymus, and these are the cells which are responsible for cell-mediated reactions (Miller and Mitchell, 1969). Such processes as rejection of skin and tumor homografts, manifestations of delayed hypersensitivity, ability to induce graft-*versus*-host reactions in appropriate recipients, response to phytohemagglutinin, and the mixed lymphocyte reaction against foreign lymphocytes, as well as antibody responses to certain antigens, are impaired following removal of the thymus early in life (Fahey, Barth, and Law, 1965; Dalmasso, Martinez, and Good, 1962; Arnason *et al.*, 1962; Miller, 1962a; Wilson, Silvers, and Nowell, 1967; Doenhoff *et al.*, 1970). The thymus appears to play a role in the development of the population of those cells which undergo cell-mediated immune reactions and those cells which collaborate with anti-body-forming cells (Roitt *et al.*, 1969), and thus it is essential during the neonatal period and in adult life under conditions requiring replenishment of the recirculating lymphocyte pool. Syngeneic thymic grafts have restored the capacity of neonatally thymectomized mice to carry out various thymus-dependent reactions (East and Parrott, 1964; Davies, 1969b), and such thymic grafts are repopulated by cells of the host soon after implantation (Metcalf and Wakonig-Vaartaja, 1964). Allogeneic thymic grafts can also restore immune functions, and in some cases they have enabled thymectomized mice to reject skin or tumor allografts obtained even from the same genetic strain as the reconstituting thymus (Dalmasso *et al.*, 1963; Leuchars, Cross, and Dukor, 1965). In addition, grafts of thymic epithelium and irradiated thymus tissue were found to restore partially lymphoid structure and function of thymectomized recipients (Hays, 1967; Miller, 1966). These findings suggest that at least part of the function of the thymus involves processing of cells produced elsewhere.

It has been demonstrated that the deficiencies caused by neonatal thymectomy of mice could be partially reversed by a diffusible factor produced by thymic tissue. Neonatally thymectomized mice implanted intraperitoneally with cell-tight Millipore diffusion chambers containing syngeneic thymic tissue did not show the degree of depletion of lympho-cytes of the blood, involution of the lymphoid organs, or characteristic signs of the wasting syndrome which accompany neonatal thymectomy (Levey, Trainin, and Law, 1963). Moreover, neonatally thymectomized mice bearing diffusion chambers containing thymic tissue regained the capacity to reject skin homografts (Osoba and Miller, 1964). While neona-tally thymectomized mice were not susceptible to the lethal effects of a lymphocytic choriomeningitis virus, those thymectomized mice implanted with cell-tight diffusion chambers containing newborn thymic tissue manifested a lethal response of a delayed hypersensitivity type to this virus, again indicating restoration of the lymphoid system by a diffusible thymic factor (Levey *et al.*, 1963). Finally, syngeneic thymic tissue in diffusion chambers restored the hemolysin response of neonatally thymectomized mice to sheep red blood cells to the same degree as did subcutaneous implants of thymic tissue (Law *et al.*, 1964). These indications of restored immunologic function by a diffusible thymic factor have been extensively reproduced by implantation of thymus-containing diffusion chambers in thymectomized mice, rats, hamsters, and rabbits (Osoba, 1965; Aisenberg and Wilkes, 1965; Wong *et al.*, 1966; Trench *et al.*, 1966).

On the basis of these early findings, we adopted the working hypothesis that thymus function is at least partially of a noncellular nature and oriented our efforts towards identifying a humoral factor which could mediate certain functions attributed to thymic activity. Extracts were prepared from thymic tissue of xenogeneic, allogeneic, and syngeneic origin, and the effects of such thymic extracts on the establishment of immunologic structure and function were tested in mice. Experiments were performed to provide insight into the immune responses which are dependent upon thymic factor, the cellular functions which are under the influence of a noncellular component of the thymus, the type of relation between these cells and the thymic factor and the level at which such a relationship is involved in the immune process, as well as the chemical nature of the active agent of thymic preparations.

6.2 Biologic properties of thymic extracts

Following the indication given by early work of Gregoire (1935) and Metcalf (1956) of a lymphocytopoietic effect of thymic extracts, in the first experiment the lymphocyte complement of thymectomized and non-thymectomized mice and signs of wasting after neonatal thymectomy were evaluated after administration of thymic preparations extracted from sheep, calves, and rabbits and injected repeatedly on the assumption that large doses would be required as long as the active principle of thymic extracts was not available in pure form (Trainin *et al.*, 1966). The results summarized in Table 6.1 indicated that thymic preparations obtained from calves, sheep, and rabbits increased the number of peripheral blood lymphocytes in intact, adult thymectomized, and neonatally thymectomized mice; control extracts of sheep liver, rabbit kidney, and calf muscle were ineffective. Histologically, enlargement of the spleen

Table 6.1. Effect of thymus extracts on wasting and on lymphocyte complement of mice

Source of extract	Rabbit, sheep, calf
Recipient mice	Intact (C57BL/6 and C3H/eb)
	Neonatally thymectomized
	(C57BL/6^a and C3H/eb^b)
	Adult thymectomized (C57BL/6^c)
Schedule of injections	22 to 35 injections twice weekly
Effect on wasting following	Reduction from 60 to 20% incidence
neonatal thymectomy	In thymectomized mice, restitution to
Percentage blood lymphocytes	normal levels; in normal mice, increase
	of 30 to 50% above normal values
Changes in lymphoid	Hyperplasia of lymphoid population;
tissue of spleen	increase in mitotic figures

^{a}Thymectomy within 24 hr.
^{b}Thymectomy at 3 days.
^{c}Thymectomy at 5 to 7 weeks.

lymphoid follicles, hyperplasia, and an increase in mitotic figures of the lymphoid tissue were observed in the spleens of intact mice, and hyperplasia and increased mitosis in the depleted areas of the spleen of thymectomized mice were noted following treatment with the various thymus extracts. Mice deprived of the thymus 12 to 18 hr after birth exhibited weight loss, lymphocyte depletion, and death, characteristic of a wasting syndrome; all of these symptoms were prevented in the majority of the thymectomized mice treated with sheep thymus extracts. In addition, the incorporation of ^{3}H-thymidine into DNA of lymph node cells was measured in either intact or adult thymectomized mice (Trainin, Burger, and Kaye, 1967). After injection of extracts prepared from calf thymus and syngeneic thymus, increased rate of incorporation of thymidine was observed, again suggesting a lymphocytopoietic effect of the thymic humoral factor (Fig. 6.1).

Taking into consideration that quantitative changes in the lymphoid population are not necessarily an expression of modified immunologic activity of the treated animals, the results of these experiments which were performed mainly with thymus extracts of nonsyngeneic origin could have been the reflection of a nonspecific type of stimulation. Thus it was considered more meaningful to measure the influence of thymus extracts in the establishment of immunologically competent animals. Experiments were then performed to evaluate the effects of thymus

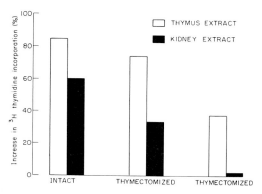

Fig. 6.1. Effect of thymus extract on the incorporation of ^{3}H-thymidine into lymph node DNA in intact and thymectomized C57BL/6 mice. The first two sets represent experiments in which bovine extracts were tested, and the last column shows the effects of syngeneic extracts. The values represent percentage increase of ^{3}H-thymidine incorporation in comparison to that of intact or thymectomized controls injected with solvent only. Extracts were injected i.p. on 3 consecutive days, and on the 4th day ^{3}H-thymidine was injected i.p. 2 hr before lymph node removal.

extracts on various immune responses known to be impaired following removal of the thymus (Trainin and Linker-Israeli, 1967; Trainin, Burger, and Linker-Israeli, 1967). The extract was prepared from calf thymus and injected repeatedly into neonatally thymectomized or adult thymectomized and sublethally irradiated mice. When the ability of these mice to reject skin homografts was evaluated, restoration of the response was observed in those mice injected with thymus extract (Table 6.2). A role of the thymic humoral factor in establishing the homograft response was again clearly indicated by restoration of the capacity of neonatally thy-

Table 6.2. Restoration of immunologic reactivity of thymectomized mice to skin homografts by thymus extracts

Source of extract	Calf
Recipient mice	Neonatally thymectomized[a] (C3H/eb)
Schedule of injections	22 to 28 injections twice weekly
Skin transplanted	(C57BL/6 × C3H/eb)F$_1$
Skin graft survival	Prolonged > 10 days in control thymectomized mice; normal pattern of rejection in 70% of mice treated with thymus extract

[a]Thymectomy at 3 days of age.

mectomized mice to reject allogeneic tumor grafts after repeated injections of calf thymus extract.

This effect was also shown in mice thymectomized as adults and irradiated sublethally, as the capacity to reject a transplanted allogeneic fibrosarcoma was similarly restored by treatment with thymus extracts (Table 6.3). These experiments indicate that establishment of the homograft rejection mechanism is dependent at some stage upon a noncellular factor which can be extracted from xenogeneic thymus tissue. In addition, these results suggest the possibility of influencing the outcome of the balance between tumor growth and host homograft rejection by means of a thymic humoral factor.

While the cells which synthesize antibody molecules have been found to develop by a thymus-independent pathway, thymus-dependent cells are also involved in the antibody response against sheep red blood cells, presumably in a nonantibody-synthesizing capacity. When the hemolysin

Table 6.3. Restoration of immunologic reactivity of thymectomized mice to allogeneic tumor grafts by injections of calf thymus extracts

Recipients	Lethal takes/no. of mice (%)		
	C57BL/6[a]	SWR/J[b]	C57BL/6[c]
Intact controls	0/15	0/9	0/17
Thymectomized	7/15 (47%)	5/6 (83%)	0/12
Thymectomized + calf kidney extract[d]		5/6 (83%)	
Thymectomized + calf thymus extract[d]	0/14	2/8 (25%)	
Thymectomized X-irradiated[e]			11/14 (78%)
Thymectomized X-irradiated[e] + calf kidney extract[d]			12/15 (80%)
Thymectomized X-irradiated[e] + calf thymus extract[d]			4/20 (20%)

[a]C57BL/6 mice thymectomized within 24 hr after birth and challenged i.m. with a C3H fibrosarcoma at 12 weeks.
[b]SWR/J thymectomized at 3 days of age and challenged i.m. with a C57BL fibrosarcoma at 16 weeks.
[c]C57BL/6 mice thymectomized at 8 weeks of age and challenged i.m. with a C3H fibrosarcoma at 18 weeks.
[d]Organ extracts injected twice weekly throughout experiment, beginning in neonatal thymectomized mice at 2 to 3 weeks of age, and in adult thymectomized mice at 13 weeks of age.
[e]X-rays, a single total-body irradiation with 550 r at 12 weeks of age.

response was measured in terms of antibody plaque-forming cells (Small and Trainin, 1967), a definite decrease was observed in neonatally thymectomized mice, and a limited restoration of the primary response was apparent after repeated injections of calf thymus extract to neonatally thymectomized mice (Fig. 6.2).

Small lymphocytes have been shown to be the mediators of cell-mediated immune responses, and one measure of the competence of these cells is the ability to induce a graft-*versus*-host type of reaction when injected into appropriate recipient animals (Gowans and McGregor,

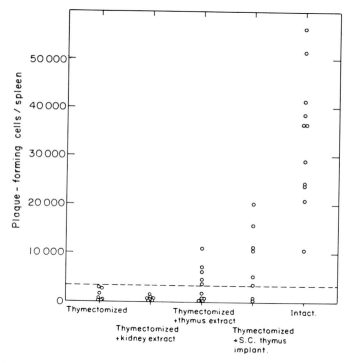

Fig. 6.2. Number of plaque-forming cells/spleen in primary hemolysin response 4 days after challenge with sheep erythrocytes. C3H/eb mice were thymectomized at 3 days of age and injected twice weekly with calf thymus or kidney extracts throughout the experiment. Extracts used were the fractions precipitated by ammonium sulfate at 20 to 40% saturation and adjusted to a protein concentration of 5 and 10 mg/ml for thymus and kidney, respectively. Antibody plaque-forming cells were estimated by the direct Jerne technique at 9 to 13 weeks of age. Animals injected with thymus extract can be compared to those that received s.c. implants of syngeneic thymus.

1965). In an assay described by Simonsen (1962), F_1 hybrid mice challenged by an inoculum of lymphoid cells from immunocompetent parental strain donors developed a splenomegaly characteristic of graft-*versus*-host disease; in a second system used to measure graft-*versus*-host activity, lymphoid cells from competent donors induced a lethal runting syndrome when injected into newborn allogeneic recipients (Billingham and Brent, 1958). The responses of lymphoid cells in both of these assays were found to be dependent upon the active agent of thymus extracts (Fig. 6.3). While splenomegaly was evident in F_1 hybrid mice challenged by parental spleen cells from intact donors, spleen enlargement was less obvious in mice challenged by spleen cell inocula from neonatally thymectomized mice. As shown in the figure, spleen cells from thymectomized mice which had previously received repeated injections of calf thymus extract were capable of inducing a graft-*versus*-host reaction manifested by significant splenomegaly (Trainin and Linker-Israeli, 1967). Also, the activity of spleen cells to initiate a lethal runting syndrome in allogeneic newborn

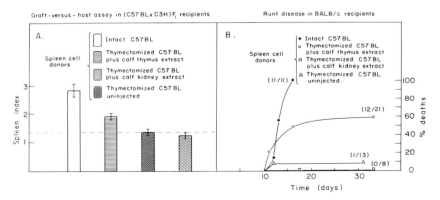

Fig. 6.3. Restoration of competence of lymphoid cells to initiate graft-*versus*-host reactions by injections of thymus extracts into neonatally thymectomized mice.

A. Simonsen assay. Index of splenomegaly of (C57BL × C3H)F_1 recipients 8 days after inoculation of 10 to 15 × 10^6 spleen cells from intact C57BL/6 mice, C57BL/6 mice thymectomized within 24 hr after birth, or neonatally thymectomized C57BL/6 mice injected with calf thymus or kidney extract twice weekly for 10 weeks. Each column represents the average spleen index of 12 to 15 recipients. The standard deviation is indicated by the vertical bar at the tip of each column.

B. Runt disease. Curve of cumulative mortality of BALB/c mice after inoculation at birth of 5 × 10^6 spleen cells from intact C57BL/6 mice, C57BL/6 mice thymectomized within 24 hr after birth, or neonatally thymectomized C57BL/6 mice injected with calf thymus or kidney extract twice weekly for 10 weeks. Figures in brackets represent number of deaths/total number of mice injected.

recipients was markedly impaired after neonatal thymectomy of the donor mice. Again, repeated injections of calf thymus extract partially restored the competence of spleen cells from neonatally thymectomized donors (Trainin et al., 1967).

Thus it was shown that a noncellular factor which can be extracted from thymic tissue influenced the homograft response to skin and tumor transplants, the hemolysin response against heterologous erythrocytes, and the induction of graft-versus-host reactions against mice differing at the locus of histocompatibility. In order to clarify the nature of the relation between the thymus factor and the cells which are ultimately reactive in an immune response, we decided to investigate the possibility of a direct interaction between thymus extracts and the cells of a particular lymphoid organ. An in vitro method of contact between thymus extracts and incompetent lymphoid cells seemed an appropriate approach to this question. Moreover, the defined requirements of in vitro techniques facilitated the use of syngeneic extracts, eliminating the possible non-specific antigenic stimulation of xenogeneic preparations. Experiments were thus designed to test the competence-inducing effect of syngeneic thymic extract on spleen cells from neonatally thymectomized mice. Immunocompetence was evaluated by the ability of the cells to induce a graft-versus-host response, which was measured according to an in vitro procedure developed by Auerbach and Globerson (1966). The relative enlargement of an F_1 newborn spleen explant 4 days after challenge by parental lymphoid cells, compared to a paired explant challenged by lymphoid cells of the same F_1 origin, reflected the response of the "host" tissue to attack by immunologically competent "graft" cells. In preliminary experiments, when spleen explants from newborn mice were exposed to an adequate number of spleen cells from intact parental young adult mice, a graft-versus-host reaction was manifested by spleen enlargement of ≥ 1.2 times the area of each corresponding spleen explant. Impaired competence of inocula containing the same number of spleen cells from neonatally thymectomized donors was evident in the failure to induce this degree of splenomegaly. It was then possible to investigate the direct effect of thymus factor upon such immunologically deficient spleen cells by addition of syngeneic thymus extract to the culture medium surrounding the pairs of F_1 spleen explants under challenge by parental spleen cells from neonatally thymectomized mice (Trainin, Small, and Globerson, 1969). Spleen cell suspensions prepared from each thymecto-mized mouse were thus divided between cultures maintained in regular medium and cultures maintained in medium supplemented with thymus extract. As can be seen in Figure 6.4, the spleen cells which were tested in the presence of thymus extract throughout the course of the 4-day test consistently exhibited the capacity to initiate a graft-*versus*-host response, indicating the ability of the thymus factor to confer reactivity by direct confrontation with suspensions of incompetent cells. When spleen cells from a single thymectomized mouse were divided between cultures containing syngeneic thymus extract and cultures containing extract of syngeneic lymph node or spleen (prepared and tested in parallel with the thymus extract), it was apparent that competence is induced by a factor of specifically thymic origin (Fig. 6.4). Moreover, when spleen cells from thymectomized mice were incubated in thymus extract and washed prior to assay of graft-*versus*-host reactivity, contact between the cells and the thymic agent for 1 hr appeared to be sufficient to enable reactivity by these cells. Thus the influence of a thymic factor in conferring immunologic reactivity appeared to be exerted prior to antigenic stimulation of the cells and did not require anatomic integrity of the lymphoid tissue. It was also evident that extrasplenic metabolic modification of the thymus factor was unnecessary and that migration of cells from other lymphoid organs was not required for the attainment of competence to carry out an *in vitro* graft-*versus*-host response. When spleen cells from neonatally thy-

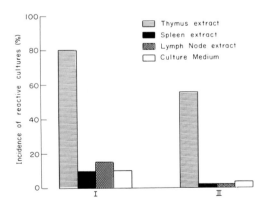

Fig. 6.4. *In vitro* graft-*versus*-host response induced by spleen cells from neonatally thymectomized C57BL/6 mice exposed to syngeneic thymus, spleen, or mesenteric lymph node extract at a concentration of 1 or 2% in culture medium. Each column represents the average of 3 to 6 assays.

I. Extracts present throughout the course of the 4-day assay.

II. Spleen cells incubated for 1 hr in the various extracts and washed prior to assay. Cultures with spleen index of ≥ 1.2 are considered reactive.

mectomized mice were assayed in the presence of thymus extract of allogeneic or xenogeneic source (Trainin and Small, 1970), the activity of these thymic preparations in conferring immunologic reactivity *in vitro* was also evident, while spleen extracts prepared and tested similarly were ineffective (Table 6.4). Thus the thymic agent which induces immune reactivity *in vitro* appears to be neither strain- nor species-specific.

Once it was shown that extracts of thymus tissue can confer immunologic competence by direct confrontation with incompetent spleen cells from neonatally thymectomized mice, it seemed of importance to determine whether these extracts have any measurable effect on normal populations of lymphoid cells obtained from intact mice (Trainin and Small, 1970). To test this possibility, similar *in vitro* assays were carried out with inocula of normal spleen cells found to contain an insufficient number of competent cells to induce a graft-*versus*-host reaction (Fig. 6.5). When such inocula were tested in the presence of thymus extract, the incidence of graft-*versus*-host response was not significantly increased, and cell suspensions prepared from explants of parental spleen tissue which were incubated with thymus extract also failed to induce a graft-*versus*-host response. When the same number of spleen cells were taken from animals given injections 1 day before with xenogeneic or syngeneic

Table 6.4. *In vitro* graft-*versus*-host response induced by spleen cells from neonatally thymectomized C57BL/6 mice in the presence of xenogeneic or allogeneic thymus extract

Extract tested[a]	Incidence of reactive cultures[b]					Cultures responding
Calf thymus	4/4	6/7	5/9	5/5	4/7	75
Calf spleen		0/5	1/7	0/9		5
(C3H × C57BL)F₁ mouse thymus		4/5	2/5	4/10		50
(C3H × C57BL)F₁ mouse spleen		0/5	0/5	0/10		0
C3H/eb mouse thymus		2/4	3/5	5/10		53
C3H/eb mouse spleen		0/5	0/5	0/10		0
SWR/J mouse thymus		4/5	3/5	5/10		60
SWR/J mouse spleen		1/5	0/5	1/10		10

[a] Extracts were tested at a concentration of 2% in the culture medium throughout the 4-day assay.
[b] Number of cultures with a spleen index ≥ 1.2 per total number of cultures tested.

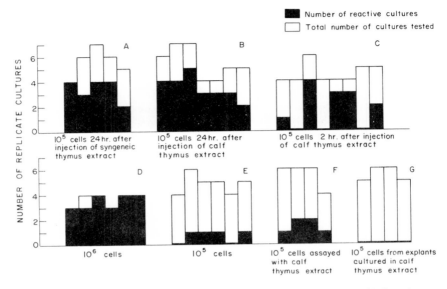

Fig. 6.5. *In vitro* graft-*versus*-host response induced by spleen cells from intact C57BL/6 mice exposed to thymus extract. Each column represents replicate cultures in a single experiment, and cultures were considered reactive when the spleen index was ≥ 1.2. While 10^6 spleen cells consistently initiated a reaction (D), 10^5 spleen cells failed to induce a significant response (E). A, B, and C represent assays performed on 10^5 spleen cells in suspension prepared after 1 ml thymus extract was injected intraperitoneally to intact mice. In F, 10^5 spleen cells were assayed in the presence of 2% thymus extract, and G represents assay of 10^5 spleen cells prepared from spleen explants cultured for 24 hr in 2% thymus extract.

thymus extract, the ability of these small inocula to induce a graft-*versus*-host response was evident. However, injection of thymus extract only 2 hr before assay of the spleen cells resulted in a less consistent effect, suggesting a gradual increase in the proportion of competent cells within the spleen under the influence of the thymus factor acting on target cells originating outside this organ.

Since evidence from several lines of investigation indicates that immunologically competent precursor cells from mouse bone marrow can acquire immune reactivity in the presence of a functioning thymus (McGregor, 1968; Micklem *et al.*, 1966; Osoba, 1968), and since the cells sensitive to thymus extract appeared to originate outside the spleen, it seemed possible that the target cells of the thymic humoral factor might be found within the bone marrow population. Thus it was decided to test the possibility that the active agent of thymic preparations might be responsible for one step in a process leading bone marrow cells toward immuno-competence (Small and Trainin, 1971). Indeed, when bone marrow cells were incubated in thymus extract and injected into syngeneic neonatally thymectomized or adult-thymectomized lethally irradiated mice, competent cells were recovered from the spleens of these animals, while spleen cells from control mice given injections of untreated bone marrow cells were without activity (Table 6.5). Immune reactivity depended upon the genetic makeup of the bone marrow cells injected. To demonstrate more conclusively that the bone marrow cells were those affected by the thymus extract, parental bone marrow cells were incubated in thymus extract and injected into F_1 recipient mice.

Twenty-four hours later, spleen cell suspensions prepared from these recipients were tested in the graft-*versus*-host assay against tissue of the

Table 6.5. *In vitro* graft-*versus*-host response induced by spleen cells from thymectomized C57BL/6 mice injected with bone marrow cells preincubated in calf thymus extract

Bone marrow cell donor	Extract[a]	C57BL recipients	Reactive cultures[b]	Incidence (%)
C57BL	Thymus	Neonatally thymectomized[c]	5/5 4/7 5/8 2/6 4/5	65
C57BL		Neonatally thymectomized[c]	1/7 1/8 0/5 1/6 0/5	10
(C3H × C57BL)F_1	Thymus	Neonatally thymectomized[c]	0/5 0/5 1/5	7
C57BL	Thymus	Adult thymectomized + 850 r irradiation[d]	3/4 3/5 4/5 4/5 4/5 2/4	71
C57BL		Adult thymectomized + 850 r irradiation[d]	0/4 0/5 1/5 0/5 0/5	4

[a]Bone marrow cells were incubated for 1 hr at 37°C either in 2% calf thymus or in culture medium.
[b]Number of cultures (C3H × C57BL)F_1 spleen explants with a spleen index ≥ 1.2 per total number of cultures tested.
[c]Twenty-four hours after i.p. injection of 50 × 10^6 bone marrow cells, 1 × 10^6 spleen cells of the neonatally thymectomized recipients were assayed.
[d]Seven to nine weeks after i.v. injection of 50 × 10^6 bone marrow cells, 1 × 10^6 spleen cells of the adult thymectomized irradiated recipients were assayed.

same F_1 origin. As can be seen in Figure 6.6, parental-type cells competent to initiate a graft-*versus*-host reaction were recovered from the spleens of those intermediate F_1 mice given injections of parental bone marrow cells previously exposed to xenogeneic or syngeneic thymus extract. Mice given injections of cells of the same parental bone marrow incubated in lymph node extract or in culture medium only did not manifest reactivity. It was thus concluded that cells originating in the bone marrow had indeed attained the capacity to initiate a graft-*versus*-host response, and a factor of specifically thymic origin was implicated in the process leading to the immunodifferentiation of the bone marrow cells. When F_1 bone marrow cells were similarly exposed to thymus extract, injected to F_1 intermediates, and assayed against tissue of the same F_1 strain, no graft-

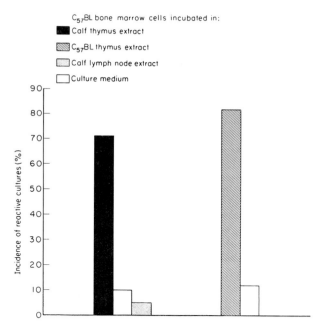

Fig. 6.6. *In vitro* graft-*versus*-host response induced by bone marrow cells from C57BL mice after incubation in 2% extract of calf or syngeneic mouse thymus and injection into (C3H × C57BL)F_1 mice. Control C57BL bone marrow cells incubated in calf lymph node extract or in culture medium alone were similarly injected. Cells recovered from the spleens of the recipient mice 24 hr after injection of the bone marrow cells were assayed against spleen explants of the same (C3H × C57BL)F_1 strain. A spleen index ≥ 1.2 was considered evidence of reactivity.

versus-host response was evident. Therefore, reactivity again depended upon the genome of the bone marrow cells, suggesting that the potential to initiate a response against foreign tissue resides in the bone marrow cells in a latent form until activated by the factors controlling further differentiation.

However, when bone marrow cells were tested directly after exposure to thymic extract, no evidence of significant graft-*versus*-host reactivity was observed (Fig. 6.7), and addition of dissociated F_1 spleen cells to the extract-treated bone marrow cells during the assay did not increase the incidence of the response. Thus an additional step appeared to be involved in the process leading to competence of the bone marrow precursor cells. To shed light upon this complementary process, parental bone marrow cells were incubated in thymus extract, and cultured *in vitro* with spleen tissue from irradiated F_1 mice, and suspensions prepared from these mixed cultures were then assayed for graft-*versus*-host activity (Fig. 6.7). The reactivity which was apparent after culture of extract-treated bone marrow cells with F_1 spleen tissue was not observed after culture of the same treated cells with F_1 thymus tissue, or after addition of dissoci-

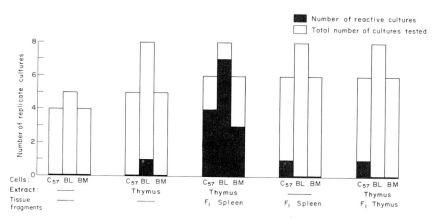

Fig. 6.7. *In vitro* graft-*versus*-host response induced by bone marrow cells from C57BL/6 donors incubated for 1 hr with 2% calf thymus extract and then cultured for 24 hr together with spleen fragments from irradiated (C3H × C57BL)F_1 mice. (C3H × C57BL)F_1 spleen explants challenged with cells from these mixed cultures were considered reactive when the spleen index ≥ 1.2. Control C57BL bone marrow cells were assayed without further treatment, or after incubation in thymus extract only, or after culture with F_1 spleen fragments without exposure to thymus extract, or after incubation in thymus extract and culture with F_1 thymus fragments.

ated F_1 spleen cells to the suspension of extract-treated bone marrow cells under assay.

From the results presented in Figure 6.7, it can be seen that three components, bone marrow cells, a thymic humoral agent, and peripheral lymphoid tissue, were sufficient as well as necessary for the differentiation of immunologically competent cells. These results, suggesting that a second step in the differentiation of cells to immunocompetence occurs in the environment provided by peripheral lymphoid tissue, were supported by experiments showing that thymus cells cultured *in vitro* together with fragments of F_1 lymph node tissue also acquired competence to induce a graft-*versus*-host response.

These experiments indicate that one step in the process by which bone marrow cells acquire competence vis-à-vis the graft-*versus*-host response depends upon a thymic agent that is noncellular and extractable and that another step in this process is under the influence of components found within the peripheral lymphoid tissue environment.

Additional experiments suggest that bone marrow cells can function in another role attributed to thymus-derived cells, as helpers in the hemolysin response to sheep erythrocytes, after a differentiation process which is triggered by the humoral factor of the thymus (Eisenthal, unpublished observation). Neonatally thymectomized mice were challenged with sheep cells injected together with suspensions of bone marrow cells incubated in thymus extracts or thymocytes, and the hemolysin response was evaluated by a modified Jerne procedure. An increased response was evident in those mice given injections of bone marrow cells incubated with thymus extract (Fig. 6.8). The magnitude of the restoration observed after injection of thymocytes suggests that only a portion of the bone marrow cells acquired the capacity to restore the response of thymectomized mice to sheep red blood cells after exposure to thymus extract.

6.3 Chemical properties of thymic extracts

The experiments described above were performed with thymus extracts prepared in the following way.

Syngeneic and allogeneic extracts were prepared from thymuses of mice of approximately 3 months of age. For each preparation, 20 thymuses were removed aseptically and homogenized in 3 ml of cold 0.1 M sodium-phosphate buffer, pH 7.4, in a conical glass tissue grinder. The homogenate was centrifuged at 35,000 g for 30 min. The supernatant was

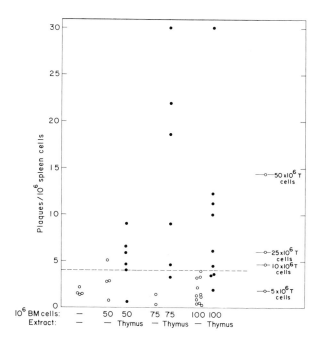

Fig. 6.8. Number of plaque-forming cells/10^6 spleen cells of neonatally thymectomized C3H/eb mice injected with sheep erythrocytes together with bone marrow cells, $\circ$,
or bone marrow cells incubated 1 hr with 10% calf thymus extract, $\bullet$. The average response
of control mice injected with sheep erythrocytes and increasing numbers of thymocytes (T)
is indicated, and in the first column the response of control mice which received sheep
erythrocytes only is also shown.

strained through gauze and diluted to contain 10 mg/ml protein according
to determination by the biuret test. Extracts were passed through Millipore filters (Millipore Filter Corp., Bedford, Mass.) of pore size 0.45μ to
sterilize and avoid contamination by cells. Extracts of spleen or mesenteric lymph node were prepared from the same mice by a similar procedure and adjusted to the same protein concentration.

Extracts of calf thymus or control organs were prepared from young
animals obtained from a local abattoir. After removal of the capsule and
blood vessels, tissues were mixed with 0.1 M sodium-phosphate buffer
pH 7.4 (w/v, 1:2) and disintegrated in a Virtis homogenizer (The Virtis
Company, Inc., Gardiner, N.Y.). The crude homogenates were centrifuged at 2500 g for 20 min, and the resulting supernatant was centrifuged
at 100,000 g for 1 or 5 hr in a Beckman Model L preparative ultracentri-

fuge (Beckman Instruments, Inc., Fullerton, Calif.). The supernatant was strained through gauze, and the extract was diluted to contain 10 mg protein/ml as determined by the biuret reaction. All procedures were carried out at 0 to 5°C with aseptic precautions. After sterilization through Millipore filters of 0.45-μ porosity, extracts were stored at $-10°C$. Extracts were prepared from rabbits and sheep according to a similar technique. In some early experiments, fractionation of xenogeneic thymus extracts with ammonium sulfate was performed, but this procedure was subsequently abandoned.

Dialysates were prepared from calf thymus or spleen extracts dialyzed against 20 volumes of 0.005 M phosphate buffer or distilled water for 60 hr at 4°C. The dialysate was then concentrated by lyophilization or flash evaporation at room temperature to dry powder which was redissolved to the original volume of the extract used for *in vitro* assay or one-half of the original volume for *in vivo* assay.

Experiments performed to measure the ability of the different samples of calf thymus extract to confer *in vitro* graft-*versus*-host reactivity indicated that higher activity was manifested after prolonging ultracentrifugation from 1 to 5 hr (Table 6.6). At this stage it is not clear whether an inhibitor is precipitated by this procedure, but this possibility is suggested since the activity of the 1-hr centrifugate is raised by dialysis. As indicated by the results in Table 6.6, the active factor is of relatively low molecular weight, since it passes through both dialysis bags and Diaflo UM-2 membranes (Amicon Ultrafiltration cell model 202, Amicon, N.Y.; The Hague, The Netherlands) which cut at about a molecular weight of 1000.

An attempt was made to extract the active material by the phenol method. Since *in vitro* graft-*versus*-host activity was found in the phenol fraction these results probably exclude a nucleic acid-like composition which was suggested earlier (Trainin and Small, 1970) and instead might suggest a protein-like structure. The possible effect of -SH agents was investigated in relation to occasional batches of thymus extract which had been found to be inactive for no apparent reason. It was found that addition of glutathione, dithiotreitol (Clelands reagent), or cysteine to an otherwise inactive preparation resulted in return of reactivity, whereas the same reagents without extract showed no activity. It is not clear if the -SH reagents activate a receptor in the cells or reactivate the thymic humoral factor.

Biochemical techniques are now in progress to elucidate the chemical nature of the active agent of thymus extracts.

Table 6.6. *In vitro* graft-*versus*-host response induced by spleen cells from neonatally thymectomized C57BL/6 mice in the presence of dialyzed extracts of calf thymus or spleen

Extract[a] tested		Incidence of reactive cultures[b]					Cultures responding
Organ	Fraction						
Thymus •		3/5	0/5	2/5	4/10	3/6	39
Spleen •		0/5	1/5	0/5	0/10	0/6	3
Thymus ○		4/4	6/7	5/9	5/5	4/7	75
Spleen ○		0/5	1/7	0/9			5
Thymus •	Dialysate	3/4	5/5	5/8	2/5		68
Thymus •	Retained in bag	1/5	1/5		0/5		13
Thymus ○	Dialysate	3/5	3/5	5/10	5/7		59
Spleen ○	Dialysate		1/4	0/10	0/6		5
Thymus	Ultrafiltrate[c]	3/5	3/5	4/6	4/5	3/5	65
		1/5	0/4	0/4	1/5	1/4	14

[a]Extracts of calf thymus or spleen centrifuged at 100,000 g for 1hr (•) or 5hr (○) were tested at a concentration of 0.2 mg protein/ml culture medium throughout the course of the 4-day assay.
[b]Number of cultures with a spleen index ≥1.2 per total number of cultures tested.
[c]Dialysate filtered through a Diaflo UM-2 membrane (retaining substances of molecular weight above 1,000).

Since evaluation of the competence-inducing activity of fractions prepared from thymus extract was performed by means of an *in vitro* assay of graft-*versus*-host reactivity, it seemed important to determine whether the activity of such fractions was reflected in other properties associated with thymus-dependent cells. An *in vivo* effect of the dialysate prepared from calf thymus extract was shown by injection of this material to neonatally thymectomized mice. Following a short schedule of injections of calf thymus (cellophane) dialysate, spleen cell suspensions prepared from the treated mice contained sufficient immunocompetent cells to initiate an *in vivo* graft-*versus*-host reaction as measured by the Simonsen procedure (Fig. 6.9). Moreover, the ability of neonatally thymectomized mice to reject transplants of an allogeneic fibrosarcoma was restored by *in vivo* administration of the dialysate of thymus extract (Table 6.7). Both the competence-inducing activity of thymic extract dialysate and the potential of bone marrow cells to attain immune competence under the influence of the thymus factor were clearly demonstrated in a further experiment (Table 6.7). Neonatally thymectomized mice given injections of bone marrow cells, or of calf thymus dialysate, or both bone marrow cells

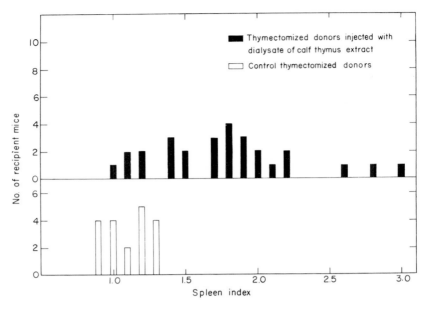

Fig. 6.9. Restoration of competence of lymphoid cells to initiate graft-*versus*-host reactions by injections of dialysate of calf thymus extract into neonatally thymectomized mice. Index of splenomegaly of (C3H × C57BL)F$_1$ recipients 8 days after inoculation of 10×10^6 spleen cells from C57BL/6 mice thymectomized within 24 hr after birth or neonatally thymectomized C57BL/6 mice injected i.p. with 0.5 ml dialysate on 5 successive days before assay by the Simonsen procedure.

and calf thymus dialysate, were challenged by an allogeneic fibrosarcoma. The results leave little doubt that the action of an agent found in the dialysate of thymus extract upon target cells located within the bone marrow population enabled the mice to reject the tumor.

6.4 Discussion of the thymic humoral factor

In the light of these experiments, the existence of a noncellular thymic factor must be taken into consideration to explain some aspects of thymic physiology. This thymic humoral factor is neither strain- nor species-specific, and although the chemical nature of the active agent has not been elucidated, activity is associated with a small dialysable molecule. The active agent of thymic extracts has been shown to serve as a substitute

Table 6.7. Restoration of immunologic reactivity of thymectomized mice against allogeneic tumor graft by injections of dialysates prepared from calf thymus extract

Mice	Treatment	Lethal takes/no of mice	%
C57BL[a]	Phosphate buffer[b]	11/20	55
C57BL[a]	Dialysate of thymus extract[b]	4/18	22
SWR[c]	Bone marrow cells[d]	9/10	90
SWR[c]	Dialysate of thymus extract[d]	5/11	45
SWR[c]	Dialysate of thymus extract + bone marrow cells[d]	1/9	11

[a]C57BL/6 mice thymectomized within 24 hr after birth and challenged i.m. with a C3H fibrosarcoma at 1 to 3 months.
[b]Injections of 0.5 ml i.p. every 2 days 5 times before the tumor challenge and 4 times following the tumor graft.
[c]SWR/J mice thymectomized at 3 days of age and challenged i.m. with a C57BL fibrosarcoma at 2 months.
[d]Syngeneic bone marrow cells (50 × 10[6]) injected i.v. and 1 ml dialysate of thymus extract injected i.p. twice on the day before the tumor challenge and the 8th day after the tumor graft.

for the thymus, thus enabling establishment of populations of lymphoid cells competent to carry out cell-mediated immune reactions. Since it has been demonstrated that the cells participating in cell-mediated responses are thymus-derived lymphocytes, the thymic humoral factor should be involved in conferring to undifferentiated cells the characteristics necessary for performance of these functions. While it is as yet unknown whether the natural interaction between a thymic factor and its target cells occurs within the thymus or outside the thymic environment, we have presented evidence that immunologically incompetent dissociated spleen cells obtained from neonatally thymectomized mice can acquire immune reactivity by direct confrontation with syngeneic thymic extracts in a closed *in vitro* system. Similar extracts from lymph node or spleen were ineffective in such a process, indicating the specificity of action of thymic extracts. Moreover, spleen cells from thymectomized mice incubated for only 1 hr with thymus extracts manifested immune reactivity, and the rapidity of this restoration points to a possible activating effect of thymus factor on cells already present within the spleen of thymectomized animals.

While the nature of this activation is still a matter of conjecture, the thymus-dependent stage required for induction of a graft-*versus*-host

response could involve the ability of the cells to recognize foreign antigens, to transform to blasts and proliferate, or to damage the host tissue.
Thus, alteration of the cell membrane, triggering of cell division, or
changes in the pattern of enzymatic processes are some alternative hy-
potheses to explain the nature of this restoration.

Although the incompetent cell which is under the influence of the
thymic humoral factor has not yet been identified, it has been possible to
demonstrate that cells of the bone marrow population can develop competence in reactions of graft-*versus*-host by a mechanism depending upon
processing by the thymic humoral factor. When bone marrow cells were
injected into mice incapable of inducing a response in the graft-*versus*-
host assay, competent cells were recovered from the spleen of the recipient mice if the bone marrow inoculum had been previously incubated in
thymus extract of xenogeneic or syngeneic source. Competent cells were
not detected in such recipients when bone marrow cells had been incubated in lymph node extract or culture medium only, indicating that a
factor present in the thymus is required to trigger immunodifferentiation
of bone marrow cells. The reactive cells were shown to be of bone marrow
origin, since immune reactivity was related to the genetic makeup of the
marrow cells rather than to that of the intermediate recipients. The interaction between a thymic factor and bone marrow cells appears to be only
one step in the process leading to immunocompetence, since contact between marrow cells and thymus extract was not sufficient *per se* to enable
graft-*versus*-host initiation by these cells. An additional process appeared
to occur within the environment provided by the peripheral lymphoid
organs, as indicated by the attainment of competence by bone marrow
cells preincubated in thymus extract and exposed to nonresponsive spleen
tissue (but not thymus tissue) *in vitro* as well as *in vivo*.

Although further investigation is required to determine whether the
target cells for the thymus extract were in fact stem cells which had never
left the bone marrow, we suggest that precursor cells could develop competence by a progressive differentiation process involving successive
steps of lymphocyte maturation occurring in separate compartments
of the lymphoid system. Thus, precursor cells from the bone marrow
could undergo changes mediated by a thymic humoral factor acting
either within the thymus or outside this organ, and additional properties acquired by the cells in the environment of the peripheral
lymphoid tissues would complete their development and enable reactivity
in cell-mediated immune responses. The finding that the number of
competent cells within the spleen of normal intact mice was increased

by an inflow of cells after activation of extrasplenic precursors by thymic extracts is compatible with such a concept. Since the mammalian lymphoid system is apparently composed of two compartments under separate control, a factor which functions in the role of the thymus should facilitate differentiation of cells along a pathway leading in particular to reactivity in cell-mediated immune reactions. Indeed, the thymus factor has increased the ability of mice to reject tumor allografts, and no enhancing effects due to circulating antibodies have been noted in the experiments involving tumor rejection. The conclusions that a dialysable factor is responsible for the activity of thymus extracts and that bone marrow cells can attain immune reactivity by a process involving their activation by such a thymic factor were confirmed by the ability of these two components to enable tumor rejection in otherwise incompetent mice.

At the present time the known physico-chemical properties of the active agent of our thymic preparation are compatible with eventual administration of such an agent to humans for the control of syndromes related to thymus agenesia or other forms of thymus insufficiency, as well as a supportive immunotherapeutic measure for the control of neoplasia. Open questions requiring further investigation include the chemical nature of the purified active agent of the thymus, the nature of the interaction between this agent and the target cells of the lymphoid system, the nature of the changes induced in these cells, and the anatomical location where such an interaction occurs naturally.

6.5 Summary of properties of the thymic humoral factor

A thymic agent that is noncellular and extractable prevented wasting in neonatally thymectomized mice.

The thymic humoral factor enhanced lymphoid cell proliferation, as indicated by increased ^{3}H-thymidine incorporation in the lymph nodes and partial reversal of lymphocyte depletion in neonatally thymectomized mice.

When injected into neonatally thymectomized mice, the thymic humoral factor restored the homograft response to allogeneic skin grafts and tumor transplants and partially restored the capacity of spleen cells from these mice to carry out a graft-*versus*-host response.

The thymic humoral factor acted directly upon cells found in the spleens of neonatally thymectomized mice and conferred upon these cells the immunologic competence to induce a graft-*versus*-host reaction. A rapid interaction between the thymic agent and the cells imparted competence to the cells in the absence of simultaneous antigenic challenge.

The active agent was demonstrated in thymus extracts of syngeneic, allogeneic, and xenogeneic origin. It was not detected in extracts prepared similarly from spleen and mesenteric lymph node tissue.

The active component of thymic extract remained in the supernatant of a 100,000 g centrifugation. It has, apparently, a low molecular weight, since it was dialysable and passed a membrane which retains molecules with molecular weight of more than 1000. It was extracted into the phenol phase by the phenol extraction method and SH groups appeared to be involved in its activity.

The thymic humoral factor enhanced the graft-*versus*-host capacity of spleen cell populations of intact mice, probably by activation of target cells originating outside the spleen.

The thymic humoral factor influenced the development of mouse bone marrow cells towards immunologic competence. The process by which bone marrow cells attained the capacity to induce a graft-*versus*-host response also depended upon additional changes in these cells which occurred within the peripheral lymphoid tissue environment.

A dialysate of thymus extracts increased the capacity of neonatally thymectomized mice to reject allogeneic tumor grafts. Tumor graft rejection was further improved by the combination of bone marrow cells administered with this factor.

7   Thymosin Reviewed

W. Gerry Robey

The thymus hormone preparation designated as thymosin by Goldstein *et al.* (1966) has been the subject of extensive characterization described herein. This review summarizes the experiments and describes the results as reported in the original literature. The extent of immunological characterization reported for thymosin has not been equaled by any of the other well characterized thymus extracts.

7.1 Identification, extraction, and purification

A calf thymus extract contained a hormone named thymosin (Goldstein *et al.*, 1966) which has been reported to have multiple functions in the conferral of cell-mediated immune responsiveness. The many functions attributed to this hormone have been reviewed (White and Goldstein, 1968; Goldstein, Asanuma, and White, 1970; Goldstein and White, 1970a, b, 1971; White and Goldstein, 1970) and evaluated (Davies, 1969a; Goldstein, 1970; Kruger, Goldstein, and Waksman, 1970). In the experiments described, adequate controls have been employed to indicate thymosin is thymus-specific.

Preliminary experiments were reported (Klein, Goldstein, and White, 1965; 1966; Goldstein *et al.*, 1966) in which a 105,000 $\times$ g supernatant of mouse, rat, or calf thymus homogenate stimulated lymphocytopoiesis and the incorporation of radioactive precursors into the DNA of mesenteric lymph nodes of adult rabbits. The rabbits were given injections of milligram quantities of the supernatant daily for 3 days prior to administration of the labeled precursor. The thymus extract increased lymph node size and DNA synthesis.

Additional purification of the thymus extract was reported and the active compound, thymosin, was partially characterized (Goldstein *et al.*, 1966). Calf thymus homogenate and supernatant were prepared as described earlier (Klein *et al.*, 1965). The supernatant (fraction 1) was heated fifteen minutes at 100° and centrifuged, and this supernatant (fraction 2) was precipitated by 90% cold acetone. The acetone precipitate was dried and designated fraction 3. Fraction 3 was the preparation used for the majority of tests described later. The acetone precipitate was chromatographed on Bio-Gel P-10 (fraction 4), followed by chromatography on DEAE-cellulose (fraction 5). Biologic activity was destroyed by digestion with trypsin and pronase, but no loss was observed after ribonuclease digestion. Thymosin (fraction 4) contained carbohydrate and had a molecular weight of approximately 10,000 based on the observation that it was slowly dialyzable.

The purification of thymosin was followed by the *in vivo* assay described earlier (Goldstein *et al.*, 1966). Thymosin (fraction 3) was active in the *in vivo* rabbit assay when milligram amounts were injected daily for 3 days. An *in vitro* assay was also described (Goldstein *et al.*, 1966) in which excised rabbit lymph nodes were incubated with fraction 3 at various concentrations. Stimulated incorporation of precursors of protein, RNA, and DNA was observed when fraction 3 was present at less than 1 mg per incubation volume. Concentrations greater than 1 mg produced a decrease in the degree of stimulation.

Further purification and characterization of thymosin have been reported (Goldstein *et al.*, 1970). The acetone precipitate (fraction 3) described earlier was redissolved, and thymosin activity was precipitated by ammonium sulfate between 25 and 50%, saturation. The ammonium sulfate precipitate was chromatographed on DEAE-cellulose and Sephadex G-100. The fraction with the highest thymosin activity was active at 25 μg per injection in the *in vivo* assay. Unfortunately, the biological activity of this preparation was not characterized further.

An inhibitor of the *in vivo* assay was removed by the acetone precipitation and was named thymostatin (Goldstein, Banerjee, and White, 1967). Additional information about the inhibitor has not been reported. The inhibitor, thymostatin, was subsequently reported lost between the DEAE-cellulose and Sephadex G-100 chromatography (Goldstein *et al.*, 1970).

Additional characterization of thymosin was included in the report by Goldstein *et al.* (1970). Thymosin was pronase-sensitive and contained less than 1% carbohydrate and a trace of lipid. The carbohydrate and lipid were not essential for biologic activity. The molecular weight of the protein was estimated to be 70,000 on the basis of the elution volume from a calibrated Sephadex G-100 column. A tendency of the molecule to aggregate was observed. Polyacrylamide gel electrophoresis showed one major and two minor bands at pH 8.3. The amount of protein per gel was not specified.

A recent report of a new isolation procedure for thymosin has appeared (Goldstein, 1971). The latest method is similar to those already described with minor exceptions. The conditions of the heat precipitation step were reduced to 15 min at 80°C and the acetone precipitate (fraction 3) was chromatographed on Sephadex G-150 followed with batch elution from an Ecteola column. The thymosin fraction was then chromatographed on Ecteola with gradient elution. The peak obtained was not symmetrical. Thirty milligrams of the most highly purified fraction was estimated to be present in 1 kg of calf thymus. Three bands were still observed after polyacrylamide gel electrophoresis at pH 8.3. The amount of protein per gel was not specified. It was stated that the bands were polymeric forms of a monomer, and the molecular weights ranged from 10,000 to 12,000 for the monomer up to 70,000 for the trimer. This explanation was based on results obtained by electrophoresis in the presence of sodium dodecyl sulfate. Ultracentrifugation studies were not reported. Purification was followed by the *in vivo* assay of Goldstein *et al.* (1966).

7.2 Biologic activity

Thymosin has been reported to reduce the incidence of wasting disease in neonatally thymectomized mice (Asanuma *et al.*, 1970). Mice were thymectomized within 12 hr of birth and treated with 0.5 to 1.0 mg of thymosin fraction 3 three times per week for 9 weeks. Thymosin treatment decreased the development of wasting disease and the rate of mortality dropped from 67 to 30%. The histology of the lymphoid tissues showed some improvement over saline-treated thymectomized mice and the leukopenia associated with neonatal thymectomy was slightly alleviated. Complete reversal of the thymoprivic condition was not observed in any test. However, limited improvement was noted in all assays.

The effects of thymosin on humoral and cell-mediated immune responsiveness have been studied in normal and immunologically deficient mice (Goldstein *et al.*, 1970a). Varying amounts of thymosin fraction 3 were tested in normal adult mice, neonatally thymectomized mice, adult lethally irradiated mice, and adult thymectomized lethally irradiated mice; the latter group was given syngeneic bone marrow cells. The effects measured in the four groups were the ability to reject skin allografts and the ability to form antibody to sheep erythrocytes as determined by the appearance of agglutinating antibody in serum and hemolytic plaque-forming cells in the spleen. Normal adult mice were injected with 4 mg of thymosin per day for 14 days and were given three injections of sheep erythrocytes during that time. No significant increase in serum agglutinating antibody was observed compared with saline-injected controls. Neonatally thymectomized mice were injected with 0.5 to 1.0 mg of thymosin three days after thymectomy and then were given three injections per week for 9 weeks. At the end of 9 weeks, allogeneic skin grafts were grafted onto those mice. The neonatally thymectomized mice rejected the grafts nearly as rapidly as intact mice. The same animals were immunized with sheep erythrocytes 91 days post-thymectomy, and their spleens were assayed for plaque-forming cells (PFC) 4 days later. The number of PFC per spleen was found to be one order of magnitude less than that of control animals; this was interpreted to be insignificant by the authors (Goldstein et al., 1970a). Adult lethally irradiated mice were injected with 4 mg of thymosin per day for 4 days and were given three injections of sheep erythrocytes during that time. The thymosin-treated mice generally had agglutination titers below those observed in saline-injected irradiated controls. Adult mice were thymectomized and injected with 3 mg of thymosin daily for 7 days prior to lethal irradiation and bone marrow administration. Daily thymosin treatment was continued for 14 days, after which the mice were immunized with sheep erythrocytes. Four days later the number of plaque-forming cells per spleen was determined. Essentially no plaque-forming cells were detected as compared with nonirradiated controls. Thus, thymosin was active in restoration of the homograft reaction but not in restoration of the antibody response to heterologous erythrocytes.

Lymphoid tissue regeneration following lethal and sublethal irradiation has been reported to be stimulated by multiple injections of milligram quantities of thymosin fraction 3 (Goldstein et al., 1970b). Adult intact mice were given lethal and sublethal doses of X-irradiation. Three milligrams of thymosin injected per day for 7 days prior to either irradiation were reported to attenuate the deleterious effects of the irradiations. Three milligrams of thymosin injected per day following irradiation were reported to accelerate recovery of the lymphoid system from the irradiation effects. The assay used was the in vivo incorporation of labeled precursors into DNA described earlier (Goldstein et al., 1966). Also, the lymphoid tissue involution due to irradiation was measured and found to be retarded by thymosin treatment. Injection of 4 mg of thymosin per day following lethal irradiation increased the survival time in mice. Histologic studies were described which indicated thymosin stimulated the proliferation of primitive and immature cell types in the thymus-dependent areas of the peripheral lymphoid tissues.

The immunologic and anatomical consequences of thymosin fraction 3 injection into rats have been reported (Kruger, Goldstein, and Waksman, 1970). Thymosin was tested in adult thymectomized rats which had been lethally irradiated and given syngeneic bone marrow cells. These rats were injected with 5 or 15 mg of thymosin per day following irradiation. Thymosin failed to restore the capability of the test animals to produce serum antibody to bovine gamma globulin, and no histologic restoration of the thymus-dependent areas of the peripheral lymphoid tissues was observed. The expected effect on regeneration of lymphoid tissue was not observed following either sublethal or lethal irradiation of rats given bone marrow. Thymosin was highly immunogenic when tested in Freund's complete adjuvant. Delayed skin reactions to thymosin were observed. When injected into adult rabbits, thymosin produced a pyrogenic effect similar to that observed following endotoxin administration. The possibility that the acceleration of skin rejection (Goldstein et al., 1970a) and the enhanced ability of spleen cells from thymosin-treated animals to elicit graft-versus-host reactions (Goldstein et al., 1971) may be due to the development of allograft sensitivity caused by microbial contaminants in the thymosin preparation was considered (Kruger, Goldstein, and Waksman, 1970).

Thymosin fraction 3 has been reported to accelerate the development of resistance of neonatal mice to murine sarcoma virus-induced tumors (Zisblatt et al., 1970). Murine sarcoma virus was shown to induce tumors which normally regressed within 2 to 3 weeks in intact adult mice. When neonatal mice were infected with the virus at 2 weeks of age, the progressive tumor growth caused death in 84% of the animals 60 days after infection. When treated with 1 mg of thymosin three times per week for 60 days, 39% of the thymosin-treated animals were alive compared with 16% of the controls. It was noted that all groups of mice developed tumors following viral infection, but the difference was the decreased susceptibility to progressive and fatal tumor growth in thymosin-treated animals. The mechanism proposed was that thymosin accelerated the ability of the intact mouse to recognize tumor-specific antigens prior to the saline-treated normal controls.

The influence of thymosin fraction 3 on the immunologic competence of spleen cells from thymectomized mice has been reported (Law, Goldstein, and White, 1968). F_1 hybrid mice were thymectomized within 24 hr of birth and injected with 1 mg of thymosin three times per week for 4 weeks. At 4 weeks of age, the spleens of the thymectomized mice were removed and reduced to cell suspensions, which were then injected into parental allogeneic hosts. Host splenomegaly was measured 7 days later to determine the presence of graft-*versus*-host reactivity. No reactivity was detected in control thymectomized mice, but reactivity was detected in 89% of the intact control mice. Spleen cells from thymosin-treated mice were able to elicit a positive graft-*versus*-host reaction in 60% of the animals in this group. These results represented a partial but significant restoration of spleen cell competence.

The acceleration of the ontogenesis of cell-mediated immunity in intact mice by thymosin fraction 3 has been reported by Goldstein *et al.* (1971). Intact neonatal mice were injected with 0.25, 2.5, or 25 μg of thymosin on the 1st and 2nd days after birth. Spleen cell suspensions were prepared at 4 days of age and injected into lethally irradiated adult hosts. Seven days later the host splenomegaly associated with a graft-*versus*-host of this type was determined. Injection of thymosin significantly accelerated the ability of the spleen cells tested to elicit a reaction at all three levels of thymosin. Spleen cells from intact mice did not elicit a reaction prior to 6 to 8 days after birth. In the same report (Goldstein *et al.*, 1971), similar observations were reported for spleen cells incubated *in vitro* with thymosin at various levels. Spleen cells from 4-day-old mice were incubated with thymosin at 1.0, 0.1, and 0.04 mg per ten million spleen cells for 1.5 hr. The spleen cells were then injected into irradiated hosts, and splenomegaly was measured seven days later. Spleen cells incubated with 1.0 and 0.1 mg, but not 0.04 mg, were significantly potentiated in their ability to elicit the graft-*versus*-host reaction. Bone marrow cells from normal adults incubated *in vitro* for 2 hr with thymosin at 100, 10, and 1 μg per one-half million cells were also shown to elicit graft-*versus*-host reactions when injected into irradiated hosts. No reaction was observed with saline-incubated bone marrow cells. It was proposed that incompetent bone marrow cells migrated to the thymosin-rich environment in the thymus, where they were made competent to mediate cellular immune reactions. These newly competent cells migrated to the thymus-dependent areas of the peripheral lymphoid tissues where they were normally found. However, it would appear that migration to the thymus was not necessarily required, according to the *in vitro* bone marrow incubation experiment.

The effects of antiserum to thymosin fraction 3 were studied in *in vitro* cultures of lymphoid cells, and the purity of the antiserum was described (Hardy *et al.*, 1969b). Antithymosin serum was made in rabbits injected with thymosin fraction 3. The antiserum contained detectable antibodies to a minimum of two components in the fraction 3 preparation. The minor component in the antiserum cross-reacted with bovine serum albumin and was removed by absorption. The purified antithymosin serum was cytotoxic to cultures of thymus cells but not lymph node or spleen cells when incubated *in vitro*. The antiserum agglutinated calf thymus cells and reacted across species barriers to agglutinate mouse and rabbit thymus cells. It appeared that the thymosin fraction 3 preparation contained a thymus specific antigen that was related to or was a part of the thymus cell membrane.

Two reports have appeared (Hardy, Quint, and State, 1969; Hardy *et al.*, 1968) that describe the effects of the antiserum to thymosin fraction 3 on skin allograft survival. Antithymosin was injected daily into intact adult mice after they had received an allogeneic skin graft. The antithymosin treatment produced a significant increase in the time required for first set and second set allograft rejection (Hardy, Quint, and State, 1969). The prolongation was not as great as that obtained when the grafted animals were treated with rabbit antimouse lymphocyte or antimouse thymocyte serum (Hardy *et al.*, 1968). In the same report, daily injections of thymosin fraction 3 were given to adult mice 1 week prior to grafting and continued after grafting. Four milligrams per day, but not 0.5 or 1.0 mg, produced an accelerated rate of first and second set allograft rejection.

Thymosin fraction 3 was reported to modify the immunosuppressive effects of rabbit antimouse lymphocyte serum (Quint, Hardy, and Monaco, 1969; Hardy *et al.*, 1969a). Thymosin accelerated skin graft rejection, and rabbit antimouse lymphocyte serum retarded graft rejection in intact adult mice. The two agents given simultaneously did not cancel their respective effects, but a slight potentiation of the rabbit antimouse lymphocyte serum was observed. Additional experiments showed that thymosin treatment initiated 7 days prior to grafting and antilymphocyte serum administration significantly increased the mean survival time for the allograft. This effect was interpreted to indicate that thymosin mobilized the target cells of the rabbit antimouse lymphocyte serum and made them more readily neutralized (Quint, Hardy, and Monaco, 1969). Adult mice injected daily with rabbit antimouse lymphocyte serum and 4 mg of thymosin for 7 days prior to skin grafting did not reject their grafts as rapidly as mice treated with rabbit antimouse lymphocyte serum alone. However, when thymosin treatment was continued after grafting, a significant decrease in the allograft mean survival time was observed relative to the group that had received only rabbit antimouse lymphocyte serum. It appeared thymosin potentiated antilymphocyte serum prior to grafting; following grafting it stimulated the differentiation of incompetent stem cells into competent lymphocytes. This was supported by the observation that continued thymosin treatment partially reversed the leukopenic condition observed in the group treated with rabbit antimouse lymphocyte serum (Hardy *et al.*, 1969a).

7.3 Comments and summary

In the literature reviewed herein, thymosin fraction 3 was active in a variety of immunologic activities. Thymosin has been shown to be thymus-specific, since equivalent preparations from lymphoid and non-lymphoid tissues have not demonstrated activity in the assays employed to describe thymosin activity. Thymosin has been shown to restore partially cell-mediated responses assayed in thymectomized mice and to accelerate or enhance those activities in intact mice. Conflicting reports about the effect of thymosin on the histologic restoration of thymus-dependent areas of the peripheral lymphoid tissues in irradiated mice and rats somewhat cloud the issue. Thymosin appeared to be unable to restore the antibody response in thymectomized mice, but published experiments have employed multiple doses in milligram quantities. Lower doses of more highly purified preparations may alter these observations.

A great deal of biologic information has accumulated on a preparation (fraction 3) that represented a 12-fold purification over the 105,000 g supernatant (Goldstein et al., 1966). Very little information has been published about the biologic activity of the preparation described as having a 240-fold purification over the 105,000 g supernatant (Goldstein et al., 1970). Due to the preliminary nature of the latest thymosin preparation described (Goldstein. 1971), the degree of purification and biologic activities are unknown. It is felt by this author that the biologic assays described for fraction 3 should be repeated using the most highly purified preparation available (Goldstein, 1971). The observation that thymosin fraction 3 contains material identical to or antigenically related to the thymus cell membrane (Hardy et al., 1969b) may be clarified by testing antiserum to the preparation described by Goldstein (1971).

Further characterization of thymosin will be eagerly awaited by those investigators who are convinced that the thymus gland exerts a humoral influence in the conferral of immunologic competence to newborn or experimentally incompetent animals.*

---

*Recently a new assay has been reported for thymosin (Bach et al., 1971) in which the in vitro incubation of thymosin fraction 3 caused normal bone marrow rosette-forming cells to acquire T-cell characteristics. Using the above assay, another paper has appeared in which the complete purification was reported (Goldstein et al., 1972). Thymosin fraction 3 was precipitated with ammonium sulfate and then chromatographed on Sephadex G-150, Exteola cellulose, and hydroxylapatite. A homogeneous protein preparation was reported that had a molecular weight of 12,600 and was named thymosin fraction 7. This was active in the rosette-forming assay in microgram quantities. The authors propose that thymosin converts B-cells into T-cells via a derepression or activation mechanism.

8   LSH, a Lymphocyte-Stimulating Hormone

T. D. Luckey, W. G. Robey, and B. J. Campbell

8.1 Activation of lymphocytopoiesis

Glimstedt (1932) noted that the lymphatic system was grossly under-developed in 2-month-old germfree guinea pigs in which other organs were normally developed. He suggested the use of this model in the study of lymphatic development and specifically the occurrence of Fleming germ centers and the effect of inoculation of germfree animals with single microbic species. Glimstedt (1933) discussed the development of the lymph nodes of germfree guinea pigs, including the Hellman reaction centers and the general development of the lymphatic system. He observed that the lymphatic system of germfree guinea pigs appeared to be atrophied, the parenchyma was rarified, and the number of lymphocytes was reduced throughout the lymphatic system. The full statement of his findings (Glimstedt, 1936) was reviewed by Luckey (1963). The quantity of lymphatic tissue in germfree animals is compared with that of classic animals in Table 8.1. The lymph nodes of most germfree mammals are only about one-third as large as those of classic mammals; the thymus is not affected. The bursa may be underdeveloped in the germfree state. Germfree animals have underdeveloped lymphatic systems because too few antigens are present to activate a full compliment of activity in their state of biologic isolation. When antigen is provided, a full titer of antibody may be expected (Luckey, 1963), and the plaque-forming cell (PFC) response is quite satisfactory (Shearer, Cudkowicz, and Wallberg, 1969).

   The effects of inoculation of specific microorganisms upon the lymphatic system and other defense elements of gnotobiotic animals have been reviewed (Luckey, 1965). The work reported in this chapter began with the observation that the earliest morphologic reaction to antigen appears to be a nonspecific reaction in the lymph nodes. This led to an attempt to determine the role of the thymus in these reactions and in antibody formation. From this base came the isolation from bovine

Table 8.1. Quantity of lymphatic tissue in germfree and classic animals[a]

Animal	Age (days)	Body Wt. (g)	Thymus (%) GF	Thymus (%) Classic	Spleen (%) GF	Spleen (%) Classic	Nodes (mg %)[b] GF	Nodes (mg %)[b] Classic	Bursa (%) GF	Bursa (%) Classic
Guinea pig	30	154	0.114	0.171	0.086	0.136	104	372		
	60	268	0.122	0.157	0.055	0.099	99.5	268		
	94		0.147	0.186	0.254	0.465	65.2	199		
Rat	30–35	370	0.314	0.455	0.090	0.165	25.5	43.2		
White Leghorn chick	14	47	0.323	0.302	0.086	0.120	60.4	66.0	0.274	0.364
White Wyandott bantam	35	133	0.373	0.313	0.133	0.215	40.5	62.6	0.193	0.288
	56	255	0.505	0.422	0.178	0.208	29.3	70.4	0.176	0.267
	141	757	0.197	0.288	0.130	0.160	20.8	38.4	0.208	0.295
	300±	874	0.115	0.083	0.132	0.150	15.8	21.4		

[a]Data are given as percentage of body *sans* ingesta and/or cecal contents (Luckey, 1963).
[b]The node weights for guinea pigs are the total weight of cervical, scapular, inguinal mesenteric, pancreatic, and bronchial nodes (Glimstedt, 1936). The chick data are the trident node; the rat data are the totals of submandibular and cecal nodes, plus Peyer's patches.

thymus of two compounds (LSH$_h$ and LSH$_r$) which have shown activity in promoting immune competence when injected into neonatal mice. The isolation of other active compounds is anticipated.

Hudson and Luckey (1964) showed that the oral inoculation of germ-free mice with one million cells of *Streptococci* sp. elicited a dramatic increase in lymph node mass and the number, size, and maturation of the cells of these nodes within 1 day. During this 24-hr period, the apical lymph patch of the cecum developed from a nonentity into a discrete body. Subsequent work indicated that the mass of lymph node doubled in approximately 13 hr (Fig. 8.1). Caster, Garner, and Luckey (1966) noted that this reaction was seen concomitant with a rise in peripheral blood lymphocytes whether the antigen was living bacteria, dead bacteria, or the soluble antigen, human gamma globulin. Such activity was known for both primary (Leduc, Coons, and Connolly, 1955) and secondary (Dutton, 1967) responses. These responses indicated that one of the first reactions to antigen was a rapid generalized proliferation of lymphocytes.

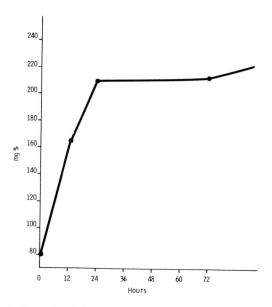

Fig. 8.1. Antigen stimulation of increased lymph node mass. The cervical lymph nodes were measured before and following oral inoculation of young adult germfree mice with *Streptococcus* sp. (Hudson and Luckey, 1964). mg% = mg wet node/100 g body weight.

This rapid response was not seen *in vitro* and was not appreciated *in vivo* according to recent concepts (Abramoff and Lavia, 1970).

Activated lymph nodes showed many small lymphocytes and many mitoses; a generation time of 4 hr beginning with 15% of the lymphocytes present would double the mass of the lymph node within a 13-hr period. It appears to be less reasonable to expect that this increase was the specific action of a single cell, clone, or prescheduled fraction of the total lymphocytes present in inverse proportion to antigen multiplicity. The data of Taliaferro and Talmage (1955) and Sterzl (1967) could detect no antibodies during this "latent" period. Therefore, it appears that large scale antibody production must accompany, if not follow, a generalized stimulation of lymphopoiesis caused by the antigen.

Gregoire (1935) and Roberts and White (1949) showed that injection of thymus extract caused lymphopoiesis. Subsequently, Metcalf (1956) showed that both mouse and human thymus contained a saline-extractable material which was a lymphocytopoietic stimulating factor (LSF) in mice. Lymph node extracts and heated thymus extracts were inactive. Gregoire and Duchateau (1956) also provided evidence that cell-free extracts of thymus activated lymphatic tissue. Confirmation of the presence of this agent was obtained about one decade ago when thymectomized animals were treated with thymus implants in diffusion chambers, as reviewed in Chapter 3 of this book. Miller and Osoba (1964) suggested the name of the humoral factor be competence-inducing factor (CIF) when they found that the active material could pass through a millipore filter. The criticism of their having used too large a pore size was negated by Barclay (1964) who, with Weissman and Kaplan, found pore sizes of 0.1 and 0.01 μ to be effective. Metcalf (1964) suggested that the intense proliferation of lymphocytes within the thymus was caused by a thymic factor, lymphopoietin. He proposed that lymphopoietin, LSF, and CIF are a single factor.

Metcalf (1959) found LSF activity in the serum of some mouse strains; thymectomy eliminated this activity. He also found LSF in the serum of patients with chronic lymphoid leukemia, of preleukemic mice, and of mice with lymphoid leukemia (Metcalf, 1956a, b, c; 1959). This evidence of the release of LSF into the serum was augmented by his reports that tissue culture fragments of thymus released the active material into the surrounding fluid and that injection of cell-free extracts of human or mouse thymus into neonatal mice stimulated lymphocytopoiesis and elevated the lymphocyte/polymorph (L/P) ratios of peripheral blood (Metcalf, 1956a). The lymphopoietic activity of thymus grafts could only be expressed when they contained medullary epithelial tissue (Metcalf, 1964). DeSomer, Denys, and Leyten (1963) and Chamblin and Bridges (1964) confirmed the Metcalf concept by showing stimulation of lympho-cytopoiesis in adult and thymectomized young rats following injection of calf thymus extracts. Calf lymph node extracts were inactive.

8.2 Isolation of pure thymic hormones

In our investigation of thymic hormones, three separate assays have been used to follow activity. A modified Metcalf assay (1959) using the L/P ratio was used for the isolation of a thymus hormone called *lymphocyte-stimulating hormone* (LSH). These studies showed that more than one protein moiety within the thymus extract was active (Hand, Caster, and Luckey, 1967). This assay also established the activity of several groupings of about fifteen specific compounds noted upon polyacrylamide gel electrophoresis of the purified preparations (methanol precipitates) at pH 4.5. Identification of the mobility of each thymus component from methanol precipitates was useful; each band had a typical mobility under standard conditions. This identification was useful to bypass biologic assays during the final isolation. Finally, the activity of two pure compounds in the LSH series was established using serum antibody level and/or the number of plaque-forming cells (PFC) in spleens of young mice following injection of sheep erythrocytes (*see also* Chapter 9).

The preliminary isolation procedure of Hand *et al.* (1967) is outlined in Figure 8.2. The L/P ratios from biologic assay of the fractions provided direction for each successive step. Saline-injected, antigen-injected (up to 250 μg of human gamma globulin), and nontreated mice had L/P ratios of less than 1.5. When appropriate extracts of thymus were injected, this ratio was two or greater. Using this technique, the activity was found to be in the saline extract of thymus and was precipitable with 20% ammonium sulfate. When this precipitate was dissolved in water, the activity could be further purified by precipitation with 75% methanol. The activity of the methanol precipitate was retained in a cellophane dialysis bag. The dialyzed residue was lyophilized and dissolved in water, and this became the standard for a variety of tests and further extraction procedures; it is the purified protein extract (PPE) of Hand *et al.* (1970). At pH 4.5, polyacrylamide gel electrophoresis gave the pattern illustrated in Figure 8.3. One of 16 gels run simultaneously was stained; the others

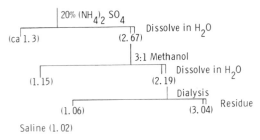

Fig. **8.2.** Chemical fractionation of bovine thymus. The biologic activity (L/P ratio) of each fraction is given in parentheses. The control values in this assay were 1.02 and 0.80 for saline and heated extract injected mice, respectively.

Intact mice were injected with 0.02 ml of test material within 12 hr of birth. The L/P ratio was determined from tail blood taken 6 days later. The methanol precipitate was dissolved in water, dialyzed, and lyophilized prior to use as the purified protein extract (PPE) (Hand, Caster, and Luckey, 1967).

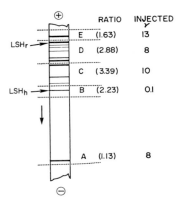

Fig. **8.3.** Gel electrophoresis of PPE from thymus. Information from the left indicates the gel pattern, the fractions taken and their alphabetical designations, the L/P ratio obtained in 6-day-old mice, and the amount of material injected 0 to 12 hr after birth (Hand, Caster, and Luckey, 1967).

were marked by pinholes, cut as indicated, combined by fraction category, and extracted overnight with water.

Compound B (later designated LSH_h) with a mobility, with respect to the ion front, of 0.49 was the most active compound (Metcalf assay) obtained by this fractionation procedure. It was active when 0.1 μg was injected into each mouse. This compound appeared to be 99% protein according to the Lowry technique. Purity was established by re-electro-phoresis, which again gave a single band. Other fractions were less pure and were given in higher quantities; thus their specific activity remained unknown. The multiple response suggested that more than one compound was active; one could also postulate that polymeric forms were present, that one compound was bound to different proteins, or that trailing occurred on the gel. Since biologic activity resided in more than one compound, different compounds were identified by their mobility in polyacrylamide gel at pH 4.5 when run in this mixture. Individual com-pounds have a higher mobility with each successive purification; when run singly, the mobility is quite different from that specified in the methanol precipitate.

The activity of this material was destroyed by heat at 56°C for 30 min. Heated material was thereafter used as the control in most of the assays. Such a control eliminates criticism regarding this assay being affected by nucleic acid, plant, or bacterial products. Normally these materials must be added in rather large quantities to demonstrate activity compared with the submicrogram quantities used in this assay. It should be noted that 0.02 ml of the test material was injected intraperitoneally into mice 6 to 12 hr following birth; 6 days later the lymphocyte/polymorph ratios of the white cells in peripheral blood were determined. The total white blood cell count was not greatly affected by the above extracts. The white blood cell counts of the untreated and saline control mice ranged between 5200 and 6600 leucocytes per millimeter, while those of thymus extract-treated mice ranged between 6500 and 7800. Since most of the properties of this compound were those ascribed by Metcalf to the humoral factor of the thymus, compound B was then named the lymphocyte stimulating hormone, LSH. In order to distinguish it from other compounds in this series, the subscript h (for Hand) will be used.

Further information (Hand, personal communication) using the Jerne PFC assay in neonatal intact mice suggested that a less pure preparation of LSH_h (Fig. 8.3) was stimulatory. PFC assay also indicated that the biologically active material was resistant to RNA nucleotidase, although it was labile to heat and to trypsin. The methanol precipitate from calf spleen was partially active, and that from calf serum was sometimes stim-ulatory. Calf kidney extract, albumin, RNA, and endotoxin were not active (Table 8.2). Further details of this work are reported in Chapter 9.

The above data were of importance in directing our future work. The band with a mobility of 0.108 caused stimulation when only 2 gamma were injected. This information provided the basis for our physical-chemical

Table 8.2. Relative activity of various extracts and materials

Mice were injected with sRBC at 11 days of age and PFC/spleen ratios were determined 4 days later.

Material	Relative activity
Control	1
Purified Protein Extract (PPE)	5.6
LSH$_h$[a]	5.3
Spleen (PPE)	2.3
Kidney (PPE)	1.6
Calf serum	0.5–1
RNA	1.2
Endotoxin	.93
BSA	1
Heated PPE	1
Trypsin treated PPE	1
Nucleotidase treated PPE	5

[a]With three minor contaminant bands, about 98% pure (not the pure material previously described) (data of Hand, unpublished).

assay. Studies were also performed on fractions made during the isolation of the band with a mobility of 0.108 from the methanol precipitate of calf thymus. Sephadex G-75 fractions of the compound with a mobility of 0.108 were observed to be active in the PFC assay (Ceglowski, Hand, and Friedman, unpublished observations). This material also increased spleen weights and total white blood cell counts (Table 8.3). Note that the methanol precipitate gave no increase in white blood cell count. This confirmed our previous finding that thymus saline extract, methanol precipitate, or LSH$_h$ gave increased L/P ratio with no significant increase in total circulating lymphocytes. This indicates a biologic difference between LSH$_h$ and this compound (LSH .108 also designated LSH$_r$).

A different fractionation method allowed the isolation of a compound having a mobility of 0.108 at pH 4.5 from the methanol precipitate; this compound is designated as LSH$_r$ (r for Robey). Details of this procedure are presented elsewhere (Robey, Campbell, and Luckey, 1972). The methanol precipitate (Fig. 8.2) was dissolved in water and charged onto a DEAE column (Fig. 8.4). Successive elutions with increased salt concentrations gave a preparation which was predominantly LSH$_r$ (Fig. 8.5). This fraction was dialyzed, lyophilized, and charged onto a Sephadex

Table 8.3. Activity of LSH$_r$[a] in neonatal BALB/c Mice

All animals (two or more sets of five mice in each group) received sRBC at 14 days of age, and these data were obtained 4 days later. The controls received nothing else. The other groups received 100 μg (i.p.) per mouse (the one indicated received only 10 μg) within 12 hr of birth. The data were obtained by collaboration with W. Ceglowski, T. Hand, and H. Freidman (personal communication, 1970).

Group	Body Wt. (g)	WBC/mm³	Spleen Wt. (mg)	PFC/ spleen	PFC/10⁶ cells
Control	7.4	9,600	86	6,440	46
Prep II-196	8.0	13,125	158	22,100	126
Prep II-196 (10 μg)	9.4	11,750	105	14,800	98
Prep II-226		10,156	133	49,100	122
PPE	8.8	7,900	110	36,300	206

[a]This preparation was about 98% pure.

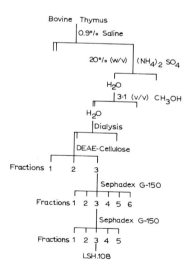

Fig. 8.4. Isolation of LSH from bovine thymus PPE. The following scheme indicates how pure LSH$_r$ was isolated using a combination of DEAE and Sephadex columns. Details are presented elsewhere (Robey, Campbell, and Luckey, in preparation).

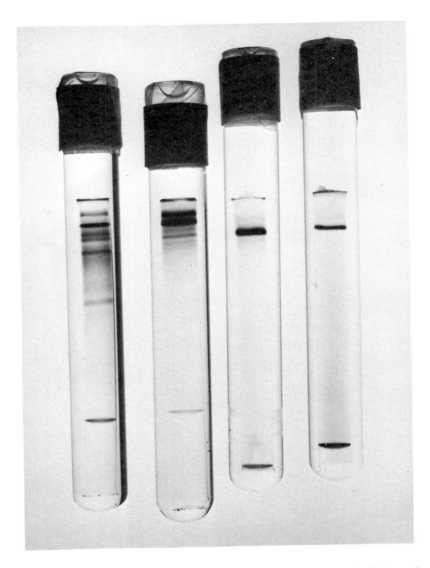

Fig. 8.5. Purification of LSH$_r$. Gel electrophoresis photographs indicate the increasing purity of LSH$_r$ as bovine thymus was processed. From left to right, the gels are made from methanol precipitate (PPE), DEAE fraction 3, and two successive Sephadex G-150 fraction 3.

G-150 column at pH 8.0. The third fraction of material from this column was almost pure LSH$_r$. The third fraction from rechromatography on Sephadex G-150 gave a single band upon gel electrophoresis. The purity of the material from each step is illustrated in Figure 8.5.

8.3 Physical-chemical characteristics of LSH$_h$ and LSH$_r$

Preliminary data from microgram quantities of LSH$_h$ were reported by Hand et al. (1967). The material is a water- and saline-soluble protein with a molecular weight of approximately 17,000. It stains with amido black 10B and is 99 + % protein by the Lowry method. It is heat labile and forms a white powder when lyophilized. Clear birefringent plates were noted in one preparation which was evaporated to near dryness; these were never seen subsequently.

Milligram quantities of LSH$_r$ have been analyzed to determine its physical and chemical characteristics (Robey, Campbell, and Luckey, 1972). It was shown to be a pure protein by producing a single band in gel electrophoresis at three different pH's and at two different concentrations and by migrating as one peak in ultracentrifuge sedimentation. A linear relationship was observed between ln C and r^2 in a sedimentation equilibrium experiment using the meniscus depletion method described by Yphantis (1964). The single band on gel electrophoresis was obtained with high quantities of protein (up to 150 gamma). Its staining characteristics on this gel, the Lowry et al. (1951) determination, and a single absorption band peaking at 280 nm showed that it was protein in nature. Pronase and trypsin digestion destroyed its biologic activity. Amino acid analysis accounted for approximately 99% of the protein; 1% of the molecule is unknown. The amino acid content of the protein moiety is given in Table 8.4. Preliminary tests for carbohydrate have been negative. Lyophilization of the pure compound provided a white fluffy powder. It was stable to heat at 60°C for 30 min. The molecular weight by ultra-centrifuge was 79,800.

8.4 Biologic activity of LSH

Hand (personal communication) found the total LSH activity to be high in mouse thymus, while calf and human thymus showed only 40% of this activity. Calf spleen showed approximately 6% of the activity of mouse

Table 8.4. Amino acid composition of the protein of LSH$_r$[a]

Amino acid	w/w (%)
Alanine	6.14
Arginine	5.72
Aspartic acid	9.70
Cysteine-cystine	1.38
Glytamic acid	16.55
Glycine	2.55
Histidine	4.46
Isoleucine	2.72
Leucine	10.34
Lysine	5.94
Methionine	1.22
Phenylalanine	5.97
Proline	6.06
Serine	5.68
Threonine	5.37
Tryptophan	+
Tyrosine	4.21
Valine	5.95
Total	100

[a]Data from collaboration with Dr. C. W. Gehrke, Director of Experiment Station Laboratories, School of Agriculture, University of Missouri, Columbia, Mo.

thymus or approximately 14% as much activity as calf thymus. Calf kidney extract showed about 1% of this activity. Electrophoresis of the methanol precipitate fractions from these organs showed no trace of either LSH$_h$ or LSH$_r$. LSH$_r$ increased the lymphocyte/polymorph ratio at least two-fold, and it doubled spleen size and increased antibody formation as measured by plaque-forming cells per 10^6 cells 4 days after the injection of sheep red blood cells into 2-week-old mice (Table 8.3). Since this material, which is a component of the methanol precipitate, increased circulating lymphocytes while methanol precipitate did not, a regulator for circulating lymphocytes must be present in the methanol precipitate, or the amount injected was not proper to elicit the response. Recent work from the Pennsylvania laboratory is presented in Chapter 9.

An experiment performed in collaboration with B. Teah of the University of Notre Dame showed that injection of a purified preparation of LSH increased the L/P ratio and the lymph node size in adult germfree mice; gamma globulin injection caused a less dramatic increased size of lymph nodes with no change in L/P ratio (Table 8.5). When pure LSH_h and gamma globulin were injected into neonatal mice (6 to 24 hr old), the results at 7 days (Table 8.6) indicated no change in total numbers of circulating lymphocytes, while the L/P ratio was increased by injection of 1.3 μg of LSH_h in the presence or absence of the human gamma globulin. These data indicate this thymic hormone increases spleen weights in young mice in the presence or absence of antigen. Antigen injection doubled both spleen and lymph node size, while LSH tripled the size of both organs. Particularly in the young adults, this suggests the amount of circulating hormone is a limiting factor in regulating the size, and presumably the cell population and cell reproduction rate, in these organs in intact animals.

Table 8.5. Effect of thymus-purified protein extract on germfree adult mice[a]

Parameter	Saline	240 μg MeOH precipitate	165 μg γ-globulin
No. of animals	6	4	4
L/P ratio average	4.34	10.2	3.8
Range	3.3–4.9	7.3–13.3	2.0–6.0
Cervical lymph nodes average (mg)	5.76	14.8	9.0
Range	3.5–8.0	13.3–18.8	7.3–11.5

[a]This experiment was performed at and by the courtesy of Lobund Laboratories at the University of Notre Dame in July 1966. Collaborators: T. Hand, P. Caster, and B. Teah.

Table 8.6. Effect of LSH_h on germfree neonatal mice[a]

Parameter	Saline	1.3 μg LSH_h	83 μg globulin	LSH_h + globulin
No. of animals	5	6	5	5
WBC average	5,250	5,030	4,890	5,420
Range	4,100–6,500	4,100–6,000	3,350–6,700	3,700–8,900
Average L/P ratio		2.53	1.5	3.3
Range		2.0–3.3	1.0–1.9	2.1–3.5
Spleen (mg average)	8.8	25.5	14.7	27.9
Range	7.6–10.7	20.0–30.6	10.2–17.1	25.5–30.9

[a]This experiment was performed at and by the courtesy of Lobund Laboratories at the University of Notre Dame in July 1966. Collaborators: T. Hand, P. Caster, and B. Teah.
[b]These animals were sacrificed 3 days before the others.

Injections of a 98% pure preparation of LSH$_r$ probably increased total circulating lymphocytes (Table 8.3). This was not usually seen after injection of the saline extract or the methanol precipitate from thymus.

The data obtained from injecting pure LSH$_r$ into two different strains of 11-day-old mice (in separate experiments) using complement lysis of sheep red blood cells (sRBC) to measure serum antibody are presented in Table 8.7. LSH$_r$ injections allowed intact neonatal mice to develop immunologic competence earlier than did saline or other control injections. Positive data noted with LSH$_r$ revealed that relatively high quantities are less active than are low quantities. Unfortunately, levels below 0.1 µg per mouse have not been tested to provide the usual dose response correlation. The data suggest that more frequent administration increases the proportion of mice which react. Quantities of 10 µg per mouse were inhibitory; higher quantities were toxic since all mice injected with 40 µg died within 3 to 4 days in another experiment.

Ceglowski et al. (1971) found that a preparation of pure LSH$_r$ gave a four-fold increase in PFC in young intact mice (Table 8.8), while neither

Table 8.7. Pure LSH$_r$ activation of immune competence

Material was injected at < 1 day of age; sRBC was injected at 10 days, and serum antibody response was determined at 17 days of age. Details are provided in Robey, Campbell, and Luckey (1972). The titer values represent the geometrical mean titer for the group.

Material injected	S-W Mice		ICR Mice	
	No. react[a]/total	Titer	No. react /total	Titer
Ringers solution	7/19	3.3	0/11	1.0
4 × Ringers solution[b]	0/4	1.7		1.0
1.0 µg BSA	2/6	2.5		
4 × 1.0 µg BSA[b]	5/6	5.7		
0.1 µg LSH$_r$	14/18	22.2	5/9	5.8
1.0 µg LSH$_r$	12/23	7.1	4/8	2.2
2 × 1.0 µg LSH$_r$			2/6	3.4
4 × 1.0 µg LSH$_r$	9/10	8.8		
10 µg LSH$_r$			2/6	2.8
1.0 µg LSH$_r$ heated	9/11	7.8	3/4	7.0
1.0 µg LSH$_r$ trypsin			2/4	1.6
1.0 µg LSH$_r$ pronase	4/8	3.4		

[a]Number of mice which reacted per total mice tested.
[b]Injections given at days 1, 2, 3, and 4, after birth.

Table 8.8. Activity of LSH$_r$ upon immune response maturation

The effect of pure LSH$_r$ on numbers of plaque-forming cells in spleens of intact neonatal ICR mice was determined on day 18 after birth. Subcutaneous injections of LSH$_r$ were given either in the 1st day of life or the 1st and 3rd day. Sheep erythrocytes were injected on the 14th day. Data of Ceglowski *et al.* (1971).

Experimental group	PFC/spleen	% of control	No. of mice
Immunized control	20,000	100	5
1.0 μg LSH$_r$	75,000	375	8
1.0 μg LSH$_r$ (2×)	60,000	300	8
3.9 μg LSH$_r$	9,200	46	7
3.9 μg LSH$_r$ (2×)	2,250	11	8
39 μg LSH$_r$	All died		4
Nonimmunized control	15	< .01	8
Nonimmunized control 3.9 μg LSH$_r$	22	< .01	6
Nonimmunized control 3.9 μg LSH$_r$ (2×)	< 10	< .01	8

this pure compound nor partially purified preparations affected the immune competence of intact adult mice.

8.5 Discussion

Although testing is far from complete, our present knowledge of LSH$_h$ shows this to be a compound which will stimulate plaque-forming cells in spleens of mice challenged with sheep erythrocytes. It also appears to increase the L/P ratio, the spleen size, and possibly the lymph node size, but it does not increase the total circulating lymphocyte count. On the other hand, LSH$_r$ appears to stimulate increased total white cells in the peripheral blood, the spleen weights, and increased plaque-forming cells and serum antibody of mice given sheep red blood cell antigen. Both compounds accelerate the maturation of competence of lymphocytes to produce antibody. These results suggest that LSH$_r$ may allow the increase of leukocytes in blood, while both compounds stimulate lymphopoiesis in nodes and spleen. Increased cell reproduction would, of course, imply increased synthesis of DNA, RNA, and protein. Assays on cell-mediated immune competence are in progess.

This work confirms data with crude extracts and thymic grafts in Millipore diffusion chambers reviewed in Chapter 3. Compounds of this series are released from thymus and can be found in serum and spleen in low quantities and in other tissues in trace quantities or not at all. Two compounds of the series have been isolated; another is probably present. The specificity of the thymus as the source of LSH active compounds, their presence in serum and spleen, and their action on lymphocytes are criteria for considering LSH a hormone. LSH_r is physiologically active at 10^{-9} M (0.1 μg/2 g mouse).

The minute quantities of LSH found in tissues other than thymus suggest that the quantity of LSH which is released would be of the stimulating concentration. The apparent inhibitory action of high quantities of this material and the finding of different protein bands in gel electrophoresis which have inhibitory action suggest the presence of more than one controlling factor in the thymus. Thymus inhibitors seem to be powerful; when both inhibitor and stimulating components are present, the results generally reveal the dominance of the inhibitor. It is possible that a low molecular weight inhibitor, *i.e.*, a steroid, would be protein-bound; however, it is doubtful that these inhibitors are comparable to thymosterin, reviewed by Potop and Milcu in Chapter 11. The combination of inhibitors present and the inhibition by excess quantities of the active hormone provide ready explanation for the difficulty of others to sustain consistent assays for the thymic hormone which promotes lymphocytopiesis.

The methods of isolation, molecular weight, and heat stability of LSH_r suggest that thymosin may be similar to it. This is particularly true since thymosin has now been reported to be nondialyzable and to have constituents up to 70,000 molecular weight (*see* Chapter 7). Until individual components of thymosin become isolated as pure compounds, it will be difficult to compare physical, chemical, or biologic properties. Particularly, the tests should be carried out by a single laboratory using the same quantities of pure materials when they become available.

8.6 Summary

The underdeveloped lymphatic systems of germfree mice were activated so rapidly with live bacteria, dead bacteria, or soluble antigen that concepts of the first reactions in antibody formation must include the nonspecific production of lymphatic cells within lymph nodes. This led us to consider the control of stem cell activity (the L/P ratio) and the maturation of immune competence in lymphocytes. A combination of three assays (L/P ratio, the activation of immune competence for serum antibody to sRBC, and gel mobility of components in purified preparations from thymus) led to information about the character of the lymphocyte stimulating hormone, LSH, and the isolation of two active proteins (LSH_h and LSH_r) from the thymus.

Both compounds were isolated from a saline extract of calf thymus which was fractionated by ammonium sulfate and methanol precipitation. Microgram quantities of pure LSH_h were obtained by elution from cut sections of analytical electrophoresis gels. Milligram quantities of pure LSH_r were obtained from the methanol precipitate by column chromatography with DEAE and Sephadex G-150. LSH_h is a heat-labile protein with a molecular weight of about 17,000; LSH_r is a heat-stable protein, and has a molecular weight of 79,800.

The concentration of LSH was estimated to be 10^{-5} in thymus, 10^{-6} in spleen, and 10^{-7} in kidney (Hand, personal communication); LSH activity was also found in serum of leukemic patients and some strains of mice.

LSH increases the size of spleen and lymph nodes in mice. LSH extracts, LSH_h and LSH_r are active in increasing the lymphocyte/polymorph ratio in white cells of peripheral blood in neonatal mice. LSH_r increases the total number of circulating lymphocytes. Both compounds accelerate and/or initiate maturation to immune competence in lymphocytes of intact mice which are too young to have developed antibody-forming capability naturally. If LSH is indeed the hormone responsible for the maturation and differentiation of the lymphocyte in immune response, we have succeeded in our goal, which was to isolate the "antibody hormone." However, other compounds have also been reported to be active. Indeed, little is presently known about either those isolated or compounds which remain to be isolated.

9 Biologic Activity of Thymic Proteins in the Maturation of the Immune Response

W. S. Ceglowski, T. L. Hand, and H. Friedman

9.1 Introduction

Within the past 20 years, and more notably in the last 10, a great deal of research has been aimed at resolving the functional significance of the thymus. A good part of the literature concerning this research is the subject of several recent books (Defendi and Metcalf, 1964; Good and Gabrielson, 1964; Metcalf, 1966b) and a number of review papers (Miller, 1964a; Good *et al.*, 1965; Miller and Osoba, 1967; White and Goldstein, 1968). The subject areas of these books and reviews cover all segments of thymic involvement from anatomical to biochemical. In spite of a great amount of research, the precise functional role of the thymus is at the present time not completely known. A number of contemporary studies have indicated that the thymus may serve as a source of cells (T cells) which are required to interact with bone marrow-derived cells (B cells), in an as yet incompletely understood manner, to effect an immune response (Claman *et al.*, 1966a, b; Miller and Mitchell, 1967; Claman, Chaperon, and Selmer, 1968).

Recent studies from a number of laboratories have suggested that the thymus may function, at least in part, as a source of humoral factors required for the development of lymphoid tissue and immunologic integrity (Miller and Osoba, 1967). A number of early studies indicated that certain thymus extracts could induce lymphocytopoesis and increase lymphoid tissue mass (Metcalf, 1966a; Miller, 1964b; Good *et al.*, 1965; Miller and Osoba, 1967; White and Goldstein, 1968). More recent reports have indicated that appropriate thymus extracts can prevent wasting disease and fatal virus infections in thymectomized mice (Klein *et al.*, 1965; Trainin *et al.*, 1966).

The considerable variation between the extracts and test systems utilized by the various investigators has been well covered by White and Goldstein (1968), and the rich and extensive literature concerning the thymus and thymus extracts is also documented (Metcalf, 1966b; Miller, 1964a; Good et al., 1965; Miller and Osoba, 1967). The concept and more particularly the evidence for humoral factors of thymic origin have also been the subject of critical review by Davies (1969b). Recent experimental evidence which reinforces the need for continuing analysis of this concept is contained in the recent report by Kruger et al. (1970). These investigators demonstrated that there was no immunologic or histologic evidence for reconstitution in thymectomized rats by thymosin, which is one of the better characterized thymic factors.

This review will make no pretense of solving the problem of whether or not the immunologic function of the thymus is mediated by humoral factors. The primary functions of this review will be a) to review the experimental work performed in our laboratories using thymus extracts prepared according to the method of Hand et al. (1967), b) to evaluate the significance of these findings relative to the observations of others, and c) to point out areas in which additional investigation might be productive and informative.

9.2 Methods

Our studies (Hand, Ceglowski, and Friedman, 1970; Hand et al., 1970) have utilized extracts and fractions of calf thymus prepared in the manner described by Hand et al. (1967) and summarized in the previous chapter.

In most of our preparations we have started with kilogram quantities of calf thymus, harvested gram quantities of crude saline extract, and obtained milligram quantities of the partially purified extract, from which we have then isolated microgram quantities of the acrylamide gel purified fractions. Following electrophoresis, two of the fractions were used for the biologic studies. The first fraction, designated "B–C" (Fig. 8.3), was previously found to contain a lymphoid cell stimulator. The second fraction, with less rapid mobility in the electrophoretic field, was designated fraction "D–E" and had been previously found to contain an inhibitory material for lymphocytopoesis (Hand et al., 1970). We have used the same fractionation scheme for calf serum, kidney, liver, and spleen in order to determine if the biologic effects we observed were specific for calf thymus or if they could be mediated by extracts of other tissues. In general, yields of partially purified extracts from these tissues were only 1 to 10% of those obtained from calf thymus.

As an assay system for biologic activity, we have utilized the newborn mouse. In all our studies, newborn mice, either random-bred Swiss (ICR) or inbred BALB/c, have been injected within 12 hr of birth with solutions of the crude thymus extract, the partially purified thymus extract, or the acrylamide gel fractions in microgram quantities. Each value is the average of three separate pooled litters. All litters of newborn mice were standardized to contain no more than eight mice. At varying time intervals thereafter, we immunized these animals by intraperitioneal inoculation of sheep erythrocytes. The test animals along with the appropriate control mice were then assayed for their ability to respond to the antigen. The immune response was assessed in two ways. The first was by performing hemagglutination assays. In brief, individual mice 2 weeks or older were bled from the retro-orbital venous plexus. Younger animals were decapitated, and blood was pooled from mice. Serum was separated from all blood specimens by clotting at room temperature and was stored at $-20°C$ until used. For serologic assay, 0.025-ml dilutions of each serum sample were prepared in microtiter plates, using calibrated wire loops and 0.025-ml volumes of physiologic saline, pH 7.2. To each dilution cup was added 0.025 ml of an 0.5% suspension of washed sheep erythrocytes. The plates were then agitated on a vibrating platform and incubated for 2 hr at $37°C$ and overnight in the cold. Serum titers were recorded as the reciprocal of the highest dilution resulting in complete hemagglutination of the added erythrocytes.

The second assay utilized was the antibody plaque-forming cell technique in agar gel. In brief, 0.1 ml of a freshly prepared mouse spleen cell suspension in Hanks' solution was rapidly mixed with 2.0 ml of melted 0.9% Noble agar containing dextran and sRBC. This mixture was then carefully poured onto the surface of a previously prepared Petri plate containing 10 ml solidified 1% Noble agar. These plates were incubated at $37°C$ for 1 hr and then treated with a 1:20 dilution of guinea pig complement. Plates were incubated for an additional 30 min at $37°C$. The resulting zones of hemolysis were regarded as being due to high efficiency 19 S hemolysins (IgM) secreted by individual antibody-forming cells. Plates were then stained with benzidine H_2O_2 solution in order to facilitate the counting of the plaques. The total number of plaques per spleen, as well as the number of plaques per 10^6 leukocytes, was calculated. Usually two to three concentrations of leukocytes were plated in duplicate or triplicate. Total leukocyte counts were determined with a hemocytometer with the use of acetic acid-methylene blue diluent, and viability was assessed by means of the Trypan blue dye exclusion technique.

9.3 Evaluation of activity

In the evaluation of the activity of thymic extracts and proteins in the neonatal mouse, it was necessary to establish the rate at which the normal untreated mouse develops the ability to form "background" antibody plaque-forming cells. This information is presented in Table 9.1. There was an increase in the number of "background" cells with time in the spleens of both the random-bred Swiss and the inbred BALB/c mice used. The administration of partially purified thymus extract appeared to have essentially no enhancing effect on the number of these cells.

Once this was established, it was then possible to assess the effect of a single inoculation at birth with the partially purified and acrylamide gel thymus fractions upon the subsequent immune response to sheep erythrocytes. A summary of these studies is presented in Table 9.2. Treatment of newborn Swiss or BALB/c mice with the partially purified thymus extract resulted in a stimulation of the immune response to sheep erythrocytes when assayed 4 days later. In the case of the Swiss mice, stimulation was observed in the immune response at 11 days of age, whereas the stimulation in the BALB/c mouse was observed at 18 days

Table 9.1. Development of background antibody plaque-forming cells (PFC) in control and thymus extract-treated mice

| Group | Age (days) | PFC/spleen (average) | |
		Swiss	BALB/c
Nonimmunized	4	1	
Control	11	3	7
	18	3	30
	32	35	55
Nonimmunized	4	1	
partially purified	11		4
thymus extract	32	30	25

Table 9.2. Effect of thymus extract and extract fractions on the immune response to sheep erythrocytes

Group treatment	Age at assay (days)	PFC expressed as ratio of control[a]	
		ICR	BALB/c
Partially purified	4	1.55	Not done
thymus extract	11	4.00	0.12
	18	1.57	5.62
	32	1.57	1.72
Stimulatory gel fraction	4	1.45	Not done
	11	14.90	1.68
	18	1.25	5.62
	32	1.48	1.74
Inhibitory gel fraction	4	1.40	Not done
	11	0.21	0.17
	18	0.04	0.28
	32	1.01	1.34

$$^a\text{Ratio} = \frac{\text{No. of PFC in immunized, treated group at day stated}}{\text{No. of PFC in immunized untreated controls at day stated}}$$

of age. When the stimulatory acrylamide gel fraction was tested, stimulation of the immune response was observed at the same time intervals as with the partially purified thymus extract. In general, results with the hemagglutination reaction were comparable to those presented herein. The inhibitory acrylamide gel fraction when administered at birth appeared to inhibit immunologic maturation in both Swiss and BALB/c at least for the first 2 to 3 weeks of life. It should be stressed that crude saline extracts have in our experimental system uniformly been without effect on immunologic maturation.

In any study of thymus extracts or fractions, an important consideration in evaluating their activity is the specificity of their site of production. For this reason extracts of other calf tissues were prepared and tested for activity in the neonatal mouse system. These results with BALB/c strain mice are summarized in Table 9.3. The calf thymus extract again stimulated the immune response to sheep erythrocytes at the 18th day of age. Extracts of calf spleen had a slight stimulatory effect at this time, while extracts of calf kidney and serum were essentially devoid of stimulatory activity in this test system over the range of times and concentrations tested. Similar results have been obtained when the

Table 9.3. Effect of extract of calf thymus, spleen, kidney, and serum on the immune response to sheep erythrocytes

Group treatment	Age of assay (days)	PFC/spleen 4 days post-imunization (ratio of treated to control)
Thymus extract	11	0.46
	18	7.18
	25	1.58
Spleen extract	11	1.61
	18	2.34
	25	0.55
Kidney extract	11	1.30
	18	1.56
	25	1.37
Calf serum extract	18	0.46
	25	0.52

extracts of organs other than thymus were administered at doses up to five times that of the thymus extract.

An additional consideration in evaluating the activity of thymus extracts is their effect on the immune competence of adult mice. In extensive studies with partially purified thymus extract, we have consistently observed no effect on the immune response to sheep erythrocytes in adult Swiss or BALB/c mice. Concentrations of partially purified thymic extract, up to 50 times that required for activity in newborn mice, have uniformly been without activity in adult mice. Additional limited studies with the polyacrylamide gel fractions, at concentrations up to three times those which are active in newborn mice, show no stimulatory or inhibitory activity in adult mice.

9.4 Discussion

We have interpreted our collective studies to indicate that appropriate extracts of calf thymus can influence immunologic maturation in newborn mice. A partially purified extract possessed the ability to enhance the maturation process. Upon acrylamide electrophoresis of this preparation, proteins were separated which had differing activities. One fraction would greatly enhance maturation, while the other fraction appeared to suppress maturation for at least the first 2 and 3 weeks of life. It should again be stressed that each of the acrylamide gel fractions (inhibitory and stimulatory) is composed of several components. The extracts have no apparent effect on either the normal development of "background" antibody-forming cells or on the immunologic responsiveness of normal adult mice. Our studies to date suggest that the activity is associated with thymic tissue, since extracts of other tissues tested have never resulted in comparable degrees of activity.

Correlation of our studies with those of other investigators is most difficult. The fractionation schemes used by the various investigators have varied greatly. The extracts utilized again vary considerably in their complexity or purity. The chemical and physical characteristics also cover a wide spectrum.

An additional complication has been the wide variation in the methods used to assess the biologic activity of thymus extracts or thymus fractions. Finally, there has been considerable variation in the dose of material administered and the frequency of administration which are required for the demonstration of biologic activity. These considerations make it, we believe, unwise to attempt at the present time to correlate the experimental evidence accumulated to date with the wide variety of thymic preparations. However, it does appear quite clear that appropriate thymic-derived materials do have striking effects on some biologic and immunologic processes. The basic question as to whether or not the thymus mediates its function through humoral factors still remains.

Future studies to determine the significance and the extent of the biologic and immunologic activities of thymus extracts would best be performed with materials which have been isolated and purified to the highest degree compatible with the retention of activity. In addition, it would appear that a number of systems for the assay of immunologic competence should be used. For example, immunologic maturation, graft rejection, graft-*versus*-host reactivity, *in vivo* and *in vitro* delayed hypersensitivity, and immunoglobulin production to particulate and soluble antigens should eventually all be examined. From the standpoint of the function of the thymus in regard to the endowment of immunocompetence, the most meaningful and rigorous test is obviously the reconstitution of immune function in a thymectomized newborn or thymectomized irradiated adult animal.

If, as our studies suggest, the thymus is the source of factors which are capable of enhancing or suppressing immunologic maturation, continued studies on the isolation and characterization of these compounds would appear to be of great interest in regard to thymus function and possible selective alterations in immunologic competence.

Acknowledgments

Studies supported in part by research grants from the Damon Runyon Memorial Fund for Cancer Research, Inc. (DRG-1037AT), the American Cancer Society, Inc. (Ethel A. Shaffer Memorial Grant No. IC-19F), and the National Science Foundation (GB-25996).

10 A Thymic Hypocalcemic Component

A. Mizutani

10.1 Early work on the thymic hypocalcemic factor

Nitschke (1928a, b; 1929a) reported that injection of an acetic acid extract of calf thymus gland into a rabbit resulted in about a 50% decrease in serum calcium levels. Scholtz (1932: 1933) and Nitzescu and Benetato (1932) found that the increased level of blood calcium produced by hyperparathyroidism in a rat could be inhibited by the administration of a calf thymus extract, with resulting recovery from fibrous ostitis. Ogata and Ito (1944) confirmed the lowering of serum calcium level in the rabbit by calf thymus extract, and Ito and Mizutani (1944) found that this extract contained a markedly high content of phosphorus compared with extracts obtained from other organs by the same method of extraction. The present series of experiments was undertaken to determine whether this product was a nucleoprotein or a mixture of nucleoprotein with active protein.

10.2 Early isolation procedures

Thymus gland was collected from a mature steer immediately after killing, and fat tissues, connective tissues, and blood clots were removed. Serum calcium was determined by the Clark and Collip (1925) method or by the chelate titration method of Bachra, Dauer, and Sobel (1958) using Dotite-NN as an indicator. Groups of six normal mature male rabbits, about 2.5 kg in body weight, were fasted for 1 day prior to the experiment. The test sample was dissolved in physiologic saline solution (0.9% NaCl) and centrifuged if necessary, and the solution was injected into the aural vein (0.5 ml/kg body weight). Blood was drawn prior to injection and 4, 5, and 6 hr after injection, and the rate of decrease in serum calcium after injection of thymus extract was compared to that before injection. The sample was considered effective when the maximum rate of decrease of one of the three time periods, expressed as the mean of six animals, was significant at the 5% level when compared to the maximum rate of decrease in the control group injected with saline.

Variation in leukocyte count was examined in rabbits prior to and 2, 4, and 6 hr after injection of the test sample. The leukocytes were counted with a Burker-Turk counting chamber after Turk or Samson staining (Mizutani *et al.*, 1968).

Since thymus is often used for preparations of nucleoprotein, the thymus gland extract was separated into a nucleoprotein fraction and a protein fraction (Mizutani *et al.*, 1970), beginning with the nucleoprotein separation method of Carter and Hall (1940).

Experiment 1. As shown in Chart 10.1, the minced gland was added to two volumes of distilled water containing a small quantity of toluene, cyanide and citrate, adjusted to pH 8.0 with 1 N NaOH, and stirred in an ice bath. The extract was added with $CaCl_2$ to give 0.1% concentration; the precipitate (including nucleoprotein) was collected and dialyzed. The dialysis residue was twice precipitated with 0.1% $CaCl_2$ and dialyzed, and the final precipitate was collected and dried with acetone. Acetone was added to the dialysate to give 50% concentration, and the precipitate was

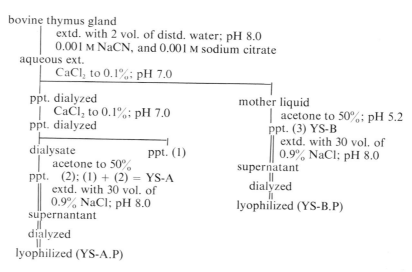

Chart 10.1. Extraction of each fraction from bovine thymus gland

collected by centrifugation and dried with acetone. These acetone-dried products were combined and designated as YS-A. The physiologic saline solution extract of YS-A was dialyzed and lyophilized, and the fraction was designated as YS-A.P. The supernatant fluid left after the initial $CaCl_2$ precipitation was adjusted to pH 5.2 with 1 NHCl, acetone was added to 50% concentration, and the precipitate was collected and dried with acetone. This fraction was designated as YS-B.P. The yield and hypocalcemic activity of these fractions are shown in Table 10.1. The yield of YS-A was 1% of the fresh gland, and it showed a hypocalcemic rate of 11.5 ± 0.5 in a dose of 1.39 mg/kg (1.39 mg of the 2.5 mg was soluble in 0.5 ml of physiologic saline solution); this was considered to be effective. The yield of YS-B was twice (1.9%) that of YS-A, but it was ineffective even in approximately double (2.46 mg/kg) the dose of YS-A, YS-A.P. was effective in a dose of 0.85 mg/kg, but YS-B.P. was ineffective.

Table 10.1. Yield of each fraction extracted with distilled water from bovine thymus gland when tested in rabbits

Material (g)	Fraction	Yield (g)	Yield (%)[a]	Dose soluble portion (mg/kg)	Dose soluble portion (mg[b])	Serum calcium decrease (%)[c] (mean ± S.E.)
600[d]	YS-A	6.2	1.0	2.5	1.39	11.5 ± 0.5[e]
	YS-B	11.35	1.9	5.0	2.46	3.2 ± 1.7
5[f]	YS-A.P	2.0	40.0 (0.4)	1.0	0.85	11.3 ± 0.5[e]
5[f]	YS-B.P	2.0	40.0 (0.76)	1.0	0.94	7.9 ± 2.0
600[d]	3-A	15.2	2.5	10.P	1.0	10.6 ± 0.6[e]
	3-B	0.8	0.1	10.0	1.0	7.4 ± 1.4
	3-C	5.0	0.8	10.0	2.0	13.5 ± 1.1[e]
500[d]	6-A	9.7	1.8	10.0	1.0	11.4 ± 2.2
	6-B	7.0	1.2	10.0	1.0	15.5 ± 1.5[e]
	6-C	5.2	1.0	7.5	1.0	6.1 ± 0.6
2[f]	6-A.R	0.138	6.9 (0.12)	1.0	1.0	8.0 ± 1.1
2[f]	6-B.R	0.94	47.0 (0.56)	1.0	1.0	15.1 ± 1.1[e]
Control (0.9% NaCl solution)				0.5ml/kg		6.5 ± 0.7

[a]Values in parentheses show percentage yield to starting materials.
[b]Saline-soluble portion of the dose expressed in milligrams of each sample per 0.5 ml solution; the nonsoluble portion was not injected.
[c]Serum calcium was estimated by the method of Clark-Collip in rabbits.
[d]The fresh gland.
[e]Significant level, $p < 0.01$.
[f]Acetone-dried powder (crude).

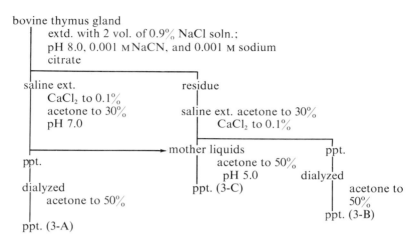

Chart 10.2. Extraction of each fraction from bovine thymus gland

Experiment 2.   As shown in Chart 10. 2, extraction of the thymus gland with physiologic saline solution (at pH 8.0) gave an extract with less viscosity, and the procedure was easier than that with water (*see above*). Then $CaCl_2$ to 0.1% and acetone to 30% concentration was added to the solution obtained by extraction with physiologic saline. The precipitate formed was treated in the same way as described above. The fraction obtained was designated as 3-A. The residue left after extraction was re-extracted with a physiologic saline-30% acetone solution, and the precipitate obtained with 0.1% $CaCl_2$ was designated as fraction 3-B. The fraction obtained by acetone precipitation of the combined supernatant fluid from the initial and final $CaCl_2$ precipitation was designated as 3-C. Fractions 3-A and 3-C had hypocalcemic activity (Table 10.1).

Experiment 3.   The procedure followed in Chart 10.2 was repeated with 0.5% $CaCl_2$. The precipitate formed from the physiologic saline extract by the addition of $CaCl_2$ to 0.5% was dialyzed, and acetone was added to a 50% concentration of the solution remaining in the dialysis bag. The fraction thereby obtained was designated as 6-A. The precipitate formed by adjusting the supernatant fluid of 0.5% $CaCl_2$ precipitation of pH 5.2 was dialyzed, acetone was added to 50% concentration to the solution inside the dialysis bag, and the fraction thereby precipitated was designated as 6-B. The mother liquor left after removal of the precipitate

at pH 5.2 was added with acetone to a final concentration of 50%; the precipitate obtained was designated as fraction 6-C. Fractions 6-A and 6-B
were each extracted with physiologic saline solution, and these fractions
were respectively designated as 6-A.R and 6-B.R. Fractions 6-B and
6-B.R showed hypocalcemic activity, while the other fractions were
inactive (Table 10.1).

It was found through experiments 1 and 2 that the hypocalcemic
principle dissolves in physiologic saline solution, and no activity remains
in the residue. The active principle does not necessarily precipitate
with 0.1% $CaCl_2$. Moreover, effectiveness was recognized in the preparation only when the soluble part was injected after removal of the
physiologic saline-insoluble materials. This fact suggests that the active
principle is different from nucleoprotein, which is sparingly soluble in
physiologic saline solution (Carter and Hall, 1940). On the other hand,
the fact that this activity was sometimes found in the precipitate formed
by 0.1% $CaCl_2$ concentration, considered to be a nucleoprotein fraction,
may be the result of coprecipitation of the active principle with nucleoprotein. It should be difficult for nucleoprotein to precipitate in 0.5%
$CaCl_2$ (experiment 3), but coprecipitation may again have caused
interference. Experiments were carried out with concentrations of
$CaCl_2$ from 0.1 to 0.6%, but there was little effect of fractionation and
reproducibility was poor.

10.3 Purification by ammonium sulfate precipitation

Since it was considered that the hypocalcemic active principle was not
a nucleoprotein, and since $CaCl_2$ precipitation did not effectively frac-
tionate the active material, purification of the active principle by
ammonium sulfate, used for the fractionation of proteins, was attempted
(Mizutani et al., 1971). Conditions necessary for purification procedure
were examined by preliminary experiments (Mizutani et al., 1969), and
fractionation was carried out in accordance with the method used for
the separation of hypocalcemic substance (Parotin) from bovine parotid
gland (Ito and Mizutani, 1952b). A crude acetone-dried powder was
prepared as shown in Chart 10.3 (Mizutani et al., 1969). Bovine thymus
gland was extracted with physiologic saline, and the precipitate obtained
by the addition of acetone to a 60% concentration (pH 5.4) was washed,
dehydrated with acetone, and dried over $CaCl_2$ in a vacuum desiccator.

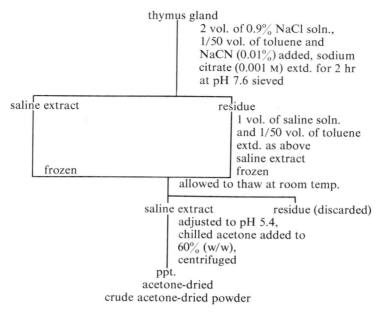

Chart 10.3. Preparation of crude acetone-dried powder

This product was designated as the acetone powder. The yield of acetone powder in triplicate experiments was about 2 to 4% of the fresh gland.

As shown in Chart 10.4, the acetone powder was extracted with physiologic saline solution, the residue was reextracted, and the supernatant was combined with the initial extract and clarified by filtration. Saturated $(NH_4)_2SO_4$ solution was added by drops to this clear filtrate to give a 25% (w/w) concentration (pH 7.0), and the mixture was allowed to stand overnight. The precipitate was collected and dialyzed in a cellulose tube against cold tap water, and the solution left in the cellulose tube was adjusted to pH 7.0 with 1 N NaOH. This solution was filtered, and the filtrate was diluted with water to bring the protein concentration to approximately 1%. Saturated $(NH_4)_2SO_4$ solution was added by drops into this solution to 15% (w/w) concentration (pH 7.0); the mixture was allowed to stand overnight, and the precipitate was collected. This precipitate was dialyzed as above, the solution in the dialysis tube was adjusted to pH 7.6 and centrifuged, and the supernatant was lyophilized. This product was designated as 15% ammonium sulfate fraction (Y-15). The supernatant fluid left after removal of the 15% $(NH_4)_2SO_4$ precipitate

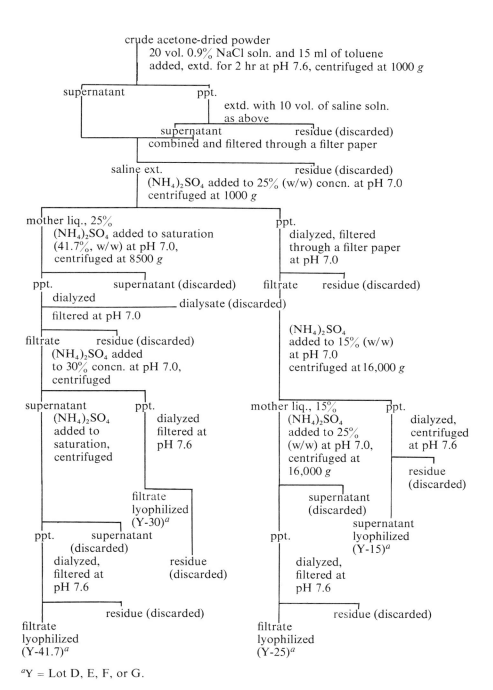

Chart 10.4. Fractionation of crude material with $(NH_4)_2SO_4$

was treated with saturated $(NH_4)_2SO_4$ solution to give 25% (w/w) concentration (pH 7.0), the precipitate was dialyzed, and the 25% $(NH_4)_2SO_4$ precipitate fraction (Y-25) was obtained from its non-dialyzable solution.

The supernatant fluid left after the initial 25% $(NH_4)_2SO_4$ precipitation was treated with powdered $(NH_4)_2SO_4$ to give a 41.7% (w/w) concentration (pH 7.0); the precipitate obtained was dialyzed, and the dialysis residue was adjusted to pH 7.0. The insoluble substance was removed by filtration. Saturated $(NH_4)_2SO_4$ solution was added to the filtrate to give 30% (w/w) concentration (pH 7.0), and the precipitate was dialyzed. The lyophilized dialysate was fraction Y-30. The 30% $(NH_4)_2SO_4$ supernatant was treated with powdered $(NH_4)_2SO_4$ to total saturation (41.7%, w/w), and the precipitate was treated as above to obtain the total $(NH_4)_2SO_4$ saturated fraction (Y-41.7).

Table 10.2. Hypocalcemic activity and percentage yield of each fraction

Fraction No.	Percent yield[a]	No. of rabbits	Percent decrease in serum Ca^{++}[b]
D-12.5[c]	0.003	6	9.9 ± 1.6
M1-12.5[d]	0.036	5	10.5 ± 2.2[e]
D-15	0.023	6	8.1 ± 1.2[e]
E-15	0.068	6	9.5 ± 1.1[f]
F-15	0.069	3	10.5 ± 1.7[f]
M1-15[g]	0.084	6	12.7 ± 1.7[f]
D-25	0.100	6	9.5 ± 1.2[f]
E-25	0.107	5	8.5 ± 0.9[e]
D-30	0.145	6	5.6 ± 1.1
E-30	0.119	6	7.8 ± 2.3
D-41.7	0.190	6	11.8 ± 1.1[f]
E-41.7	0.161	5	11.5 ± 2.2[e]
Control		6+	4.5 ± 0.9

[a] Percentage yield of the crude material.

[b] Serum calcium was estimated by the method of Bachra et al.

[c] The dose was 1 mg/kg body weight, excepting D-12.5, where due to poor solubility only 0.56 mg/kg was injected.

[d] M1-Fractions were prepared from a mixture of lots D, E, and F.

[e] Significantly different from control, $p < 0.05$.

[f] Signigcantly different from control, $p < 0.01$.

[g] M2-Fractions were prepared from mixture of lots F and G.

Yields of each fraction and their hypocalcemic activities are shown in Table 10.2. Activity was found in the fractions precipitated at 15, 12.5, 25, and 41.7% saturation of $(NH_4)_2SO_4$, and none was found in the 30% fraction. The polyacrylamide gel electrophoresis shown in Figure 10.1 indicated that the 41.7% fraction contained a larger percentage of components with large mobility than did the 15% fraction. Consequently, it seems possible that the active principle contained in the 41.7% fraction is different from that contained in the 15% fraction. They have different absorption spectra (Fig. 10.2). It is probable that the active principle contained in the 15% fraction is included in the 25% fraction, but considering the fractionation procedures it would be extremely small in the 30% fraction. For the same reason, the active principle of the 41.7% fraction did not mix with the 30% fraction, and the active principle may be considered to have been separated into the 15% and 41.7% fractions, with the 30% fraction as the boundary.

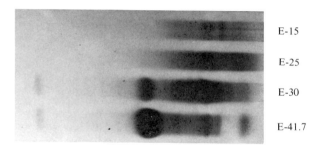

E-15

E-25

E-30

E-41.7

Fig. 10.1. Electrophoretic pattern of E fractions. Gel, 5% polyacrylamide; buffer, Tris-EDTA-borate, pH 8.91; constant current, 6.7 mA/cm², 6 hr; anode to the left, cathode to the right; arrow, origin.

Testing of most fractions showed no correlation between the effect on leukocytes and hypocalcemic activity in rabbits. However, one experiment with mice showed a significant increase in the lymphocyte/polymorph ratio at 6 days following injection of these fractions.

10.4 Discussion

The effect on leukocytes differed considerably between fractions obtained by $CaCl_2$ precipitation and $(NH_4)_2SO_4$ fractionation. In the $(NH_4)_2SO_4$

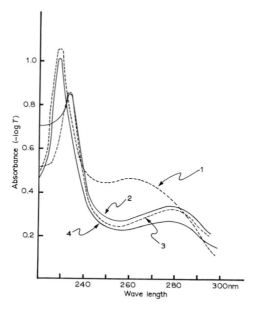

Fig. 10.2. Ultraviolet absorption spectra of E fractions. 1: E-41.7; 2: E-15; 3: E-25; 4: E-30. Each solution contains 200 µg/ml of sample in Tris-EDTA-borate buffer of pH 8.91.

fractionation, the starting acetone powder had no activity against leuko-cytes (not reported here), and the possibility cannot be excluded that the activity was lost during the preparation of the crude powder. However, great care was taken in the preparation of crude powder and the sub-sequent $(NH_4)_2SO_4$ fractionation; there seems to have been small chance of losing this activity. Another interpretation is that the leukocyte activity is essentially absent, and the activity is produced during the procedure by contamination of a foreign substance. At any rate, no conclusion can be drawn at present.

Hand *et al.* (1967) reported the isolation of a substance from calf thymus gland which increased the lymphocytes-to-polymorph ratio. The present data cannot be compared *per se* with their data since the animals used and measurements of leukocytes are different. There seems to be a great difference in the size of molecules of their product and the product reported here.

When the product extracted from the thymus gland by the method of

Nitschke (1928b) was intravenously injected into a rabbit, in a dose of 245 mg, calculated as the fresh gland weight per kilogram of body weight, the hypocalcemic rate was 15.3 ± 4.0 (mean of six animals), whereas the effective quantity of the crude acetone powder obtained in this study corresponded to 74 mg of fresh gland. In our experiments there was no evidence of 50% lowering in serum calcium level, as was reported by Nitschke (1927a).

The result of polyacrylamide gel electrophoresis (Tris-EDTA-borate buffer, pH 8.90) suggested that the product obtained by the procedure of Nitschke was a polypeptide containing a large quantity of a component (nucleohistone) which moved toward the cathode. The product obtained in the present series of experiments moved toward the anode and showed a maximum absorption at about 278 nm in its ultraviolet absorption spectrum (Fig. 10.2, products E-15 and E-25), indicating the usual characteristics of a protein. However, the fraction obtained with total saturation (41.7%) of $(NH_4)_2SO_4$ showed a maximum absorption at about 261 nm, and the presence of a substance related to nucleic acids may be considered.

The crude thymus extract of Ito et al. (1952a) contained about 3.46% of phosphorus, a value much higher than that obtained from bovine parotid gland. Determination of phosphorus by the method of Fiske and Subbarow (1925), after wet combustion of the products obtained in the study (method of Allen, 1940), gave the value of 0.86% in 6-B and 1.09% in one sample of 15% $(NH_4)_2SO_4$ fraction. Lowering of phosphorus content inversely with increasing activity by purification is not contrary to the above interpretation.

Thyrocalcitonin, the hypocalcemic substance, is now known to be a polypeptide with a molecular weight of 4,000 (Potts et al., 1967). This hypocalcemic activity has been found in human thymus by Galante et al. (1968). Thymosin components have 10,000 to 70,000 molecular weights; one of them has calcitonin activity, according to A. Goldstein (unpublished workshop on thymic hormones at the First International Congress of Immunology, 1971). Thymosin and the TP of Milcu and Potop (Chapter 5) appear to be smaller molecules than those studied by us. The hypocalcemic factor studied by our group is expected to be a very large molecule, since it is barely retarded by Sephadex G-200 but is retarded by Sepharose 4B (unpublished data).

The appearance of the 15% $(NH_4)_2SO_4$ precipitate was very similar to that of the 12.1% $(NH_4)_2SO_4$ precipitate obtained from the bovine parotid gland by Ito et al. (1952b), and there was a close similarity between these two products in their hypocalcemic activity and their behavior to gel filtration (unpublished data). Nothing definite can be said at this point as to their identity.

10.5 Summary

Substances having the ability to lower serum calcium levels have been extracted from salivary gland, thyroid, and other organs. We have studied the hypocalcemic factor of thymus in relationship to the studies of bovine patotid gland. The thymus was extracted with physiologic saline solution at pH 8.0, and the extract was fractionated with ammonium sulfate. Our thymus extracts may be related to other hypocalcemic substances on further purification. Significant activity was found when the materials were injected into the aural vein of rabbits at a dose of 1 mg per kilogram body weight. These fractions also had some activity in increasing the lymphocyte-polymorph ratio. Further examination of their leukopoietic activity is planned. The present product extracted from the thymus of a mature steer may give different results than those obtained from calf thymus.

11 Isolation, Biologic Activity, and Structure of Thymic Lipids and Thymosterin

I. Potop and S. M. Milcu

11.1 Review

The discoveries in the past few decades on the effects of neonatal thymectomy have given rise to new concepts of the role of the thymus in immunity. The work of Miller (1961a) created much enthusiasm for scientists in a field which had been almost completely abandoned by most researchers. This is reviewed in previous chapters.

Various active compounds have been isolated from the thymus, but only rarely have they been identified. According to recent data in the literature, there are some features suggesting the presence in the thymus of factors with a hormone-like action, such as Metcalf's (1958) lymphocytosis-stimulating factor, Miller's (1965a) competence-inducing factor, Rowentree, Clark, and Hanson's (1934) growth-stimulating factor, Szent-Györgyi et al.'s (1962) growth-stimulating factor and tumor growth-inhibiting factor, some metabolic active insulin-like factors of Pansky et al. (1965), calcitonin (Galante et al., 1968), thymosin (Goldstein et al., 1966), which restores immune competence of lymphoid cells in thymectomized mice (Law et al., 1968), and those developed in this book.

Thymectomy, thymus grafts, and administration of a number of active extracts were used to study the function of the thymus. Among the isolated factors which were characterized and identified are Comsa's (1971) and Bernardi and Comsa's (1965a, b) factor, which is a glycopeptide, retine and promine, isolated by Szent-Györgyi, Együd, and McLaughlin (1967), who found retine to be a methylglyoxal derivative from many tissues, and LSH, isolated by Hand et al. (1967) as a pure basic protein.

Most extracts derived from the thymus were of protein nature; only occasionally were they lipid in nature. Some workers in this century (Thurner, Torda, and Wolff, cited by Comsa, 1959a) prepared lipid extracts on the basis of their variable solubility in different solvents. Bomskov (1940) and Bomskov, Kaulla, and Maurath (1941) isolated a complex lipid compound from the thymus using ethyl alcohol and acetone as solvents. The authors claimed that the extract contained a steroid-like thymus hormone which was active in carbohydrate metabolism. Administration of this substance induced glycosuria and a fall in liver and heart glycogen levels. Its action may be similar to that of the diabetogenic hormone of the pituitary gland, which in the authors' view may be analogous to the thymòtropic hormone. Thymic hormone may impair thyroid activity. Impairment of oxidation in intermediary metabolism may be an effect characteristic of thymic hormones. Bomskov's extract, which was not analyzed chemically, has been disregarded since 1942; however, Abraham (1971) has recently shown steroid synthesis in the thymus using radioactive acetate and cholesterol.

11.2 Isolation and characterization of thymic lipid fractions

Our experiments on thymic lipid extracts were initiated in 1959. Starting with the finding that the total lipid extract derived from thymus, when administered to rats bearing methylcholanthrene-induced tumors, had a stronger antitumor activity that the polypeptide fraction TP (fraction TP is presented in Chapter 5), special attention was paid to lipid extracts (Potop, Juvina, and Lupulescu, 1961). This complex extract includes an antitumor factor. We endeavored to isolate it and to determine its chemical structure.

Elucidation of the chemical isolation of factor B

A total lipid extract was separated using various solvents at low temperatures, and, subsequently, a range of increasingly purified thymus fractions was analyzed and tested for antiproliferative activity. We used an original procedure adopted and modified from several other methods.

By exhaustive extraction of the thymus with various solvents, a total lipid extract was obtained. Fractionation difficulties associated with solubility were overcome by a pertinent choice of solvents; as far as possible, we used methods of extraction at freezing or slightly elevated temperatures and avoided degrading exposure to air and light. In order to insure the most satisfactory extraction of the lipids from the biologic material, minced fresh-frozen material was totally dehydrated at low temperature with acetone (Loiseleur, 1954).

The total lipid extract (TL) was obtained by dehydration of the frozen minced thymus with technical acetone at about 20°C, repeated total extraction with acetone during 72 hr, and total lipid extraction from the dry residue with ethyl ether. The pooled acetone and ether residue was evaporated in vacuum at a temperature of approximately 55°C, thus yielding the total lipid extract which was analyzed (Potop, Boeru and Mreana, 1963).

Thomas and Reymond's method (1958) for separating various types of brain lipids as modified by us was used for isolating fraction B. Thus, four fractions were isolated which contained various types of lipids. The extraction of factor B was performed according to the following scheme:

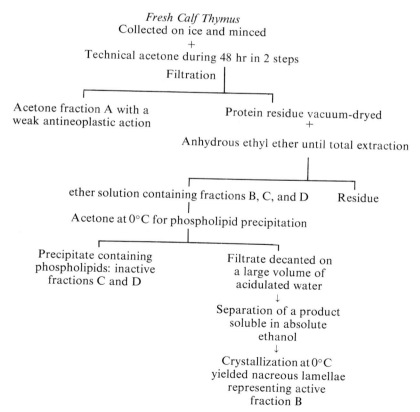

Fresh Calf Thymus
Collected on ice and minced
+
Technical acetone during 48 hr in 2 steps

Filtration

Acetone fraction A with a
weak antineoplastic action

Protein residue vacuum-dried
+
Anhydrous ethyl ether until total extraction

ether solution containing fractions B, C, and D   Residue

Acetone at 0°C for phospholipid precipitation

Precipitate containing
phospholipids: inactive
fractions C and D

Filtrate decanted on
a large volume of
acidulated water
↓
Separation of a product
soluble in absolute
ethanol
↓
Crystallization at 0°C
yielded nacreous lamellae
representing active
fraction B

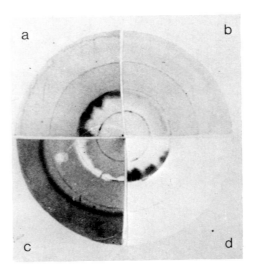

Fig. 11.1. Circular paper chromatography, using Whatmann paper No. 1 with the following solvent system: for the first migration, chloroform-methanol (4:1); for the second migration, acetone; for the third migration, methanol. Paper disk chromatography of fraction B. Staining with Sudan black (a), Sudan II (b); rhodamine (c), and osmic acid (d).

Chemical and chromatographic analyses revealed the complex nature of fraction B. Figure 11.1 presents the paper chromatograph of fraction B by the Hack method according to the indications of Horacek and Cernikova (1959) and Block, Durrum, and Zweig (1958).

Gas chromatography showed fraction B to contain nine identified and four unidentified fatty acids following saponification and extraction. There was a high percentage of oleic, palmitic, and stearic acids present (Fig. 11.2).

Isolation of fractions I B, II B, and III B from fraction B

Starting from fraction B, three fractions with different effects on tumor development were obtained using Bush's method (1952) for separating blood steroids; they were inactive I B, II B, which had a stronger antineoplastic activity when compared with TL or B, and III B, which had a stimulating activity on tumor growth (Potop *et al.* 1967a, b).

The extraction scheme for fractions I B, II B, and III B was as follows:

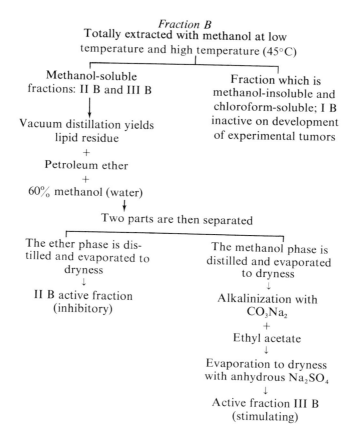

Fraction B
Totally extracted with methanol at low
temperature and high temperature (45°C)

Methanol-soluble
fractions: II B and III B

Fraction which is
methanol-insoluble and
chloroform-soluble; I B
inactive on development
of experimental tumors

Vacuum distillation yields
lipid residue
+
Petroleum ether
+
60% methanol (water)

Two parts are then separated

The ether phase is dis-
tilled and evaporated to
dryness

II B active fraction
(inhibitory)

The methanol phase is
distilled and evaporated
to dryness

Alkalinization with
CO_3Na_2
+
Ethyl acetate

Evaporation to dryness
with anhydrous Na_2SO_4

Active fraction III B
(stimulating)

The analysis of fraction II B by gas chromatography (Table 11.1) demonstrated that the proportion of saturated fatty acids, and especially of oleic, palmitic, and stearic acids, was comparable to that of fraction B. In contrast, fraction II B had a higher content of linoleic acid, 5.19%, compared with 3.53% in fraction B. A further difference was that fraction II B contained no eicosenoic acid. Chemical analysis showed marked dissimilarities between fractions II B and III B (Table 11.2); fraction II B contained much cholesterol, while fraction III B had only trace quantities.

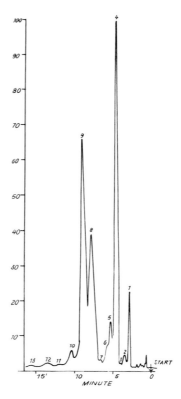

Fig. 11.2. Gas chromatography with the Fractovap B/f apparatus. In the graphic representation, $y = f(x)$. Identification of fatty acids in the thymic fractions was made and compared with a standard mixture of pure fatty acids. Quantitative determination was made by the method of peak measurement. Analysis of free fatty acids in fraction B by gas chromatography, as acids: 1, myristic; 2 and 3, unidentified; 4, palmitic; 5, palmitoleic; 6 and 7, unidentified; 8, stearic; 9, oleic; 10, linoleic; 11, arachic; 12, linolenic; and 13, eicosenoic.

Preliminary analysis demonstrated that fraction III B contained lipid compounds which move to the same position as the various control steroids used in the experiment (deoxycorticosterone, andosterone, estrone). Concurrent staining of the different steroids and chromatographic analyses of fraction III B failed to disclose the presence of any androgen or estrogen. Tetrazol blue staining for corticoids yielded a weak, unstable reaction which disappeared rapidly, reducing the dye. This fact may

Table 11.1. Fatty acid concentration in thymus fractions IIB and B measured by gas-chromatography, given in relative percent of lipids

No.	Fatty acids	II B	B
1	Myristic acid	2.78	2.31
2	Unidentified	1.29	1.27
3	Unidentified	Traces	Traces
4	Palmitic acid	26.02	26.12
5	Palmitoleic acid	3.60	3.37
6	Unidentified	0.06	0.44
7	Unidentified	0.23	0.25
8	Stearic acid	18.13	19.14
9	Oleic acid	41.68	42.33
10	Linoleic acid	5.19	3.53
11	Arachidic acid	0.54	0.74
12	Linolenic acid	0.50	0.50
13	Eicosanoic acid	Absent	2.22

Table 11.2. Concentration in free fatty acids and cholesterol of fraction II B and III B isolated from the thymus

Thymus fraction	Free fatty acids (μEq/g)	Cholesterol (mg/g)
II B	312	58
III B	236	Traces

indicate that fraction III B contained compounds which were too active when compared with known steroids, thus hampering color development, or that the fraction contained only lipids having a dye-reducing ability.

Isolation of fractions II B$_2$, II B$_3$, and II B$_4$ from fraction II B

Fraction II B had a complex nature; therefore, we attempted to separate its different components by silica gel column chromatography (Milcu et al., 1969). Analyses of the resulting compounds by thin-layer chromatography were performed using standard techniques (Crieder et al., 1964). Our results were coincident with those obtained by Crieder, with very slight differences which presumably could be ascribed to the use of different reagents.

The various subfractions (II B$_2$, II B$_3$, and II B$_4$) derived from fraction II B had a distinctly different antineoplastic activity when tested on KB tumor cell cultures.

Fraction II B$_3$ had a stronger antiproliferative activity than did fraction II B, while fractions II B$_2$ and II B$_4$ had weak and moderate activities, respectively (Milcu *et al.*, 1969).

Analysis of fraction II B$_3$ and separation of fraction S

The physical-chemical analysis of fraction II B$_3$ showed this fraction to be only slightly soluble in ethanol, but to be soluble in chloroform and very soluble in ethyl ether. The melting point of fraction II B$_3$ ranged from as low as 28 to 30°C up to 132 to 135°C, indicating a complex chemical mixture. Infrared spectral analysis of fraction II B$_3$ showed the presence of a steroid nucleus, which was indicated by the presence of bands at 1470 cm^{-1}, 1038 cm^{-1}, 970 cm^{-1}, and 850 cm^{-1}, as well as an absorption range of 3000 to 2800 cm^{-1}. The bands at 1720 cm^{-1} and 1750 cm^{-1} indicated the presence of 12 alpha-acetoxy-11-ketones, which always present two absorption peaks in this region. The 1038 cm^{-1} band may be ascribed to the methyl groups of the chain at C-21 and C-28.

11.3 Isolation of factor S

Factor S was obtained from fraction II B$_3$ according to a procedure described in an earlier work by Potop and Milcu (1970). Factor S was isolated by thin-layer chromatography. Originally, 0.25-mm silica gel plates were used; then plates of 0.5-mm thickness were used. The chromatographic silica gel plates were moderately activated for 60 min at 105°C. The sample (II B$_3$) was dissolved in chloroform. The solvent system used was cyclohexane-ethyl acetate-chloroform (40:10:1). Chromatography of fraction II B$_3$ separates some four spots possessing different rf values. The spot with the lowest rf which quantitatively represented 10 to 50% of the total extract depending on the raw material was subjected to further analysis. This is fraction S. Chromatography of the spot with the second system in benzene-acetic acid (60:10) again gave a single spot.

Factor S was identified by chromatography in a cyclohexane-ethyl acetate-chloroform system after spraying with concentrated H$_2$SO$_4$ and examination in UV light. After H$_2$SO$_4$ treatment, the spot S became orange and in UV light appeared to be red. The other spots developed no

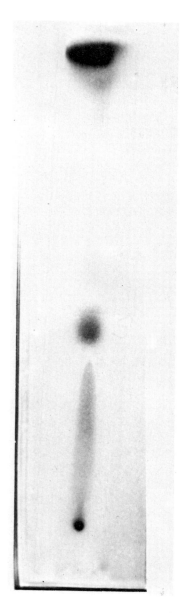

Fig. 11.3. Thin-layer chromatography of fraction II B$_3$ on silica gel H plates moderately activated at 105°C for 60 min for separation of factor S. The sample was dissolved in chloroform. The solvent system was cyclohexane-ethyl acetate-chloroform (40:10:1). The plates to be photographed were developed by exposure to an atmosphere of osmic acid vapors during 2 hr.

color reaction, either orange or red (Fig. 11.3). The spot S was taken up from a plate and extracted with ethyl ether with repeated shaking and filtration through small pore filters. Following evaporation of the ethyl ether, a white material was obtained.

Isolation of fraction S was reproducible and its antiproliferative action was subsequently confirmed in every sample analyzed. Moreover, the spot in the immediate vicinity of S was inactive. The spot S proved to be responsible for the biologic activity after its extraction from the chromatographic plate, as tested on tumor cell cultures.

Elution of the given spot with ethyl ether from a large number of chromatograms allowed the accumulation of a sufficient amount of material to test its activity on tumor cell cultures and to use for physical chemical analysis.

On further chromatography in various developing substances (benzene-acetic acid, benzene-ethyl acetate, cyclohexane-ethyl acetate-chloroform), factor S behaved as a single substance (Fig. 11.4a, b). Its relationship to other fractions is given in Figure 11.5.

11.4 Determination of the structure of factor S

The pure factor S gave a positive Lieberman-Burchard test. The infrared spectrum of the isolated substance was recorded in a chloroform solution in the 4000 to 700 cm^{-1} field (Fig. 11.6). Absorption peaks at 1470 cm^{-1}, 1038 cm^{-1}, 988 cm^{-1}, 970 cm^{-1}, and 860 cm^{-1}, as well as in the 3050 to 2860 cm^{-1} field suggested the existence of a perhydrocyclopentanophenanthrene ring. Although the 3000 to 2800 cm^{-1} zone furnishes no essential information to correlate with the rest of the absorption peaks, it supplements the possibilities of ascribing the bands observed in the spectrum. Absorption in 1670 cm^{-1} may be ascribed to the C=C vibration in position Δ^5; the 1380 cm^{-1} band may be ascribed to the methyl groups in the chain at C-21 and C-28, a fact which is reinforced by the existence of an absorption area between 1250 and 1170 cm^{-1}, indicating the existence of some groups of the $(CH_3)_2CH$ or $(CH_3)_3C'$ type.

The study of the other absorptions revealed the presence of an ester. Thus, the strong band at 1735 cm^{-1} may be ascribed to ketone or acetate carbonyl vibrations (Jones, Herling, and Katzenellenbogen, 1955; Jones and Herling, 1956), the maximum at 1350 cm^{-1} to the vibration of the methyl group bound to the acetate groups, and the 1240 cm^{-1} band to C−O vibrations of the acetate group bound to a steroid ring. Absorption

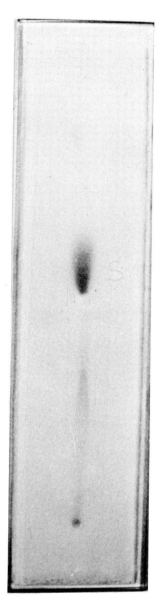

Fig. 11.4a. Rechromatography of factor S in the benzene-ethyl acetate system.

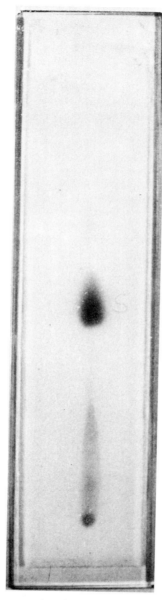

Fig. 11.4b. Rechromatography of factor S in cyclohexane-ethyl acetate-chloroform system.

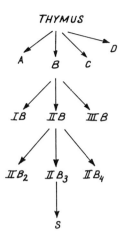

Fig. 11.5. Scheme of extraction of pure factor S from fraction B.

in the 1155 to 1135 cm^{-1} field is characteristic of ether groups in the case of steroids. The brief preliminary study did not allow the location and determination of the number of ether groups. The presence of a single band at 3615 cm^{-1} indicates the existence of a hydroxyl group bound to a steroid nucleus. Figure 11.7 shows the spectrum of nuclear paramagnetic resonance of thymosterin; the presence of the cyclopentanophenanthrene ring is confirmed. The substance analyzed demonstrated a remarkable antiproliferative activity, as discussed below.

In view of the chemical structure of factor S, we proposed to designate it "thymosterin."

11.5 Antiproliferative activity of thymus lipid fractions

The KB line of tumor cells originally derived from a carcinoma of the human buccal epithelium was employed. The cells, in a 1×10^3 or 10^4/ml concentration, were suspended in Hanks' medium with lactalbumin hydrolysate supplemented with 2.5% calf serum and 2.5% N-16 medium. The cell suspension was distributed into tubes containing coverslips, 1.5 ml being placed in each tube. The substance under investigation was dissolved in 0.05 ml of acetone and added to the nutritive medium at the beginning at concentrations of 0.3, 0.2, 0.1, and 0.05 mg per tube.

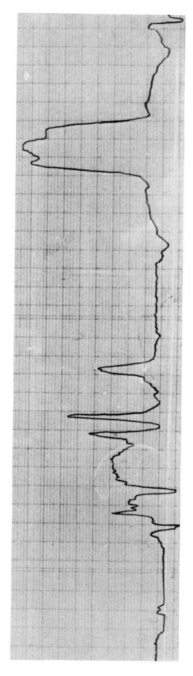

Fig. 11.6. Infrared spectrum analysis of factor S. 10 K Zeiss Jena infrared apparatus in the 4000 cm^{-1} to 400 cm^{-1} region. Presence of a perhydrocyclopentanophenathrene ring. This material was shown to have antiproliferative activity.

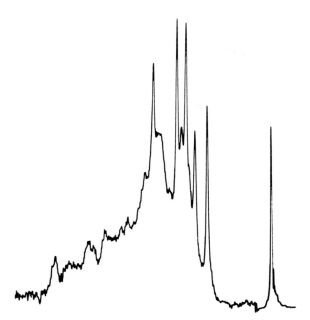

Fig. 11.7. Nuclear paramagnetic resonance spectrum of factor S. A 60 *A* NMR Spectrum, Varian form. Spectrum made in deuterochloroform with interval tetramethylsylan standard. This material had intense antiproliferative activity.

Fifteen tubes were used for each group. The tubes were put in a thermostat at 37°C. After 24 hr of incubation, which is necessary for the adherence of the cells to the glass walls, the culture began to develop. At this time the tubes were put in a roller and rotated at 16 rph, a condition which stimulates the development of the culture.

In the control cultures, the cells covered the surface of the glass as a monolayer in 5 days. The difference in growth between the groups was evaluated by cell counts (Sanford's method), protein content, for which the Folin-Ciocalteau reagent was used (Lowry's method), and the examination of smears stained with Giemsa.

The above method was routinely used since too little of some fractions were obtained for *in vivo* testing. The demonstration of an antiblastic effect *in vitro* constitutes a valuable indication for *in vivo* experiments. Whenever enough extract was available, *in vivo* results in tumor-bearing animals and chick embryos were in harmony with those obtained *in vitro*

with tumor cell cultures. They confirm the presence in the thymus extracts
of an active inhibitory factor of tumor growth.

The antiproliferative activity of the thymic fractions and of factor S
was tested using as parameters the number of cells in the culture, protein
concentration and morphologic pattern of the cultures treated or not
treated with thymus fractions, and control extracts. The first studies on
KB tumor cell cultures showed fraction B to have an inhibitory action
(Milcu *et al.*, 1965).

Testing the antiproliferative activity of thymus fraction II B

By testing the antiproliferative effect of fraction II B on KB tumor cell
cultures (Milcu *et al.*, 1966) (Table 11.3) and thyroid cancer (Table 11.4),
it was shown that the partly purified fraction II B had an antiproliferative
action on KB tumor and thyroid cancer cell cultures (Potop *et al.*, 1971),
manifested by a reduction in the number of cells and a diminution in
protein concentration. It is noteworthy that the antiproliferative effect
is in direct proportion to the dose of extract employed. It was seen that
the control extract II B prepared from skeletal muscle had no inhibitory
action; lower doses of II B (muscle) actually exhibited a slight stimulating
effect. This fact demonstrates that the activity of thymus fraction B does
not lack in specificity.

Morphologically, there was no evidence of cellular and nuclear polymorphism with frequent mitoses in the control cultures (Fig. 11.8a), while
in cultures treated with fraction II B there was evidence of proliferation
inhibition, degenerative lesions, and nuclei with angular or wrinkled
borders (Fig. 11.8b). In the culture treated with extract II B in a two-fold
concentration, there were greater changes (Fig. 11.8c).

After 5 days, the pathologic pattern of thyroid tumor (adenocarcinoma
type) cultures showed that untreated monolayer control cell cultures contained groups of giant cells (Fig. 11.9a). In cultures treated with 0.3 mg of
fraction II B, rarifaction of the cell population, equalization in shape and
size, and absence of cytotoxic lesions (Fig. 11.9b) were seen.

Testing for fraction II B$_3$ activity

Potop and Milcu (1970) showed that administration of fraction II B$_3$
induced a significant decrease in cell counts, coincident with a reduction
in protein concentration (Table 11.5). The reduced cell population and
the decreased protein concentration were in direct proportion to the dose

Table 11.3. Effect of fraction II B (thymus) and II B (muscle) on proliferation of tumor (KB) cell cultures

Dose of B	Proteins[a,b]			No. of cells[b,c]		
	0.5 mg	0.1 mg	0.05 mg	0.5 mg	0.1 mg	0.05 mg
Control		37.5 ± 1.89			734 ± 37.42	
Fraction II B muscle	35.5 ± 4.12 $p > 0.05$ (5%)	37.9 ± 2.66 $p > 0.05$ (0%)	38.3 ± 2.80 $p > 0.05$ (−1%)	678 ± 11.18 $p > 0.05$ (8%)	716 ± 43.39 $p > 0.05$ (2%)	740 ± 29.83 $p > 0.05$ (0%)
Fraction II B thymus	25.8 ± 2.96 $p < 0.05$ (31%)	31.0 ± 1.37 $p < 0.05$ (17%)	34.5 ± 0.70 $p < 0.05$ (8%)	442 ± 24.80 $p < 0.05$ (40%)	452 ± 27.20 $p < 0.05$ (38%)	676 ± 25.50 $p < 0.05$ (8%)

[a] Quantity of protein per 1.5 ml culture. In mg obtained using the figures from table (y) and by the formula:

$$x = (Y - 2)/114.3.$$

[b] Average per group ± S.D. and percentage variation in comparison with controls. The figures also indicate the statistically significant differences as compared with controls.

[c] Average number of cells per tube.

Table 11.4. Effect of fraction II B (thymus) on growth of human thyroid cancer cells *in vitro* (adenocarcinoma)

Fraction II B (mg/1.5 ml)	Protein[a]	p	Varia-tions (%)[b]	No. of cells ×10³	p	Varia-tions (%)
Dose	48.9 ± 45			162.8 ± 2.90		
0.05	33.5 ± 71	<0.001	31	108.0 ± 3.56	<0.001	33
0.1	29.6 ± 0.71	<0.001	39	95.2 ± 7.21	<0.001	42
0.3	23.5 ± 0.59	<0.001	52	71.5 ± 1.18	<0.001	56

[a]Average protein content of each culture.
[b]Percentage change from control.

of fraction II B$_3$ used. It should be emphasized that the results were reproducible. The morphologic examination of Giemsa-stained untreated cultures revealed a high cell density and anisokaryocytochromia (Fig. 11.10a). Large doses of fraction II B$_3$ resulted in an inhibition of proliferation with degenerative lesions in the nuclei, pycnosis, or irregular and serrated contour. At times the cellular pattern showed a disruptive tendency. In the cultures, cell density varied with the amount of thymus fraction used. As a rule, proliferation of the cultures was progressively impaired with increasing concentrations of fraction II B$_3$ (Fig. 11.10b, c, d).

Factors causing variability in the neoplastic activity of thymic extracts

On testing thymus fraction B activity in KB tumor cell cultures, this fraction was found to be dependent upon a variety of factors, such as age of the cattle at the time of removal of the thymus, physiologic and nutritional conditions, and season of the year (Potop *et al.*, 1971).

The results given in Table 11.6 show that the greatest activity was exhibited by the fractions isolated from thymus of calves under 1 year of age, bred under physiologic conditions without growth stimulation, and fed a normal diet. Likewise, the thymus obtained in spring and summer had more activity than that obtained in autumn and winter. It should be stressed that the activity was maintained for a relatively long period when the fractions were stored in the refrigerator away from light and air.

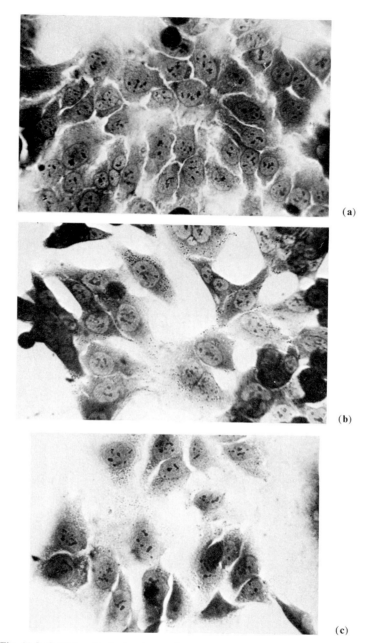

Fig. 11.8 a) Histopathologic picture of untreated KB cell cultures. b) CB cell culture treated with thymic fraction II B in dose of 0.1 mg. c) KB culture treated with thymic fraction II B in dose of 0.2 mg.

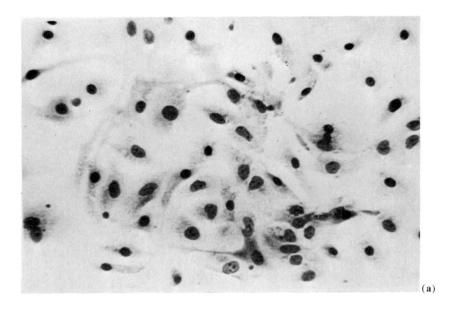

(a)

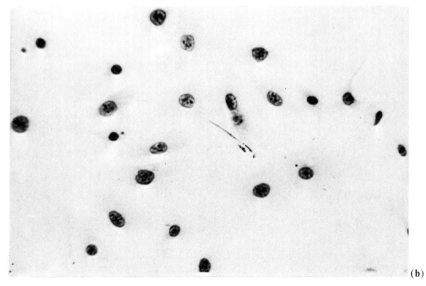

(b)

Fig. 11.9. a) Histopathologic examination of untreated thyroid cancer cultures. b) Histopathologic examination of thyroid cancer cultures treated with thymus fraction B.

Table 11.5. Effect of fraction II B₃ (thymus) on proliferation of tumor (KB) cell cultures

Fraction II B₃ (mg/culture)	Protein[a]	p	No. of cells × 10³	p
Dose	30.76 ± 1.20		215.4 ± 18.41	
0.1	16.66 ± 0.35	<0.001	98.92 ± 9.89	<0.001
0.3	12.11 ± 0.45	<0.001	57.00 ± 3.44	<0.001

[a]See Table 11.3 for determining the protein content of each 1.5-ml culture tube.

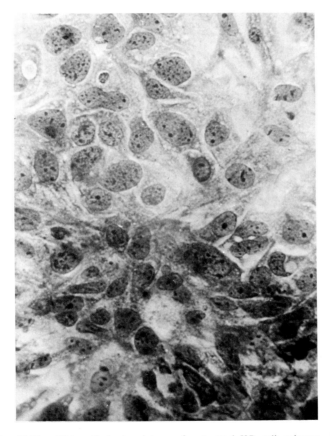

Fig. 11.10a. Histopathologic picture of untreated KB cell cultures. A marked density is seen in the cell population and the process of an isokaryocytochromia (Giemsa, ×400).

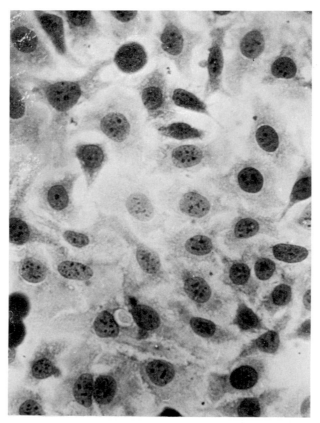

Fig. 11.10b. Histopathologic examination of KB cultures treated with 0.05 mg 11 B₃. Slightly reduced anisokaryocytochromia, tendency towards a decreased cell density (Giemsa, ×400).

Morphologic variations of the thymus in terms of age are reported in the literature. Cesarini, Benkoel, and Bonneau (1969) demonstrated the ultrastructure of the thymus in young and adult hamsters. Some of the features found in the young hamster were no longer present in the adult. The lymphocyte activity likewise disappeared in the aged thymus.

Antiproliferative action of a thymic extract B prepared from human thymus

The results of recent preliminary experiments (Potop *et al.*, 1971) demonstrated that the total lipid extract (TL) prepared from alcad obstetrical trauma infant thymus exhibited an antiproliferative activity when tested

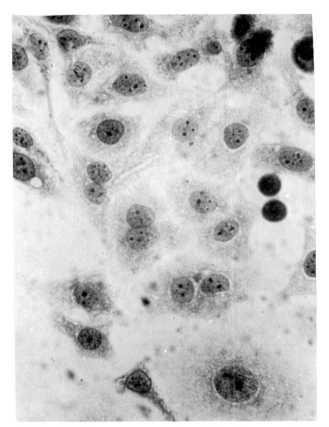

Fig. 11.10c. Histopathologic examination of KB cultures treated with 0.1 mg II B₁.
Decreased anisokaryocytochromia. Presence of nuclear twinning. Slightly increased cell
density. Some nuclei are pyenotic and tachychromatic (Giemsa, ×400).

on KB tumor cell cultures. The first results suggested that the activity of
the total lipid extract, while still in the impurified crude form, was
greater than that of thymic protein extract TP (Table 11.7).

11.6 Antiproliferative activity of thymosterin

The antiproliferative activity of thymosterin (factor S) was greater
than that of the other thymus extracts (B, II B, and II B₃) when tested
in KB tumor cell cultures. The inhibitory action on tumor growth was
expressed in the cultures by a parallel and gradual reduction in both cell

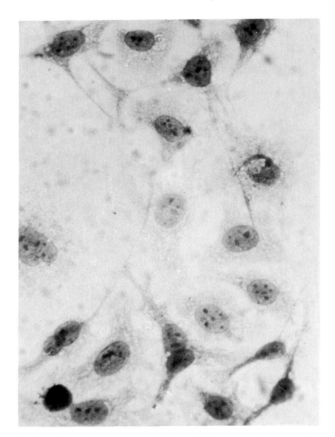

Fig. 11.10d. Histopathologic examination of KB cultures treated with 0.5 mg II B₁. Degenerative lesions are found. Karyocytoplasmatic vacuolization and nuclear pycnosis. Marked decrease in cell density (Giemsa, ×400).

Table 11.6a. Influence of thymus fraction B prepared from young cattle (under 1 yr of age) in physiologic and usual nutritional conditions on KB cell culture proliferation *in vitro*

Group	Fraction B (mg/tube)	No. of cells × 10⁴	p	Varia-tions (%)	Protein[a]	p	Varia-tions (%)
1	Dose	170.6 ± 7.17			40.42 ± 1.12		
2	0.05	118.8 ± 4.85	<0.001	−31	32.80 ± 1.14	<0.001	−19
3	0.2	98.5 ± 2.55	<0.001	−43	28.24 ± 1.16	<0.001	−32

[a]See Table 11.3.

Table 11.6b. Influence of thymus fraction B prepared from young cattle with stimulated growth on KB cell culture proliferation *in vitro*

Group	Fraction B (mg/tube)	No. of cells × 10⁴	p	Varia-tions (%)	Protein[a]	p	Varia-tions (%)
1	Dose	232.0 ± 7.00			43.26 ± 0.45		
2	0.05	192.2 ± 6.19	<0.001	−17	37.14 ± 0.55	<0.001	−14
3	0.2	177.6 ± 4.99	<0.001	−23	35.34 ± 0.59	<0.001	−19

[a]See Table 11.3.

Table 11.6c. Influence of thymus fraction B prepared from aged cattle (more than 3 years old) on KB cell culture proliferation *in vitro*

Group	Fraction B (mg/tube)	No. of cells × 10⁴	p	Variations (%)
1	Dose	232.0 ± 7		
2	0.05	236.8 ± 5.75	>0.32	+1
3	0.2	224.6 ± 7.32	>0.32	−3

population and protein concentration (Table 11.8). The antiproliferative activity of thymic extracts on tumor cell cultures was impressive (Potop and Milcu, 1970). The activity of thymic fractions increased with the degree of purification (Fig. 11.11). A direct dose-response relationship was found with thymosterin (Fig. 11.12). It is noteworthy that the antiproliferative effect of various thymus preparations was reproducible.

The antiproliferative effect of thymus extracts did not lack in specificity. This was shown when compared with control preparations from muscle in similar conditions (Fig. 11.13).

Table 11.7. Action of some thymic extracts prepared from newborn child thymus on proliferation of KB cell cultures

Group	Material (mg)	No. of cells × 10³	p	Variations (%)	Protein[a]	p	Variations (%)
1. Control		170.6 ± 7.17			40.42 ± 1.12		
2. TL	0.05	134.0 ± 8.19	<0.003	21	32.72 ± 0.67	<0.001	19
3. TL	0.2	118.0 ± 7.60	<0.001	31	30.60 ± 0.87	<0.001	24
4. TP	0.05	154.4 ± 6.78	<0.05	10	38.58 ± 1.00	>0.13	5
5. TP	0.2	146.0 ± 5.57	<0.01	14	37.06 ± 0.89	<0.05	8

[a]See Table 11.3.

Table 11.8. Influence of the thymus factor S on proliferation *in vitro* of a culture of KB tumor cells[a]. Three experiments.

Dose	No. of cells $\pm$ E.S. (average per tube $\times 10^4$)	p	Varia-tions (%)	Protein[a] (average/ tube)	p	Varia-tions (%)
Control	109.6 $\pm$ 3.74			32.56 $\pm$ 0.92		
0.2 mg	24.0 $\pm$ 3.60	<0.003	77	11.14 $\pm$ 0.32	<0.001	66
0.1 mg	28.0 $\pm$ 2.75	<0.001	75	12.34 $\pm$ 0.32	<0.001	62
0.05 mg	41.0 $\pm$ 2.79	<0.003	63	20.60 $\pm$ 0.32	<0.001	36
Control	18.8 $\pm$ 0.371					
0.2 mg	6.2 $\pm$ 0.499	<0.001	67			
0.05 mg	14.4 $\pm$ 0.575	<0.05	23			
Control	135.0 $\pm$ 1.01					
0.02 mg	26.8 $\pm$ 0.42	<0.001	80			
0.05 mg	56.1 $\pm$ 1.11	<0.001	58			

[a]See Table 11.3 for explanation of parameters.

These findings demonstrated the presence of an antiblastic factor with a pharmacodynamic hormone-like action in the thymus (Milcu and Potop, 1971).

11.7 Biochemical testing of thymus fraction B activity

The amount of fraction B obtained was sufficient for *in vivo* testing in metabolic pathways. Activity was tested on the basis of changes induced in glucose-6-phosphatase activity and lactic acid levels in rat liver (Potop, Juvina, and Mreana, 1970).

The experimental data showed a particularly high lability of some enzymatic activities under the influence of thymus extracts of lipid nature. Fraction B induced a rise in glucose-6-phosphatase activity which paralleled a decrease in liver lactic acid. A direct relationship was found between the dose of extract B and the effect produced in both glucose-6-phosphatase and lactic acid (Fig. 11.14). Administration of fraction B in short-term experiments (24 hr) produced the most significant modifications of these parameters 12 hr following administration; these returned to normal values within 24 hr (Figs. 11.15 and 11.16).

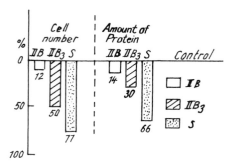

Fig. 11.11. Effect of degree of purification of thymus fractions on inhibition of cell (KB) proliferation and total protein content *in vitro*.

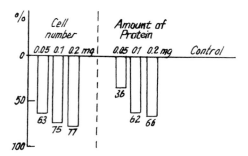

Fig. 11.12. Antiproliferative effect on KB tumor cell cultures of pure thymic factor S, thymosterin, in terms of the dose administered.

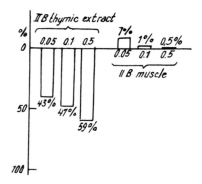

Fig. 11.13. Inhibitory effect of thymus fraction II B on proliferation of KB tumor cell cultures *in vitro* as compared with that of a control fraction II B prepared from skeletal muscle.

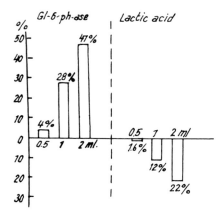

Fig. 11.14. Administration to male mice (weight about 30 g) of progressive doses of thymic extract B: 0.5 ml, 1 ml, and 2 ml per animal. Determination of glucose-6-phosphatase activity and of lactic acid 12 hr after thymic extract administration. Concentration of the extract administered: 1 g fraction B/30 ml corn oil. Percent variations of glucose-6-phosphatase and of lactic acid in the rat liver, compared to administered B extract doses.

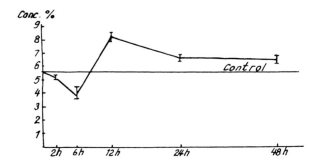

Fig. 11.15. Kinetics of change in glucose-6-phosphatase activity in the liver of mice treated with 2 ml of fraction B (in mg P released/g of tissue/15 min). Dose injected, 2 ml containing 0.066 g thymic extract B.

Our findings demonstrate the involvement of the thymus in glucose-6-phosphatase activity and in hepatic lactic acid concentrations. Hence, these parameters may be useful for testing of fraction B. It is interesting that in previous experiments we had established that thymus fraction B has no toxic effect when given in progressive doses (0.15 to 2 ml/100 g) along a protracted time interval (30 to 45 days).

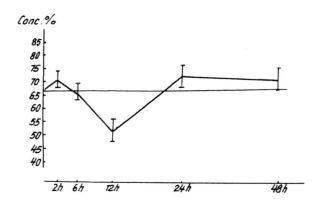

Fig. 11.16. Kinetics of change in concentration of lactic acid in mouse liver following injection of 2 ml thymus fraction B (mg of lactic acid/100 g tissue).

11.8 Antineoplastic action of thymus lipid extracts in vivo

The antineoplastic effect of the thymus and thymic extracts was reported in the first half of the present century by Hanson (cited by Davies, 1969a), Ficchera (1933), and others. In the past decade, research on the thymus was extended especially into the field of immunity and oncology. The research centered on establishing the role of the thymus or the immune response of the body in the neoplastic process. Recent work has demonstrated the role of the thymus in the regulation of the immune response and in tumor graft rejection. According to Miller, Marshall, and White (1962), the thymus may be involved in immunologic homeostasis which would permit the body to monitor cell integrity to eliminate the cancerous, that is, foreign, lines before they expand. This hypothesis has not been invalidated by other authors.

Accordingly, evidence obtained by current investigations will be reviewed to indicate that the association between immune incompetence and tumor growth is a common event.

Both thymectomy in newborn and irradiation of adult animals cause lymphopenia, immune deficiency, and growth of various types of tumors (Miller, 1967; Osoba, 1968). A greater incidence of 3–4,benzopyrene-induced tumors was found in the thymectomized animals *versus* sham-thymectomized controls (MacDonald, 1963), as well as a shortening of the latency period and an elevated incidence of polyoma virus tumors (Law, 1965; Miller, Ting, and Law, 1964; Allison and Taylor, 1967; Taylor, 1963).

The immunologic function of the thymus was restored by implantation of neonatal thymus grafts or by diffusion in a Millipore chamber (Osoba, 1965a) in both neonatally thymectomized mice and adult rats with low immunologic potential brought about by neonatal thymectomy or irradiation (Leuchars, Cross, and Dukov, 1965; Nettensheim, Williams, and Hammons, 1969). It was shown that leukopenia induced by total body irradiation in neonatally thymectomized rats may be alleviated by administration of thymus protein extracts (Trainin and Linker-Israeli, 1967). The transplanted thymus cells had a synergistic action with those of the bone marrow in producing immune competence in the X-irradiated animals.

In 1935, Parhon and Milcu (unpublished) suggested the idea of the inhibitory action of the thymus in neoplastic processes which was subsequently confirmed by our own findings and by those from data in the literature. The comparative study of thymus polypeptide and lipid fractions on tumor growth (Potop, Juvina et al., 1961) proved the antineoplastic action of the total lipid thymus extract to be more significant. This statement was based on the study of tumor incidence, development of tumors, pathologic appearance of the tumor, and nucleic acid levels in liver and tumor tissues.

Later we investigated the action of thymus fraction B, II B, and III B in rats, mice, and chick embryos in vivo. The antineoplastic action was studied on various types of tumors induced by chemical carcinogens (methylcholanthrene and diazobenzene) (Potop et al., 1960; Potop, Biener, and Lupulescu, 1960; Potop, Biener et al., 1961), by Guerin tumor grafts (Potop et al., 1961; Potop et al., 1969), Walker tumor (Potop et al., 1969; Potop, 1966a; Potop and Juvina, 1966), Jensen and Crocker 180 tumor (Potop, Mreana, and Juvina, 1969), Ehrlich tumor (Potop et al., 1966; Potop, 1966b; Potop et al., 1967) and experimental leukemia (Potop et al., 1967). We also extended our studies to the influence of fraction B on X-irradiated rats.

The antineoplastic action of thymus extracts was tested in tumor tissue and in the tumor-bearing organism. Some experiments were made to elucidate the action of thymus extracts in young, thymectomized tumor-bearing rats (Potop et al., 1969). The effect of thymus extracts on biologic parameters and metabolic pattern was studied. The major results in our experiments formed the object of a comprehensive report (Milcu and Potop, 1970).

Examples of the antineoplastic effect of thymus fractions B and II B *in vivo* are presented. The antineoplastic action studied in biologic parameters demonstrated a reduced tumor incidence (Fig. 11.17), weight (Fig. 11.18), and growth dynamics (Fig. 11.19, 11.20 and 11.21), and lengthening of the survival rate (Fig. 11.22). Morphologically, there was a decreased degree of malignancy in tumor structure which demonstrated the protective action in the neoplastic process. Significantly, fraction B from spleen gave no protective action (Fig. 11.21), while fraction B from thymus was inhibitory. Upon pathologic examination of a methylcholanthrene-induced tumor (Fig. 11.23a), a fusocellular sarcoma was found. Its structure was composed of atypical polygonal cell cords invading the adjacent tissue. The cytoplasm was intensely basophilic, and the nucleus was polymorphous. Multipolar atypical mitoses were frequent. Monstrous giant nuclei were also present. In animals given fraction B (Fig. 11.23b), there was a dislocation and separation of the tumor structure by large zones of necrosis and fibrosis. The cell cords, no longer compact with tumor cells, were disposed in clusters surrounded by hemorrhagic areas. Cell atypia was reduced, and there were frequent mitonecroses. Collagen fibroses were often seen about the tumor cords. Throughout the tumor there was a dislocation of the tissue, which became loose and

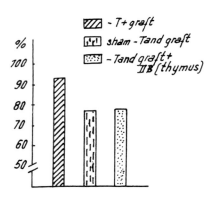

Fig. 11.17. Influence of the thymus fraction II B on the incidence of Walker carcinosarcoma in thymectomized rats. − T, thymectomized; − T + graft, thymectomized and grafted; Sham − T + graft, sham thymectomy + graft; − T and graft + II B (thymus).

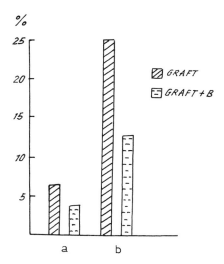

Fig. 11.18. Weight variations in the rats bearing Ehrlich ascites tumor following treatment with thymus fraction B: a, weight gain 10 days after inoculation; b, weight gain 20 days after inoculation.

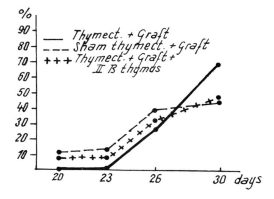

Fig. 11.19. Dynamics of the tumor development of a Walker carcinosarcoma in thymectomized rats treated by fraction II B.

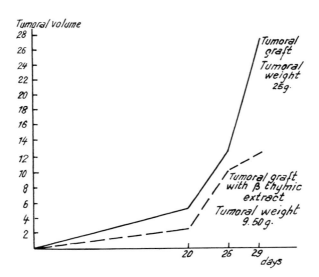

Fig. 11.20. Dynamics of tumor development and variations of tumor weight in rats with Guerin implant, after administration of thymic fraction B.

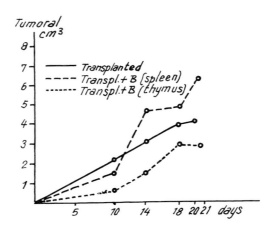

Fig. 11.21. Dynamics of development of a Crocker 180 sarcoma in mice treated with thymus fraction B, as compared with a control fraction B prepared from the spleen.

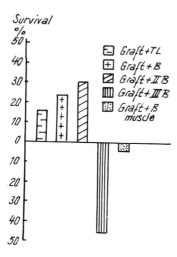

Fig. 11.22. Percent variations of the mean of survival time in mice with Ehrlich transplant, treated with control and thymic fractions.

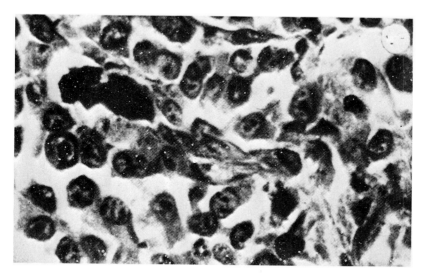

Fig. 11.23a. Fusocellular sarcoma (methylcholanthrene), untreated. Frequent antypical mitoses, giant nuclei.

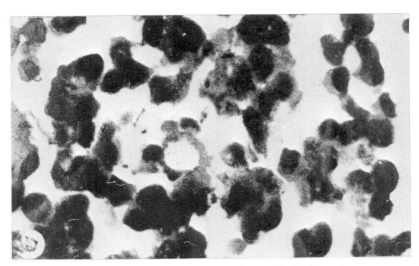

Fig. 11.23b. Sarcoma treated with thymic fraction B. Dislocated structure, separated by large areas of necrosis and fibrosis. The cellular and nuclear atypic forms reduced.

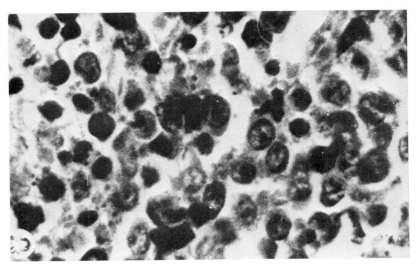

Fig. 11.23c. Sarcoma treated with control fraction B prepared from the spleen. No change in the structure of the tumor is noted.

presented no solid structure as ordinarily found in untreated tumors. Accordingly, from the pathologic standpoint, there was a marked inhibition of methylcholanthrene-induced sarcoma by fraction B administration. Administration of a control extract B derived from the spleen failed to yield similar inhibitory changes (Fig. 11.23c).

The effect of fraction B in Guerin tumor-bearing rats was illustrated by a decreased tumor cell incidence and volume (Fig. 11.24a, b) and by alterations in its structure. In animals given fraction B, an advanced process of necrosis characterized by alteration of the cytoplasm and cell nuclei was seen. The process was conspicuous both at the periphery and in the center of the tumor. In control animals, a proliferation of tumor cells predominantly around the neovessels and polyedrical cells with large nuclei disposed in a circular array around the tributary vessel were noted.

The morphology of the liver after administration of fraction B in DAB-treated rats fed a carcinogenic diet demonstrated a moderate inhibition of hepatoma growth (Potop, Biener, *et al.* 1960; Potop, Biener *et al*, 1961). A number of successive investigations centered on the study of various isolated lipid thymus fractions on the growth of Ehrlich ascites carcinoma in mice were attempted (Potop *et al.*, 1966; Potop, 1966a, b; Potop *et al.*, 1967). It was shown primarily that the survival rate of inoculated mice was lower in untreated *versus* TL, B, and II B-treated mice (Table 11.9). Interestingly enough, the action of III B was expressed by a decrease in the mean survival time and increase in tumor incidence and death rate. This indicated the stimulating action of that fraction on Ehrlich ascites carcinoma growth. Particularly striking results were obtained with a highly active Jensen tumor, resistant to other treatments, in Sprague rats selected and checked since birth (unpublished). On reaching the weight of approximately 40 g, the animals were treated with fraction B for 48 days. After grafting the tumor, they were further treated for another 32 days. Originally, all the animals, either treated or not, developed tumors within 5 days. The size of the tumor started to decrease gradually until complete disappearance in treated animals; in untreated animals, the weight of the tumor ranged from 52 to 105 g (Fig. 11.25a, b, c). Mortality in untreated animals was 100%, while in animals treated with fraction B there was 100% survival.

Pathologic examination showed the untreated tumor to be a sarcoma of predominantly polymorphous appearance, with rare fusocellular areas. The cellular elements were unequal in size and showed marked anisokaryochromia. Relatively frequent mitoses and numerous vascular lacunae were present. Sarcoma proliferation of variable

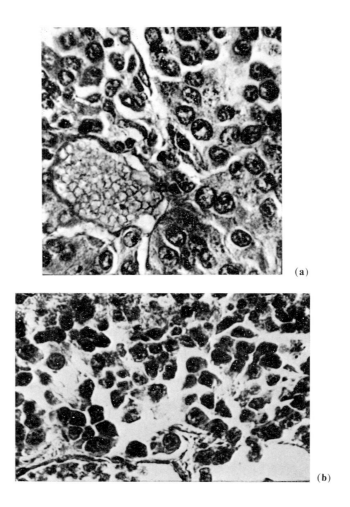

(a)

(b)

Fig. 11.24. a) Histopathologic picture of Guerin tumor graft in nontreated rats. Marked proliferation of tumor cells. b) Histopathologic picture of Guerin tumor graft in rats treated with thymus fraction B. Advanced necrotic process alteration of the cytoplasma and of the nuclei of perivascular cells.

Table 11.9. The mean survival rate in Ehrlich ascites tumor-bearing animals following administration of thymus extracts TL, B, II B, and III B[a]

Parameter	Inoculated	Inoculated + TL	Inoculated + B (thymus)	Inoculated + B (muscle)	Inoculated + II B	Inoculated + III B
Survival days[b]	14.5 ± 0.30 (60 animals)	17 ± 0.97 (20 animals)	18 ± 0.3 (60 animals)	13.8 ± 1.2 (20 animals)	19 ± 0.5 (30 animals)	9 ± 0.45 (15 animals)
Tumor incidence after 10 days	100%	80%	74%	100%	70%	100%
Death rate after 10 days	59%	43%	28%	42%	10%	100%

[a]After implantation, 0.2 ml of extract was injected every other day. During 10 days, each mouse received 33 mg of extract in 0.1 ml corn oil.
[b]The survival mean was calculated starting from the time when the animals started dying until their death in proportion of 50%, according to the method of Strack *et al.* (1961).

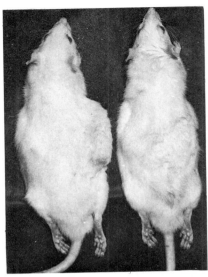

Fig. 11.25a. Development of Jensen sarcoma in control rats treated with oil (*left*), as compared with that in rats given thymic fraction B (*right*) 5 days after transplantation.

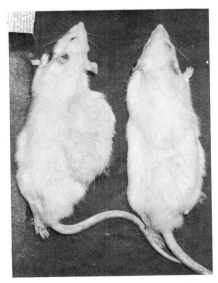

Fig. 11.25b. Development of Jensen sarcoma in control rats treated with oil (*left*), as compared with that in rats given thymus fraction B (*right*) 32 days after transplant.

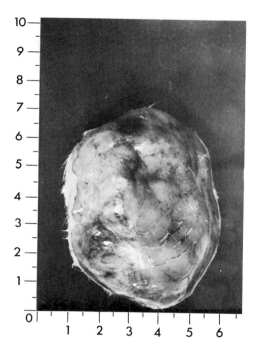

Fig. 11.25c. Size of Jensen sarcoma in control rats nontreated with thymus fraction B. Weight of the tumor, 52 g.

degrees and areas of great cell density were also found with cells separated by loose stroma. Also areas of necrobiosis may be observed (Fig. 11.26a). In the small remnant fragment of the fraction B-treated tumor, the neoplastic tissue is replaced by a tissue exhibiting lympho-polyblastic elements and numerous cells with a vacuolized cytoplasm (Fig. 11.26b).

These results are in harmony with the work of Perri *et al.* (1963). These authors obtained a greater development of the Jensen sarcoma in thymectomized animals when compared with intact controls, due to a decline in immunologic reactions.

The results obtained in young thymectomized rats in which Walker carcinosarcoma had been grafted and were subsequently treated with

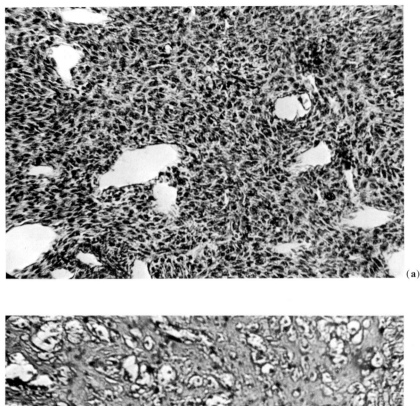

(a)

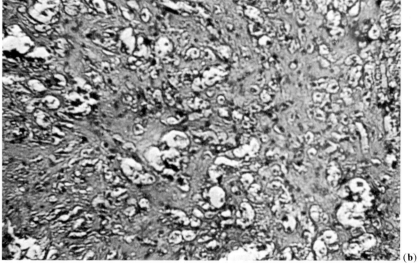

(b)

Fig. 11.26. a) Histopathologic examination of the Jensen sarcoma, Predominantly polymorphous appearance with rare zones of fusocellular aspect. b) Examination of the remnant fragment of the Jensen sarcoma in rats treated with thymus fraction B. Tumor elements are no longer present.

fraction II B (Potop *et al.*, 1969) revealed a higher tumor incidence in thymectomized and grafted rats than either sham-thymectomized and grafted rats or rats grafted and given thymus fraction II B. Thymectomy resulted in a concurrent increase of tumor volume. The results obtained emphasize the stimulating action of thymectomy on Walker carcinosarcoma growth and its inhibition by fraction II B administration.

It was found that administration of thymus fraction B and II B did not inhibit the development of leukemic ascites in mice (Potop *et al.*, 1967). It was also noted that following fraction II B administration there was some reduction in the amount of ascites fluid in treated animals and at the same time a slight decrease in the survival rate (Table 11.10). Treatment with thymus fraction II B did not modify the RNA content in ascites cells, but induced a rise in their DNA content. The data obtained confirm those found in the literature. It is a familiar fact that thymectomy decreases the incidence of lymphoid leukemia in rats injected with Gross and Molony viruses (Gross, 1959); in AK mice which develop a spontaneous lymphoid leukemia, Cazal (1969) reported that thymectomy reduces the incidence of this condition.

Our biologic research demonstrated that administration of thymus fractions caused a reduction in tumor incidence and a lengthening of the latency period, a reduction in weight and in dynamics of tumor mass growth, and a lower malignancy in the structure of the tumor; these facts all point to the protective role of the thymus in the neoplastic process. The results obtained have shown a variety of facets proving the part played by the thymus in immunologic reactions associated with the neoplastic process. Thus, it was also established that neonatal thymectomy in mice shortens the latency and increases the incidence of polyoma virus tumors (Allison and Taylor, 1967; Law, 1965; Potop, 1970). The role of the thymus in viral carcinogensis was demonstrated by the fact that rats thymectomized at birth and inoculated at various ages are more prone to develop tumors due to the impaired immunologic response (Monnerot-Dumaine, 1965). Grant and Miller (1962) and Miller *et al.* (1963) showed latency to be shorter and the incidence of skin tumors and 3,4-benzopyrene-induced fibrosarcomata to be higher in neonatally thymectomized rats. Maisin (1963: 1964) reported on the role of the thymus in immune defense based on his experiments with thymus grafts. In grafted animals, the incidence and expansion of 20-methylcholanthrene-induced tumors was reduced.

Actually, there is relatively little conflicting evidence. Yashuhira (1969) considers that the immune mechanism affects carcinoma induc-

Table 11.10. Influence of thymus fraction B on some physiologic parameters and on biochemical parameters in RAP mice with leukemic ascites

Groups	No. of animals	Positive graft (%)	Difference in body wt. (%)	Ascites volume	No. of cells	Mean survival rate	RNA (mg P/100 mg cells)	DNA (mg P/100 mg cells)
Inoculated leukemic controls	44	75	+20.4	5.16	54,166	7	120 ± 5.20	8 ± 0.60
Inoculated animals treated with II B (thymus, 12 injections)	20	37.5	−14	2.00	1,400,000	3.6		
Inoculated animals treated with II B (muscle)	20	22.2	−20	2.40	1,200,000	7.0		
Inoculated animals treated with B (thymus)	44	72	+2.6	5.90	425,300	7.0	120 ± 7.60 $p > 0.05$	13 ± 0.50 $p < 0.05$
Inoculated animals treated with B (muscle)	44	69.6	−0.5	7.16	410,530	6.4	110 ± 6.06 $p > 0.05$	11.8 ± 0.70 $p < 0.05$
Inoculated animals treated with oil	20	43	−6.	10.00	1,380,000	6.8		

tion only and not that of papilloma. Balner and Dersjant (1966) failed to demonstrate any significant effect of thymectomy on latency, induction, and incidence of methylcholanthrene-induced neoplasms, and we found no antitumor effect of cholesterol in methylcholanthrene-injected rats.

11.9 Metabolic changes in experimental cancer caused by thymic lipid fractions

The host's metabolic pattern in carcinogenesis furnishes a valuable indication of the origin of the tumor process on the basis of correlations with metabolic exchanges. The experimental data indicated that metabolic changes lay at the base of the process of becoming malignant by modifying the properties of the tissue. The cancer cell constitutes a clear evidence of metabolic alterations. Recognition of metabolic peculiarities will contribute to the elucidation of the problem of neoplastic development. The biochemical study of tumors and of the tumor-bearing organism forms the object of a large number of works in world literature, yet works devoted to the role of the thymus in cancer metabolism are virtually nonexistent.

Concurrently with biologic alterations, the thymic extracts induce metabolic modifications in the tumor tissue and in the recipient animal, establishing biochemical tumor/host correlations. The thymus tends to restore the abnormal metabolism of the host to normal metabolism.

In the neoplastic tissue at the hepatic level, thymic fractions reduce the synthesis and metabolism of nucleic acids, which are essential for tumor growth (Potop, Biener et al., 1960; Potop et al., 1969; Potop, Juvina, and Mreana, 1963) (Tables 11.11 and 11.12). The modifications in nucleic acids are less significant after treatment with fraction B when compared with polypeptide fraction TP treatment, according to the results obtained in our experiments.

The electrophoretic investigations made on serum protein fractions in Guerin tumor-bearing rats treated with fraction B revealed significant modifications (Table 11.13) when compared with the untreated controls.

A change noted in the presence of tumors was an enhanced glycolysis and a decreased O_2 consumption in the recipient animal. The thymic fraction B induces a decrease in glycolysis, a rise in glycogen levels, and a fall in lactic acid concentration simultaneously with an increase in enzymatic activities which are significantly lower in untreated tumor-

Table 11.11. Concentration in RNA and DNA in the liver of three rats bearing Guerin tumors, treated with fraction B

Group	RNA	Modif. (%)	p	DNA[a]	Modif. (%)	p
Normal control	729 ± 22.56			199 ± 1.26		
Transplanted and treated with corn oil	1022 ± 69.50	40.1/N	<0.001	254 ± 12.76	27.60/N	<0.001
Transplanted and treated with extract B	868 ± 27.34	15.05/Tr.	$\simeq 0.05$	235 ± 7.07	7.48/Tr.	>0.13

[a]mg/100 g fresh tissue.

Table 11.12. Incorporation of ^{32}P into RNA and DNA in the liver of mice bearing Ehrlich ascites carcinoma, treated with thymic fraction B[a]

Group	No.	^{32}P into RNA	p	^{32}P into DNA	p	^{32}P into total nucleic acids	p
Control grafted	20	29.3 ± 2.1	–	18 ± 1.3	–	47.3 ± 1.5	–
Grafted, treated with B (thymus)	30	30.0 ± 1.6	unsig.[b]	11.6 ± 1	sig.[c]	41.6 ± 1.6	sig.
Grafted, treated with B (muscle)	15	30.2 ± 2.4	unsig.	21.4 ± 1.6	unsig.	52.0 ± 2	unsig.

[a]Counts per gram per second.
[b]$R_1 - R_2 < 2_r$; unsignificant.
[c]$R_1 - R_2 > 2_r$; significant.

Table 11.13. Electrophoresis of serum proteins of Guerin carcinoma-bearing rats treated with fraction B (relative values %)

Group	Albumins	Globulins α_1	α_2	β	γ	Albumin /globulin
Normal control	46.45	12.23	5.94	24.90	19.69	2.35
Grafted and treated with corn oil	15.66	19.29	17.13	31.94	15.68	0.99
Grafted and treated with B in corn oil	26.90	23.03	14.37	28.38	18.57	1.44

bearing animals than in experimental animals. (Figs. 11.27–11.31, Table 11.14). The modifications of enzymatic activity in mouse and rat tumors parallel the antitumor action of thymic fractions. This suggests that these alterations at the hepatic level can be regarded as a biochemical index of the evolution of the neoplastic process.

The study of some enzymatic activities in KB tumor cell cultures *in vitro* demonstrated a decay in the activity of β-glucuronidase, glucose-6-phosphate dehydrogenase, and malate dehydrogenase by treatment with thymus fraction II B_3 when compared with controls (Figs. 11.32–37). Galactosidase activity undergoes no changes under the influence of fraction II B_3. The decreased enzymatic activity in KB tumor cell cultures treated with thymus could be related to the inhibition of proliferation

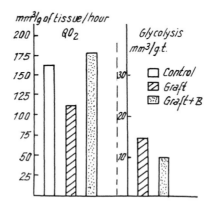

Fig. 11.27. QO$_2$ and glycolisis variations in the liver of rats bearing a methylcholanthrene-induced tumor and treated with thymic fraction B.

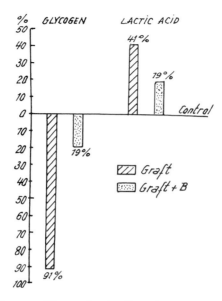

Fig. 11.28 Influence of thymus fraction B on glycogen and lactic acid levels in the liver of rats with methylcholanthrene-induced tumor.

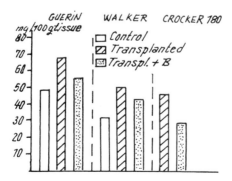

Fig. 11.29. Variations of lactic acid levels in the liver of rats bearing various types of tumor (Guerin carcinoma, Walker carcinosarcoma, Crocker 180 carcinoma) after treatment with thymus fraction B.

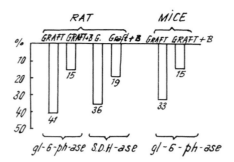

Fig. 11.30. Influence of thymus fraction B on glucose-6-phosphatase and succinic dehydrogenase in rats with Guerin carcinoma and in mice with Ehrlich ascitic carcinoma.

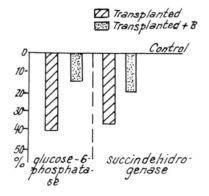

Fig. 11.31. Percentage variations of glucose-6-phosphatase and succinic dehydrogenase activity in rats bearing Guerin tumors treated with thymus fraction B.

Table 11.14. Changes in glucose-6-phosphatase and fructose-1,6-diphosphatase activity in Ehrlich ascites carcinoma-bearing rats treated with thymic fraction B

Groups	Glucose-6-phosphatase (mg of P released/g/ 20 min)	p	Fructose-1,6-diphosphatase (mg of P released/ g/tissue/20 min)	p
Normal control	7.32 ± 0.31		3.80 ± 0.047	
Implanted	5.84 ± 0.20	< 0.05	2.52 ± 0.16	< 0.05
Implanted + B (thymus)	6.80 ± 0.23/impl.	< 0.05	3.70 ± 0.10/impl.	> 0.05

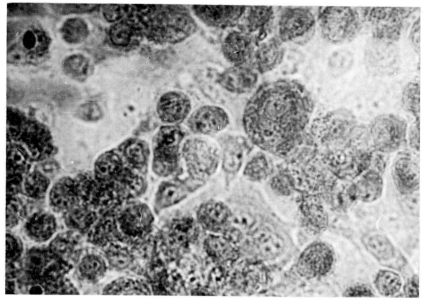

Fig. 11.32. Control KB cell culture, glucose-6-phosphate dehydrogenase activity visualized by rather abundant granules ($\times$ 200).

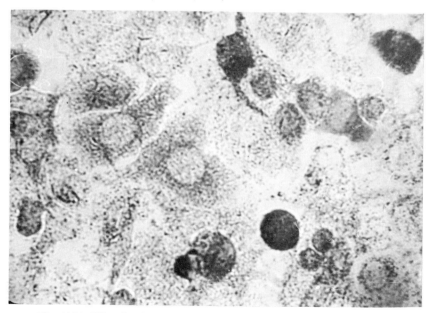

Fig. 11.33. KB cell culture treated with 0.1 mg fraction II B$_3$. Glucose-6-phosphate dehydrogenase generally diminished. In some isolated cells, activity of this enzyme persists, as may be seen from confluent granules ($\times$ 200).

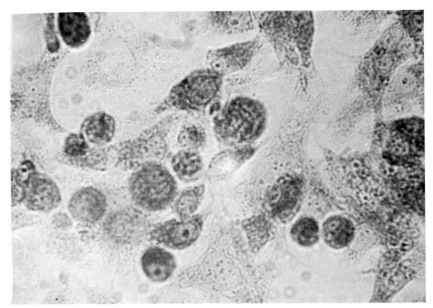

Fig. 11.34. KB cell culture treated with 0.1 mg of fraction II B$_3$. β-glucuronidase activity visualized by black granules in cytoplasma ($\times$ 200).

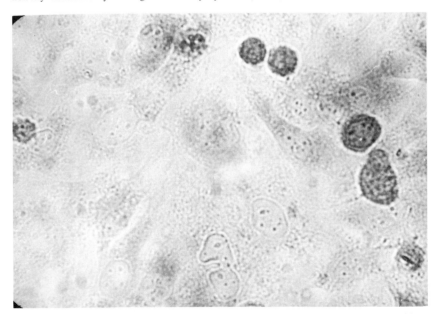

Fig. 11.35. KB cell culture treated with 0.5 mg of fraction II B$_3$. β-glucuronidase activity generally diminishes as compared to previous dose ($\times$ 200).

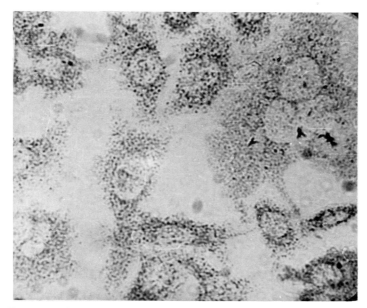

Fig. 11.36. Control KB cell culture. Malic dehydrogenase activity visible in cytoplasm as scattered black granules ($\times$ 2200).

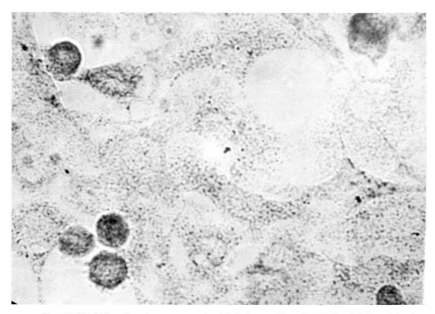

Fig. 11.37. KB cell cultures treated with 0.5 mg of fraction II B$_3$. Malate dehydrogenase activity diminished ($\times$ 200).

caused by thymus extracts. In this sense, Cristofalo, Kabakjian, and Kritchevsloy (1967) found a two-fold increase of lactic dehydrogenase activity in the tumors as compared with normal cultures.

The difference in enzymatic activity can be ascribed to the degree of proliferation of the malignant cells. It is interesting that the decrease in enzymatic activity demonstrated in our laboratory is related to the enzymes pertaining to the Krebs cycle, the hexosephosphate shunt, and the group of lysosomal enzymes. The decrease in lysosomal enzymes might be interpreted as a consequence of the stabilization of lysosomes exerted by the thymic extracts.

In general, we should emphasize the high sensitivity of some enzymatic activities brought about by the administration of thymus fraction B series (B, II B, and II B_3) both *in vivo* and *in vitro*.

11.10 Metabolic changes in intact and thymectomized animals

The results of experiments in which thymus extract TL and B were administered in certain species of animals demonstrated the metabolic action of these compounds. There were no significant weight variations in either rats or chick embryos following fraction B administration (Fig. 11.38). The water content of the thymus following fraction B administration exhibited significant elevations (Potop, Boeru et al., 1970) (Fig. 11.39).

Fraction B significantly increases Ca and P fixation at the level of the tibia in the treated chick embryos (Table 11.15) when compared with controls (Potop et al., 1962). Extract TL increases Ca concentration and decreases P_i concentration in the serum of thymectomized rabbits (Potop, Boeru et al., 1966) in which a drop in Ca and a rise in serum P_i were noted

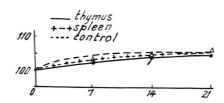

Fig. 11.38. Weight curve related to the initial overall mean weight in hybrid albino mice treated with thymic fraction B, as compared with those given a control fraction prepared from spleen.

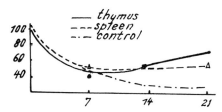

Fig. 11.39. Relative values of the water content of thymus tissue in hybrid albino mice treated with thymic fraction B, as compared with a control fraction B derived from spleen.

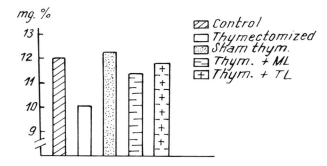

Fig. 11.40. Calcium concentration in serum of thymectomized rabbits before and after injection of thymus extract TL and control extract ML.

Table 11.15. P and Ca concentration in the bone (tibia) of chick embryo (Rhode Island) treated with thymic extract TL and thymic fraction B

Thymic fraction administered	Relative weight (mg bony tissue/ 100 g embryo weight)	P in g/100 g moist tissue	Ca in g/100 g moist tissue
Control	570 ± 18	1.22 ± 0.04	2.31 ± 0.08
Treated with TL	510 ± 18 unsig.[a]	1.38 ± 0.11 unsig.	2.62 ± 0.19 sig.[b]
Treated with B	480 ± 26 sig.	1.61 ± 0.3 sig.	3.15 ± 0.16 sig.

[a] $\overline{R}_1 - \overline{R}_2 < 2_r$; unsignificant.

[b] $R_1 - R_2 > 2_r$; significant.

(Figs. 11.40 and 11.41). The action of the extract is relatively unspecific, since muscle lipids were also active.

In order to study the involvement of the thymus in energy metabolism, we investigated the action of extract TL on brain ATP and P/O in some vertebrate forms (Potop, Mreana, and Neascu, 1963: 1967). Extract TL produced changes in ATP content and simultaneously the incorporation of ^{32}P into ATP. It also affected O_2 consumption (Fig. 11.42) and in some vertebrates influenced the P/O ratio as a result of energy and oxidative metabolism changes (Fig. 11.43). Extract TL decreases the P/O ratio in mammals and increases it in amphibians. It is interesting that there is an essential and specific action of fraction B on thymus alkaline phosphatase activity in contrast to the control fraction B prepared from the spleen (Fig. 11.44).

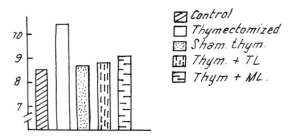

Fig. 11.41. Inorganic phosphate concentrations in serum of thymectomized rabbits before and after injection of thymus extract TL and control extract ML prepared from calf skeletal muscle.

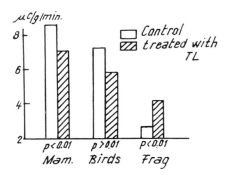

Fig. 11.42. Variations in O_2 consumption (QO_2) in vertebrates treated with thymus extract TL.

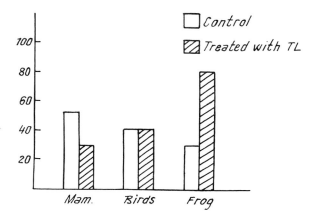

Fig. 11.43. Variations of the P/O ratio in brain tissues in vertebrates treated with thymus total lipid extract (TL). Ordinate provides relative units.

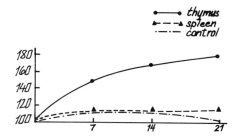

Fig. 11.44. Variations in alkaline phosphatase activity in the thymus of hybrid albino mice treated with fraction B, compared to a control and a fraction prepared from spleen.

As was shown above, an interesting fact was the influence exerted by thymus extracts of lipid nature on some enzymatic activities both in the intact and in the thymectomized animal, as well as in animals bearing various types of tumors.

11.11 Radioprotective action of thymus fraction B

The morphologic and functional modifications of the endocrine glands following irradiation, suggesting an endocrine imbalance as well as a protective mechanism of the hormones, are well known from the literature. Comsa (1965d, e) demonstrated that, while the pituitary growth hormone, the thymus hormone and deoxycorticosteroids lengthen the survival time in the irradiated animal, it is shortened by adrenaline. Thymus radio-protection in regaining immunologic competency was demonstrated. Thus thymus extract restores the immune response in CBA mice irradi-ated with lethal doses of X-ray (Aisenberg and Davies, 1968). The radio-protective ability found in the young mouse disappears within 3 to 12 weeks (Schneiberg, Joneko, and Bartinikowa, 1968). Thymectomy performed prior to irradiation enhanced the reducing effect on immuno-logic competence, and thymus tissue transplant partially restored this ability (Rosenthal, 1969). Regaining of the immune capacity following X-irradiation may also be generated in the adult thymectomized animal by thymus cells (Braun, 1968).

Potop *et al.* (1967) studied the effect of fraction B on Wistar rats sub-jected to whole body X-irradiation. Under our experimental conditions, irradiation produces a statistically significant decrease of ^{32}P incorpora-tion into liver RNA and a simultaneous decrease in β-glucuronidase ac-tivity and protein concentration in the thymus. The decreased absolute and relative weights of the thymus noted with irradiation suggest that this organ undergoes a process of involution (Table 11.16). Administra-tion of fraction B significantly raises ^{32}P incorporation into liver RNA and parallels the activity of β-glucuronidase and of protein levels in the thymus. These effects were less specific than those in which fraction B caused the thymus relative and absolute weights to increase.

The biologic radioprotective action of the thymus fraction is illus-trated by normalization in thymus weight and in the biochemical paramenters under consideration. Likewise, it was found that the mean survival time in irradiated animals treated with fraction B is higher when compared with untreated animals. The results obtained are in harmony with some of the data found in the literature; irradiation with sublethal doses results in an involution of the thymus, establishing a direct gland weight/pycnotic lymphocyte relationship. Toro (Toro, Bacsy, and Oros, 1968) noted that whole body irradiation induces a destruction of most of the thymocytes.

Experiments performed in tumor-bearing rats

The radioprotective effect of fraction B was investigated in the X-irradi-ated rat in which a Guerin carcinoma had been grafted (Potop *et al.*, 1969).

Table 11.16. Variations in ^{32}P incorporated into liver nucleic acids and variations of proteins and of β-glucuronidase in thymus of X-irradiated rat treated with fraction B

Groups	^{32}P incorporated into nucleic acids (P/g/s)[a]	Proteins (g/100 g tissue)	Activity of β-glucuronidase (phenolphtalein /1 g protein/hr)	Absolute weight of the thymus (mg)	Relative weight (%)
Normal control	61 ±15	10.2 ±0.4	22.6 ±1.56	62.3 ±5.47	260
X-irradiated	45 ±1.1 $p < 0.01$ (N)	7.6 ±0.4 $p < 0.05$ (N)	14.2 ±0.09 $p < 0.01$ (N)	26.5 ±2.80	108
Irradiated + B (thymus)	60 ±2.8 $p > 0.01$ (N)	8.1 ±0.6 $p < 0.05$ (N)	22.3 ±3.47 $p < 0.01$ (Ir)	37.5 ±4.28	159
Irradiated + B (muscle-control)		7.9 ±0.4 $p < 0.05$ (N)	20.7 ±2.27 $p < 0.01$ (Ir)	28.8 ±3.98	125

[a]This column is data from liver; all other data are from thymus.

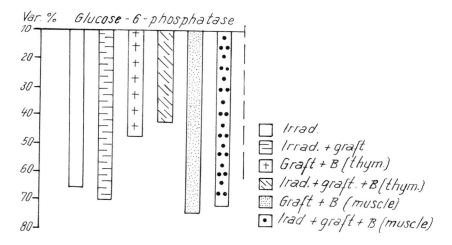

Fig. 11.45. Variations of glucose-6-phosphatase activity in irradiated rats bearing Guerin tumors and treated with thymus fraction B or muscle fraction B.

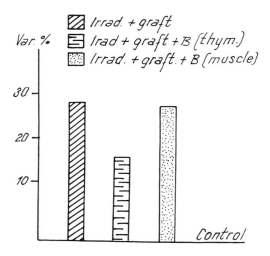

Fig. 11.46. Lactic acid concentration in livers of irradiated rats bearing Guerin carcinoma and treated with thymus fraction B.

Investigation of liver glucose-6-phosphatase and succinic dehydrogenase activities disclosed that the presence of the tumor in irradiated animals decreased the activity of this enzyme when compared to nonirradiated hosts and normal controls (Fig. 11.45). At the same time, there was an elevated concentration of lactic acid (Fig. 11.46). Fraction B administration increased glucose-6-phosphatase activity in irradiated, tumor-bearing animals when compared with untreated animals. Lactic acid levels increased both in the irradiated and tumor-bearing animal. Fraction B decreased lactic acid concentration in the liver of the irradiated rat and in irradiated tumor-bearing rats. The lack of response from muscle fraction B showed that the effect of thymus fraction B was specific. The results obtained indicate a biologic radioprotective action of fraction B in tumor-bearing animals, reflected by carbohydrate metabolism changes and reduction of tumor size (Fig. 11.47). It is noteworthy that there was good agreement between the results obtained regarding the modifications of biochemical parameters and tumor growth.

Our own experiments as well as those of other workers suggest a high lability of some enzymatic activities under the influence of thymus fractions associated with irradiation. Moreover, at present it is known that the thymus possesses a rich enzymatic supply (Ogier, Bastide and

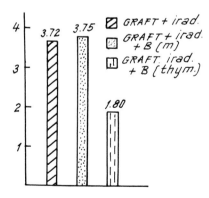

Fig. 11.47. Influence of thymus fraction B on the volume of the Guerin tumor in irradiated rats. Tumor volume calculated according to the formula where A and B are cell diameters in two directions:

$$V = \frac{4}{3}\pi \cdot \frac{A}{2}\left(\frac{B}{2}\right).$$

Dastique, 1966), a fact which might partly contribute to an explanation for the multiple functions of the thymus.

The metabolic changes associated with irradiation have been high-lighted by various authors. Thus, fructose-1,6-diphosphate accumulates in X-irradiated thymocytes concurrently with an inhibition of respiration and QO_2, depending on X-ray dose (Yamata and Ohyama, 1968). Like-wise, a rise is noted in lactate production and in phosphofructokinase activity in *in vitro* thymocyte suspensions in the whole-body irradiated rat (Yamada, Ohyama, and Kumatori, 1969). The mechanism of reduction in enzymatic activity noted under conditions of irradiation, although dif-ficult to explain, could be influenced by the S−S and H bonds, by pH changes induced by ionization, by the modification of ionic force, by conformational change of enzyme structural proteins, and by other factors which could stimulate or inhibit enzyme synthesis.

Our own findings reinforce data from the literature showing that the thymus exerts a radioprotective action in irradiated animals, whether tumor-bearing or not, which is reflected by nucleic acid metabolism changes, rise in enzyme activity, drop in blood sugar levels, increased weight of the thymus, lengthening of the survival time in animals with or without tumors, or inhibition of tumor growth. Recent reports in the literature demonstrate the radioprotective action of the thymus on the basis of the synergistic reaction of thymus cells, with those prepared from bone marrow bringing about an immunologic competence in irradiated animals (Delbez and Haot, 1969; Davis and Cole, 1969).

11.12 Stimulating action of thymus fraction B on antibody formation, hemoglobin, and serum leukocytes

By virtue of its fundamental function in immunologic events, the thymus dominates the study of reactions taking place in this field. At the same time, much work has accumulated pointing to the role played by the entire lymphoid system in the immune mechanism. Miller *et al.* (1967) demonstrated that lymphocyte increase is dependent on the normal functioning of the thymus. In animals thymectomized at birth, a marked reduction in the number of circulating lymphocytes and in the amount of cells able to react with histocompatible antigens and to respond to sheep erythrocytes was noted.

Immune reactivity following thymectomy was restored by thymus grafts (Yunis *et al.*, 1969), lymphocyte transfusion (Agnew, 1967), subcutaneous implant of isologous thymus (Parrot and East, 1964a, b), and by thymus extract administration (Trainin and Linker-Israeli, 1967). These subjects are reviewed in Chapter 3. It was seen that immune reactivity is not restored by thymus tumor grafts in animals (Vanderputte, 1967).

In a series of experiments of major importance, Miller has attempted to explain the mechanism whereby immunologic responsiveness is restored following thymectomy. The recognition that neonatal thymectomy reduces the immune response in mammals opens up new concepts with which to analyze the role of immunity in oncogenesis. In a previous work and in Chapter 5, we demonstrated the potentiating effect of polypeptide fraction TP isolated from calf thymus on antiviral antibody genesis (Babes *et al.*, 1970).

In a recent study (Babes *et al.*, 1971, in press) we investigated the stimulating effect of thymus fraction B on antibody-forming spleen cells. A kinetic study was performed on spleen cells and serum hemolytic antibodies in hybrid mice immunized with sheep red blood cells and hyperthymized. Demonstration of hemolytic plaque-forming cells was done according to the technique described by Jerne-Nordin. The results of this study (Figs. 11.48 and 11.49) indicated that the administration of

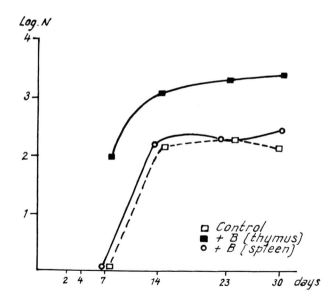

Fig. 11.48. Kinetics of serum hemolytic antibodies in mice treated with thymic fraction B. Ordinate provides a measure of the highest dilution or titer.

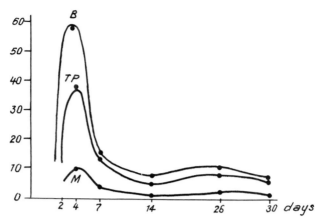

Fig. 11.49. Kinetics of the number of hemolytic plaques following treatment with thymus fraction B.

thymus fraction B during active immunization with heterologous red blood cells increased the occurrence of hemolytic plaque-forming cells as well as serum antibodies in significantly larger amounts than immunized but untreated controls. It should be emphasized that the graphs from groups of animals treated with thymus fraction demonstrate a similar kinetics, but quantitatively the values in the two groups (those treated with fraction B compared with those treated with thymus fraction TP or fraction B from spleen) demonstrate a major rise at the beginning of the experiment. It should be remembered that the group injected with fraction B has a much more increasing slope, as compared with the group given the polypeptide fraction TP, and that spleen fraction B was inactive.

Of the two thymic fractions tested, fraction B exhibited the stronger immunostimulating action. Secondary antigen stimulus resulted in a moderate rise in the number of hemolytic plaques, whereas the curve of serum hemolysis showed an obvious upward slope. In Figure 11.48, the kinetics of serum hemolytic antibodies is illustrated, and Figure 11.49 illustrates the kinetics of the average number of hemolytic plaques in the different groups.

Results obtained in this study suggest the hypothesis that stimulation with thymus fractions could operate via an effect on the precursors of immunologically competent cells. The results agree with those of Small and Trainin (1967), which show that thymic treatment increases the number of antisheep hemolysin-forming cells.

Action of thymus fraction B on hemoglobin and serum leukocytes

The action of the thymus and of thymectomy on the red and white blood cells was reported in various works in the literature. In a work published by Potop and Boeru (1951), it was shown that administration of a thymic polypeptide fraction induced an increase in the number of erythrocytes and lymphocytes in rabbits, and that thymus X-irradiation decreased these values. The results obtained in recent works (Potop, Boeru et al., 1970; Potop, Manitescu et al., 1971) demonstrated a major rise in hemoglobin levels in the peripheral blood following treatment with fraction B in the hybrid albino mouse (Fig. 11.50). This fact, which points to the part played by the thymus in erythropoiesis, was reported by various authors.

Following thymus fraction B administration, there is a significant increase in the blood leukocyte count. These investigations bear out our earlier results. The importance of the thymus in white blood cells and especially in lymphocyte genesis and its role in immunologic reactions was demonstrated by a large number of workers. According to Maisin (1963), the thymus is the source of competent immunologic cells.

To date it has been ascertained that the thymus has a hemato- and lymphopoietic function during embryonic life. It should be stressed that the action of fraction B prepared from calf thymus does not seem to lack in specificity, since a control extract prepared from spleen under the same conditions has no influence on the parameters under consideration.

11.13 Discussion

The activity of the thymus fractions of steroid nature deserves a few comments. Originally, our study dealt with the inhibitory activity of the thymus on neoplastic processes postulated by Parhon and Milcu in 1935

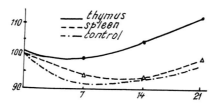

Fig. 11.50. Relative values of hemoglobin (related to the initial overall mean) in mice treated with thymus fraction B.

(unpublished). As work progressed, other biologic activities of the extracts were also investigated, since the extracts were found to have multiple effects.

From the variety of fractions which we isolated and purified from the lipid complex of thymus, we finally isolated a pure steroid factor which proved to have antiproliferative action. By means of thin-layer chromatography, several spots were separated. The one spot we analyzed, which was quantitatively the largest portion (10 to 50% of the total), exhibited a high antiproliferative activity, whereas one of the immediately adjacent spots was inactive. Presumably, thymosterin is made in the thymus, since other tissues were inactive, and Abraham (1971) has shown steroid synthesis to occur in rat thymus.

As seen from data in the literature, apart from the identified chemical factors (Bernardi and Comsa, 1965a, b; Hand, Caster, and Luckey 1967), there are a large number of thymus preparations, notably of protein nature, which have various biologic activities. To our knowledge there is no evidence in the literature with which our results on lipid fractions and particularly their antineoplastic effect could be corroborated. The total lipid extract prepared by Bomskov (1940) and Bomskov and Holscher (1942), while being endowed by the author with a variety of metabolic effects, is still of obscure chemical structure.

The fact that the extracts we prepared are not all equally active deserves some emphasis. We investigated a number of factors, including age, physiologic and nutritional conditions of the animal supplying the thymus, and the season in which the thymus was collected, which influence the activity of the extracts. Another factor which contributes to the successful outcome of the experiments is the purity of the solvents used; in the course of the relatively elaborate handling during separation, the active factor could be carried away, with the fraction being removed. Also, the biologic activity of fraction B could be decided by the relative amount of the two fractions with opposite effects on tumor growth (II B, inhibitory, and III B, stimulating) in the initial fraction B.

An interesting factor in our experiments was that the same extract, in the same preparation, simultaneously exhibits antitumoral, metabolic, and antibody-stimulating activities. The fraction inactive on tumor growth will not influence the metabolic status. Our research demonstrates the presence in the thymus of a hormone-like active factor of steroid nature. The study of the thymus is an intricate problem with several unknown elements still to be elucidated by further accurate investigations.

11.14 Conclusions

By using solubility in different solvents and column and thin-layer chromatography, we isolated a range of thymic fractions, consecutively deriving one from the other (B, II B, III B, and III B$_3$), as well as a factor S in the pure state. The research regarding the structure of these compounds by infrared spectral analysis showed them to be of steroid nature. Pure factor S was named thymosterin.

The spectral analysis of fraction II B$_3$ which yielded factor S attests the presence of a steroid ring and of a 12-acetoxy-11 ketone group and of methyl groups of the chain in C$_{21}$ through C$_{28}$.

The infrared spectrum of isolated substance S supports the existence of the perhydrocyclopentanophenanthrene ring. The presence of some (CH$_3$)$_2$ or (CH$_3$)$_3$ types of groups and of an ether group in the case of the steroids was demonstrated. In addition, the presence of an OH group bound to the steroid ring was found.

Investigations carried out on the thymic fractions isolated in our laboratory demonstrated their significant biologic action on tumor development *in vitro* and *in vivo*, on the metabolism of normal or thymectomized, tumor-bearing, or X-irradiated animals and on immune phenomena and blood morphology of neonatal animals.

Testing for the antiproliferative action of the various fractions of the thymus on tumor cell cultures *in vitro* allows the following conclusions to be drawn. Fraction B, II B, and II B$_3$, and factor S inhibited the development of tumor cell cultures, evidenced by the reduction of cell population and of protein concentration in the culture and, from the histopathologic viewpoint, by a decline in malignancy. The antiproliferative activity increased with higher degrees of purification of the thymic fraction; thymosterin exhibits the most intense activity. There is a direct dose-effect relationship of antiproliferative activity. The antiproliferative effect is specific, as shown by comparison with control fractions prepared from muscle and spleen. It was established that the age of the animal from which the thymus was obtained and its physiologic and nutritional conditions determine a variability in the antitumor action of the thymic extracts. Likewise, the antiproliferative effect of a lipid extract from child thymus (obstetrical trauma) was established.

The antiproliferative activity tested on the basis of histochemical studies revealed the effect of fraction II B$_3$ on the enzymatic activities of glucose-6-phosphatase, succinic dehydrogenase, and β-glucuronidase. The activity of fraction B was tested on the basis of biochemical variables at the hepatic level; glucose-6-phosphatase activity and the concentration of lactic acid showed a direct dose-response relationship.

The investigations concerning the biologic activity of thymus fractions B, II B, and III B in rats, mice, and chick embryos allow us to draw the following conclusions. Thymus fractions B and II B inhibit the development of various types of tumor induced by chemical carcinogens or by implantation of tumor grafts, acting on tumor tissue and on the recipient organism. The inhibitory action is disclosed by a reduced tumor incidence, decreased tumor weight and dynamics of tumor growth, modification of tumor structure in the sense of a lower malignancy, complete retrogression of some types of tumor following long-term treatment made prior to transplantation (Jensen sarcoma), and increased survival time. The interference of the thymus is evidenced by the altered metabolism of the cancer cell and of the host, which tends to be restored to normal by thymic lipid fractions.

Thymic lipid fractions reduce nucleic acid synthesis and metabolism and protein metabolism, which are increased in the presence of tumors; they increase liver glycogen synthesis, decrease glycolysis parallel with elevation of O_2 consumption, and induce major changes in the activity of some enzymes (glucose-6-phosphatase, succinic dehydrogenase), etc. It is noteworthy that the results *in vivo* can be superimposed on those obtained *in vitro*.

Thymic fraction B has a protective role in the processes induced by X-irradiation manifested by a rise in ^{32}P incorporation into liver RNA coincidental with the increase in protein concentration, β-glucuronidase activity, and weight of the thymus. In Guerin tumor-bearing animals, fraction B causes alterations in carbohydrate metabolism and a reduction in tumor volume.

Thymectomy induces a stimulation in tumor growth which is a totally opposite effect to that of thymus fraction II B administration. However, thymus fraction III B isolated from fraction B stimulates tumor growth by reducing the time of survival, increasing tumor volume, and reducing the latency period; these effects are antagonistic with those of fraction II B.

Our investigations of metabolism in intact and thymectomized animals and chick embryo support the following conclusions. The total lipid extract (TL) reduces inorganic serum phosphorus levels and increases serum calcium levels in the thymectomized rabbit. Extract TL influences energy metabolism and oxidative metabolism modifying oxidative phosphorylation in the brain of various classes of vertebrates; different classes of vertebrates react differently. Fraction B enhances calcium and phosphorus fixation in chick embryo tibia. Fractions B and II B modify the activity of glucose-6-phosphatase, succinic dehydrogenase, and alkaline phosphatase.

Research on the role of thymic fraction B in the immune phenomena allows certain conclusions. Fraction B stimulates antibody formation in mice as measured following heterologous red blood cell immunization by the elaboration of antibodies which form hemolytic plaques and by serum antibodies. Administration of fraction B induces a significant rise in hemoglobulin and in leukocyte counts in the peripheral blood.

The way in which the isolated thymic fractions interfere with various biologic processes is shown by the dose-effect relationship, the action opposing the response following thymectomy and administration of the fractions, correction for the absence of the gland by thymus extracts and fractions, correlations with other organs and endocrine glands, and the degree of specificity exhibited by the fractions. The total of our results supports the concept of the production by the thymus of a hormone-like substance. We proposed to designate factor S by the term thymosterin.

Acknowledgments

We acknowledge, with gratitude, the help of many co-workers: V. Pelloni, V. Boeru, M. Olteneaunu, and M. Elian in the early extraction procedures; and A. Lupu, G. Mreana, and C. Tasca for unpublished tumor work.

12 Perspective of Thymic Hormones

T. D. Luckey

12.1 Introduction

This perspective of thymic hormones will summarize the physical-chemical-biologic characteristics of known compounds. It will explore how adequately the criteria for hormones have been satisfied. Concepts of thymic activators and inhibitors will be presented. A hypothesis of thymic hormone control of immune and other systems within the context of generalized hormone action will be presented. Insight from concepts derived from the study of thymic hormones suggests a generalized hypothesis regarding the induction of recognition by molecular imprinting. The function of molecular imprinting in a variety of communication phenomena is suggested. Our first intimate view of the unique molecules of the thymus suggests that important new concepts and applications will result from continued work on the thymus during the next decade.

Summary of active compounds

Comparison of the characteristics of the compounds described in the previous chapters (Table 12.1) allows some understanding of the variety of compounds produced by the thymus; these provide special activities not produced by other tissues, excepting perhaps by the bursa and its mammalian equivalent. The compounds described by Mizutani (see Chapter 10), Milcu and Potop (see Chapter 5), G. Goldstein and Hofmann (1969), and Tallberg and coworkers (1966, 1968) have nebulous characteristics.

Thymosterin of Potop and Milcu (see Chapter 11) differs strikingly from all the others by being a steroid. Although the exact structure is undetermined, it is not a known steroid. This material inhibits tumor growth both *in vitro* and *in vivo*. It has also been noted to inhibit lymphocytopoiesis. Further characterization and possibilities of utility should

Table 12.1. Comparison of thymic hormones and inhibitors

Identification[a]	LSH$_r$	LSH$_h$	Thymosin	HTH
Laboratory	Luckey	Luckey	White	Comsa
Purity	+ + +	+ +	+ + +	+
Chemistry	Protein	Protein	Protein	Peptide
Mol. wt.	80,000	17,000[b]	12,600	2,000
	±1%	±10%	±2%	± 10%
Heat stability	+	−	+	+
Occurrence				
Thymus/g[b]	10 µg	25 µg	15 µg	3 mg
Spleen	±	1/10	−	+→−
Lymph node		1/50	−	+→−
Serum		−	+→−	+→−
Urine				+−
Others	−[c]	−[c]	−[d]	−[e]
Prevents wasting			+	+
Activates skin graft rejection			+	+
Lymphopoietic	+	±	+	
L/P ratio	↑	↑		
Antibody production competence	+	+	−	+
Cell-mediated response			+	
Graft-host reaction			+	
Antitumor			+	

[a]LSH, lymphocyte-stimulating hormone; HTH, homeostatic thymus hormone; THF, thymic humoral factor; TP, thymic protein; CaC, hypocalcemic component; and TSA, thymic specific antigen.

[b]Rough estimates from isolation data.

[c]Not in muscle or kidney. Unpublished data from my laboratory (B. Lenoble) indicates chick bursa to have LSH$_h$ in larger quantities than LSH$_r$.

[d]Not found in muscle or kidney.

[e]Not found in muscle, kidney, liver, lung, or testes.

be of great importance. The remaining entities are readily soluble in water and saline and are protein in nature, with the possible exception of the material of Trainin (thymic humoral factor, THF) which has a molecular weight of less than 1,000. HTH (homeostatic thymic hormone) contains sugar derivatives and may contain nucleic acid (see the absorption spectrum, Fig. 3.1). Thymosin, previously thought to be a dialyzable glycoprotein, is a nondialyzable protein.

The contrasting sizes of the different compounds are remarkable. The molecular weight of HTH is approximately 2,000, LSH$_h$ (lymphocyte stimulating hormone) is approximately 17,000, and the thymus-specific antigen compound (TSA) of Tallberg is approximately 70,000, while LSH$_r$

THF	TP	CaC	TSA	Thymin	Thymo-toxin	Thymo-sterin
Trainin	Milcu	Mizutani	Tallberg	Goldstein	Goldstein	Potop
−	−	+	+	+ +	+ +	+ +
Peptide <1,000[b]	Peptides 1,000[b]	Protein 200,000[b]	Protein 70,000[b]	Proteinaceous 6,000[b]	Proteinaceous 7,000[b]	Steroid 400[b]
+	+		−	+	+	+
+	+	+	+	15 μg/g	+	+
			+			
−			−			
+						
+			+			↓
+			↓			+
+						
			+			+

is 80,000. Thymosin* is 12,600 (Guha, Goldstein, and White, 1972).
Trainin and coworkers have shown that the thymus humoral factor (THF)
increased mitosis, but did not cause release of lymphocytes from the
central lymphatic organs at the concentrations used thus far. Dieter

---

*A recent abstract (Goldstein et al., 1972) reveals how the chameleon character of thymosin has allowed it to approach the properties previously ascribed to LSH_h (Hand et al., 1967). Comparable properties are outlined in table form:

Characteristic	Thymosin		LSH 1967
	Early	Recent	
Amount injected	mg	μg	μg
Chemistry	glycoprotein	protein	protein
Dialysis	+	−	−
Molecular wt. $\times 10^3$	10	13	12–22
$(NH_4)_2SO_4$ pptn.	not used	25–50%	20%

These similarities are great enough to permit the question of whether or not the low molecular weight component of thymosin recently isolated is LSH_h. Since both ammonium sulfate and Sephadex G-150 are useful in the final purification, might the high molecular weight component of thymosin be LSH_r?

(1971) suggests the quantity of THF varies directly with the vitamin C content of tissues.

All of the compounds considered occur in the thymus and may be expected to have diminished concentrations under conditions of genetic defect, prolonged thymic involution from old age, stresses, certain diseases, or toxicities such as radiation or excess glucocorticoids or testosterone. Little systematic information is available about the occurrence of this series of compounds in other tissues. The spleen has low quantities of HTH and LSH. Many lymphocytes migrate through the thymus; this would allow a cytocrine effect. Wasting disease and death of thymectomized animals have been prevented by injections of HTH, thymosin, or THF. Unfortunately, pure compounds like LSH have not yet been tested for this activity. The lymphocyte-polymorphonuclear cell ratio was increased by HTH or either component of LSH. LSH also increased spleen and lymph node weights following injection into germ-free animals. However, LSH$_h$ administration did not cause an increase in circulating white blood cells, while injection of LSH$_r$, TSA, or THF gave an increased circulation of total white blood cells. Both LSH$_h$ and LSH$_r$ activate antibody formation in neonatal mice. THF also induces antibody formation *in vitro*, as illustrated in Chapter 6. Pure thymosin has not been obtained; this might preclude its being in this list of compounds which increase antibody formation. Purified thymosin and THF stimulate cell-mediated immunity; this response has not been examined with HTH and LSH compounds. These are the known compounds of the thymus.

There appears to be an equal number of less well identified compounds. However, once the major hormone becomes readily available, the many apparent compounds will probably fall into a simple perspective. The thymus functions in immune responsiveness, differentiation, and hormonal regulation. The inhibitory activity of a given compound on one of these functions may be as important as its stimulatory activity.

Inhibitors of the thymus

Historically, inhibitors have interfered with the bioassay of the stimulating compounds of the thymus. This interference has thwarted individual, laboratory, and industrial attempts to isolate the compounds which evoked immune competence in lymphocytes. Clinical and industrial emphasis has now changed from an interest in stimulators to an interest in inhibitors for transplantation and cancer therapy. Confirmation of inhibitor interference was seen during the isolation of LSH$_h$. Compounds with characteristics similar to LSH $_r$ are noted in Fig. 8.3. When the purified protein extract was developed on gel electrophoresis and material from different parts were eluted and injected into newborn mice, the antibody-forming ability, according to Hand (personal communication, 1970), was stimulated by LSH-active compounds, while it was inhibited by material which does not migrate during electrophoresis. A second strong inhibitor was found with a mobility somewhat less than that of LSH $_h$. In the concentrations that occur during isolation, the inhibitors are definitely stronger than the stimulating compounds. The success of our laboratory in isolating a thymic hormone may be attributed to the consistent use of small quantities of injected material. This may dilute the inhibitors to the extent that they are no longer active or they may react differently when provided in dilute concentration. The fact that these inhibitors coprecipitated with the stimulating compounds through the ammonium sulfate and methanol precipitation and were nondialyzable show their similarity in chemical characteristics to LSH. One of these inhibitors may be the impure thymostatin of A. L. Goldstein et al. (1967), which inhibits DNA and RNA synthesis.

The first class of inhibitors to be discussed are the compounds and extracts of the thymus which have been followed using biologic assays involving inhibition. The best characterized of the inhibitors is thymosterin, which is described in detail by Potop and Milcu in Chapter 11. This steroid inhibits tumor formation both *in vivo* and *in vitro*. A tumor inhibitor of protein nature, pursued by Milcu and Potop, is discussed in Chapter 5. Although this material is biologically active in many tests and occurs only in thymus, it has not been obtained in sufficient purity to compare it with other compounds described in this book.

Equally exciting and equally little known is the work of Tallberg and coworkers (1966; 1968) who used a thymic deficiency disease to provide an immunologic approach to isolate and partially purify a thymus-specific antigen (TSA) from human fetal thymus. It was not found in other normal human tissues. This leukocyte-control factor is apparently a heat-labile protein of approximately 70,000 molecular weight. Thymuses of persons with lymphatic leukemia or Burkitt's lymphoma have little or none of this compound, although it apparently can be detected in the spleens of these patients (Luckey, 1971). Since it is antagonistic to anti-lymphocyte serum, synergistic with phytohemagglutinin and increases uridine incorporation in normoblasts of tumor patients, it must be considered an inhibitor of leukocyte survival and a stimulator by other parameters.

Tallberg, Nordling, and Cautell (1968) noted a second human thymus antigen which was partially specific for thymus but was also found in different parts of the ileojejunal tract. No other species, excepting monkeys, has this material. Since it was found in no other tissue, they suggest this may be the mammalian equivalent of the bursa of Fabricius.

G. Goldstein (1968) and Goldstein and Mackay (1967) reviewed the status of thymin, a thymic hormone which depresses neuromuscular transmission. It is thought to be released in excess in autoimmune thymitis and to cause the neuromuscular block in myasthenia gravis. Goldstein reported the isolation of thymin at the First International Congress for Immunology, August, 1971. Closely associated with thymin is the myasthenia-promoting substance which Goldstein called thymotoxin. It has not been isolated in pure form. His information is incorporated into Table 12.1 in order to present a complete comparison of thymic hormones.

Bedo et al. (1971) reported the presence of one fraction from beef thymus which shortened generation times in a variety of enteric bacteria and another fraction which inhibited the growth of bacteria and Ehrlich sarcoma in mice. The stimulation-inhibition concept is reinforced by this study and by the opposite effects of thymus lipid (Chapter 11) and thymic hypocalcemic factor (Chapter 10) on serum calcium.

The second class of thymic inhibitors are the compounds which were studied as stimulators. Although the exact role of each of the multiple compounds characteristic of the thymus is not known, it is obvious that some of these compounds are stimulatory at very low levels and inhibitory at higher levels, whereas those discussed above are inhibitory without being stimulatory at any level tested. All biologically active compounds and particularly hormones are harmful if given in excessive quantity. The usual dose-response curve seen with hormone administration covers a very limited range of the total biologic activity spectrum of those compounds. A generalized activity spectrum over a wide range is illustrated in Figure 12.1. From this broad viewpoint, hormones are a special class of compounds in hormology (Luckey, 1959). This concept is particularly appropriate when one considers a dose-response curve (Fig. 12.2) of the raw data available on LSH_r at this time; only the inhibitory aspect of the curve has been tested. Even during LSH isolation, we were testing quantities which are on the descending or back side of the dose-response curve. These data parallel those from LSH_h; relatively low quantities of this series of compounds are toxic to young mice.

Thus, the thymus could balance activation and inhibition either by the quantity of a compound released or by the balance between different

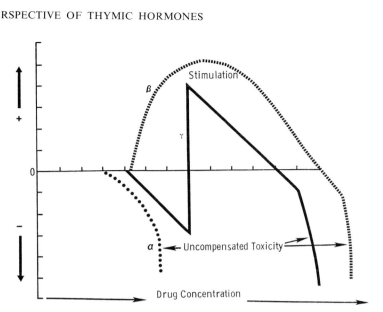

Fig. 12.1. General dose-response curves. Data taken from classic pharmacology (Townsend and Luckey, 1960).

compounds released at any given time. Details of this phenomenon should provide exciting areas of future research.

Combinations of stimulators may produce inhibition. Both tri-adeny-late and phytohemagglutinin stimulate adenyl cyclase activity; when added together in the same concentration, they inhibit cAMP formation (Braun et al., 1971).

Another area to be considered is the antagonistic effect of thymic extracts upon the action of other hormones. These have been summarized by Comsa in Chapter 4. Opposing reactions between thymic hormones and glucocorticoids have been noted in lymphocytosis (Metcalf, 1959), DNA and protein synthesis (Klein et al., 1965), and homograft rejections (Miller et al., 1965). Rushing (1968) observed a direct antagonism in an assay for radioactive amino acid incorporation involving either micro-somal or ribosomal preparations from spleens of rats which had previous-ly received four injections of LSH_h or methanol precipitate (PPE) during the 4 days prior to sacrifice. These unconfirmed experiments are most interesting because the methanol precipitate completely overcame any inhibition by hydrocortisone (Table 12.2). These data suggest a major

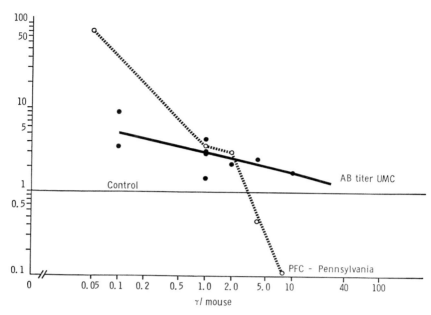

Fig. 12.2. Laboratory data for LSH activity. Collaborative study in progress with Drs. G. Robey and W. Ceglowski at Pennsylvania State University Department of Microbiology. The ordinate gives the geometric antibody (AB) titer (*solid line*) and the change in plaque-forming cells (PFC, *dotted line*) compared to the saline-injected control per 10⁶ spleen cells. Injection at lower levels than indicated have not been used. Quantities higher than indicated are harmful to newborn mice. The advice and help of Dr. John McKenna is acknowledged for the UMC work. Each point represents the average from four or more mice.

control exists for excess glucocorticoids. This antagonism could explain why young rats, 3 to 10 days of age, show no effect from hydrocortisone and have no demonstrable synthesis of inducible enzymes such as tryptophan oxidase. The finding (Whitfield, MacManus, and Rixon, 1970; Whitfield *et al.*, 1971) that low concentrations (10^{-9} M) of cortisol stimulate rat thymocyte proliferation while concentrations higher than 10^{-7} M inhibit it is a specific example of the generalization described in the previous paragraph and suggests how thymic hormones and glucocorticoids could act in concert. A suggestion of the balance required between these two antagonists is the finding that *in vitro* antibody formation increased with 0.01 to 1.0 μg of hydrocortisone per ml incubation fluid (Ambrose, 1964). Physiological levels were not active in this experiment.

Table 12.2. Effect of LSH and hydrocortisone upon *in vitro* amino acid incorporation into protein

Rat spleen microsomes and ribosomes are compared using beef serum albumin (BSA) injected rats as the control. BSA was given in the same quantity as LSH$_h$. Heated methanol precipitate was the control for the other groups. Four rats per group were used. Spleens were pooled when needed.

Material	Injections (mg)	Experiments	Amino acid incorporation % of control (range)
BSA	0.01–0.07	3	100
Hydrocortisone	5.0	1	68[a]
LSH$_h$	0.01–0.07	3	134 (118–145)
MeOH PPT.	0.25	2	126 (122–130)
MEOH PPT. plus hydrocortisone	As above	3	140 (109–170)

[a]This value is much higher than previous results with hydrocortosione; it is the only value obtained during this series of experiments.

12.2 Possible action of thymic hormones

Hormonal character of thymic compounds

What general characteristics of a hormone can be applied to thymic hormones? First noted are changes following thymus extirpation; these changes are described in Chapter 1 without consideration of how many thymic hormones may be deleted by this operation. It should be noted particularly that thymectomy shortly after birth will give characteristic deficiency symptoms, while thymectomy of mice at 1 week or older gives no quickly discernable sign of deficiency. Thymectomy in older animals shows no overt effect for many weeks. Within the developing thymus are materials which dramatically affect the host; thymic hormones act fast, and their immunologic effects are long-lasting. From this viewpoint, thymic hormones act more like differentiation factors, reminiscent of thyroxine or ecdysone, than hydrocortisone, erythropoietin, or gastrointestinal hormones.

The second criterion for a hormone is that material from one specific organ should have replacement value following extirpation of that organ. These experiments were performed a decade ago, as outlined in Chapter 3. Thymus grafts had full replacement value. Small remnants left after

284 T. D. LUCKEY

thymectomy were fully effective in restoring immunologic competence in the rat (Steward, 1971). Replacement has been obtained by implantation of thymus tissue in diffusion chambers, cell-free extracts, purified extracts, and, finally, pure compounds. All the compounds reported herein are active when injected. The specificity of these compounds for the thymus has been verified and is summarized in Table 12.1. Implantation and extracts of other organs have generally been of no value following thymectomy. Tissues in which thymus hormone activity is negligible include liver, muscle, kidney, lung, and testes. The low activity noted in the spleen, lymph nodes, urine, and serum disappears within a few days following thymectomy (Comsa, Chapter 1; Hand, personal communication, 1970; Metcalf, 1959). Chicken bursa contains five times more LSH_r and LSH_h than chicken thymus; it contains about two-thirds as much LSH_r as does calf thymus, according to recent experiments by R. Lenoble and R. LeGrand (unpublished data from our laboratory, 1971).

Are one or more compounds carried by body fluids from the thymus to the place of action? Following extirpation of the thymus, the activity found in low quantities in the spleen and in lesser quantities in other organs, serum, and urine decreased to zero in a few days. However, small lymphocytes are active for a long time following thymectomy in adult animals. Therefore, the rapid disappearance of hormone from spleen is significant. Thymic hormones may induce maturation of lymphocytes residing in the spleen, but they apparently do not stay in the cells. The activity of thymus fragments implanted into diffusion chambers in thymectomized or irradiated animals provides evidence that a cell-free material, produced by the surviving reticular cells, affects host lymphocytes. The bursa also releases a factor which restores antibody-forming capability through a diffusion chamber (Pierre and Ackerman, 1965). Further evidence that thymic hormones which raise immune competence are carried through the blood is provided in the experiment of Osoba (1965b); neonatally thymectomized mice were reared to maturity, and pregnant females had an increased immune competence at parturition. The discrepancy between this phenomenon and immune incompetence in newborn mice has yet to be resolved. Perhaps, as the data of Sussdorf (1971) indicate, the gut equivalent to the thymus is more active than the thymus in neonatal animals. Jolley and Hinshaw (1965) give further evidence of the transfer of peptides from thymus to lymph nodes. Injection of extracts and finally pure compounds shows that thymic hormones can act through the usual avenues of administration. In addition to evidence of thymus specificity and humoral transport of material from it to other organs, speculatively, lymphocytes may obtain cytocrines during migration through the thymus; such material could be transported throughout the body and appear in direct clones of the emigrant cells.

Modern concepts would suggest another characterization of many hormones; protein hormones might be expected to be effective via a second (nonspecific) messenger. Cyclic AMP and cyclic GMP stimulate reproduction of white blood cells *in vitro* (Braun *et al.*, 1971) and *in vivo* (Rixon, Whitfield, and MacManus, 1970). Cyclic GMP increases lymphocytopoiesis and cyclic AMP content of cells by two means; in low concentrations (10^{-11} M), it may stimulate adenyl cyclase, and at high concentrations (10^{-6} M), it may inhibit the esterase degradation (Whitefield *et al.*, 1971). Cyclic AMP is a reasonable choice as a second messenger within thymocytes and mature lymphocytes following stimulation by antigen. It will be important to test cyclic nucleotides during stem cell differentiation and maturation of immune competence. Wilson and Weissman (1971) and Cooper and Ginsburg (1971) summarize work showing that within 10 min of the addition of mitogen to lymphocytes, adenyl cyclase activity was increased, and cyclic AMP content was increased and subsequently fell to unstimulated levels as the esterase catalyzed the formation of AMP. Low concentrations of cyclic AMP were reported to stimulate lymphocytes; concentrations greater than 10^{-4} M inhibit lymphocyte activation. Trainin and Small (1970b) found cyclic AMP did not confer immune competence *in vitro*. However, Ishizuka, Gafni, and Braun (1970) and Braun *et al.* (1971) report that administration

Table 12.3. Possible parallels between cyclase-mediated hormonal and antigen reactions.

Process	Endocrinology	Immunology
Switch	Stimulus	Thymic hormone
Transmitter	Endocrine gland	Environment
Signal	Hormone	Antigen
Discriminator	Membrane site	Membrane site
Converter	Cyclase	Cyclase
Preamp	cAMP	cAMP
Amplifier (Cascade)	Kinases	Kinases
Transcription selector	Derepressor	Derepressor
Master transcriptor	DNA	DNA
Translator	mRNA	mRNA
Production	Protein, enzymes, etc.	Antibody ± membrane bound

of cyclic AMP *in vivo* and *in vitro* enhanced antibody formation. Cyclic AMP content of macrophages increased three-fold during the first 5 min of phagocytosis (Park *et al.*, 1971). This generalized action is summarized in Table 12.3.

Finally, identification of a target organ, tissues, or cells is important. Stem cells appear to be affected, and bone marrow cells are one important target for this hormone in immunology. There is little doubt that compounds produced by the thymus confer immune competence to bone marrow cells. The spleen contains the highest quantity of exported thymic hormone. Approximately one-half of the spleen leukocytes may be thymocytes (T cells). Other target cells are suggested below.

Generalized hormone actions

A diagrammatic concept of the action of a protein hormone (Fig. 12.3 and Table 12.3) is helpful in suggesting possible places of action for the diversity of compounds isolated from the thymus. In this generalized flow of hormonal interactions, most components are comparable to those suggested by Tepperman (1968). A unified hypothetical view incorporating the active molecules with their disparity of molecular sizes follows. In a mature system (*i.e.*, in the presence of the enabling thymic hormone), injection of antigen (the environmental stimulus) rapidly activates white blood cell proliferation. The fact that injected antigen affects lymph nodes in the region of injection suggests that the direct action of the antigen on the cells residing in the area is more intensive than any centralized activity. This concept is strengthened by the finding that the full complement of thymocytes is produced by thymuses of germfree rats which have only about one-third as many circulating leukocytes as do classic rats. Actually, there is no experimental evidence that antigen directly affects the flow of thymic hormones. Thymic hormone is increased in lymphoma; except for this and pituitary interaction, the epithelial thymus appears to have its own time clock and may be responsible for other development changes. Its development and hormonal release appear to be species-specific.

Although the diagram suggests the central nervous system is the usual input for external stimuli, this may be bypassed, since antigen represents the outside environment which is carried into the host. Nevertheless, it would be irrational to suggest that the thymic hormone has no central nervous system or hypothalmic control. Indeed the striking responses noted by Comsa (Chapter 3) to extirpation of either the thymus

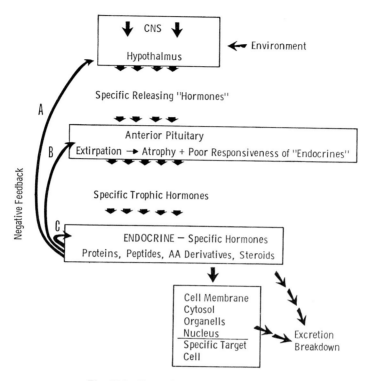

Fig. 12.3. Generalized endocrine actions.

or the pituitary suggest an interplay between these two organs. The hypertrophy of the thymus caused by hypophysectomy suggests a restrictive control of thymic activity by the pituitary, perhaps mediated through adrenal corticotrophic hormone (ACTH) and the corticosteroids of the adrenal gland. Thymectomy caused hypertrophy of other endocrines, followed by a state of exhaustion, which suggests that there is a negative feedback of the thymus upon the pituitary and thus other organs. This feedback could be expected to go through the hypothalamus and/or directly to the anterior pituitary, as indicated by lines A and B in the diagram. This negative feedback of other endocrines appears to be mediated through the thymus. However, when Metcalf (1964) grafted up to 24 neonatal thymuses into one isologous mouse, lymphocyte production increased but no deleterious effects were noted.

There is obviously an activation of lymphocytes within the thymus; their prodigious and prodigal reproduction within the thymus is not well understood. Since the character of the cell which leaves the thymus is quite different than that of bone marrow cells, the thymus must also be considered a cytocrine gland with specific and effective action on transient cells within it; immunologically, this may be as important as its action on cells and tissues affected by secreted thymic hormones.

The target cell may be expected to react as diagrammed in Table 12.3. In this general scheme, any molecule coming into the environment of the cell may have indirect effects on the cell membrane due to polarity sites expressed by the macromolecule relative to the cell, the osmotic environment, or the attraction or adsorption of small molecules including substrate. Such changes in the pico (micro-micro) environment could allow a degree of discrimination by the cell membrane without direct interaction between the macromolecule and the cell membrane. Mosaic patterns in the plasma membrane might allow as many as 10^4 unit reactions of the membrane; this estimate is based on the number of penicillin molecules bound to bacteria (10^3) and the electron microscopic appearance of cells charged with virus antibody.

The double membrane of a cell suggests a dozen discrete parts (Fig. 12.4) which could contain or react with available molecules. From the

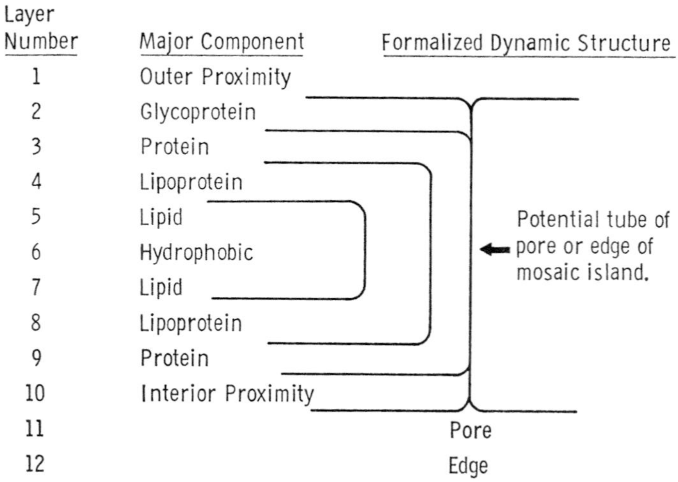

Layer Number	Major Component	Formalized Dynamic Structure
1	Outer Proximity	
2	Glycoprotein	
3	Protein	
4	Lipoprotein	
5	Lipid	
6	Hydrophobic	Potential tube of pore or edge of mosaic island.
7	Lipid	
8	Lipoprotein	
9	Protein	
10	Interior Proximity	
11		Pore
12		Edge

Fig. 12.4. Cell membrane layers.

outer coat to the interior they could be designated as: 1) outer proximity; 2) glycoprotein; 3) protein; 4) lipoprotein; 5) lipid; 6) hydrophobic; 7) lipid; 8) lipoprotein; 9) protein; 10) interior proximity; 11) pore; and 12) edge. Unless a molecule is engulfed during endocytosis, every molecule entering the cell must affect the cell membrane at least during a fleeting instant when it slips through a pore in the membrane; the effect may be dramatic even though passage is fast. If attracted, a nonspecific molecule could be adsorbed or bound to the membrane with a given equilibrium and with little subsequent effect on the cell. Thus, any of the outer components of the membrane could have a general attraction to or repulsion of any molecule or a specific site for a macromolecule. If the attracted molecule is the hormone for which that cell was the target, the cell membrane must have specific recognition sites to accept this particular message. One of these sites may be visualized molecularly as a binding affinity of the hormone to an active site within the membrane. This fitting of molecules provides a meaningful contact which immediately changes the membrane and the total cell. Mechanistically, this would appear more easily accomplished in a pore or at the edge of the mosaic rather than through the double membrane lipid-lipid layers. Perhaps a new mosaic pattern or pore is triggered. Most messages must affect the inner membrane where their reception is translated into action at the inner membrane. Classically (see Litwack, 1970; Rassmussen, 1970; Pastan and Perlman, 1971), this translation leads to the activation of a cyclase for amplification of the signal. Membrane-bound inactive adenyl cyclase is activated by the sequence of events started by the arrival of the hormone message within this cell type. The message is specific for the cell; the translation starts a nonspecific action. The cyclic AMP or other second messenger provides a variety of third messages: decreased potassium, depolarization of the area, increased calcium, increased AMP, and protein kinase activation. Esterase quickly reduces free cAMP to near zero. One mechanism for the last is the release of fully active kinase when cAMP binds to the receptor protein component of the inactive kinase complex (Gill and Garren, 1971). Each of these third messengers can again provide multiple nonspecific actions. Both the cyclase and kinases provide amplification of the initial message received. Cyclic AMP interacts with a number of proteins within the cell, and the final result depends upon the affinity (Jest and Rickenberg, 1971) and the compartmentalization of each with respect to the source of cAMP-protein. Protein kinase is activated when free cAMP combines reversibly with the regulatory kinase subunit R to free the catalytic subunit C as shown by Reimann *et al.* (1971):

$$R\text{-}C + cAMP \xrightarrow[\text{ATP}]{Mg^{++}} R\text{-}cAMP + C.$$

The protein kinases cascade with greatly increased amplification to affect a specific protein in the nucleus which then could provide an activated area of DNA in chromosomes. This activation could come from phosphorylated histones, as summarized by Greengaard and Costac (1970); present concepts suggest that phosphorylation of more acidic protein is necessary to provide specificity.

If a molecule activated the cell from the outside to increase pinocytosis, the vacuole would transport the molecule into the cell and activate the classic sequence with release of second and third messages near the nucleus. However, in order to move out of the vacuole before a lysosome merges with it, the hormone presumably goes through the "cell membrane" and should have the same effect even though it is inside the cell. The short existence of free cAMP due to esterase activity might be more effective if this message were released near the nucleus.

Another means of entering the cell or the nucleus appears to be through the endoplasmic reticulum. These tubes may reach from outside the cell, have interplay with the cell interior, and lead directly to the nucleus. Although this is a relatively long pathway, pulsation or other action in a dynamic cell could provide an effective transport system. This could be augmented by the rotation of the nucleus, slowly revolving in one direction while rotating along the cell membrane in the opposite direction. This action, noted in time-lapse photographs, could provide a pumping action by which material could be brought into or pushed out of the nucleus through the pores of the nuclear membrane and possibly through the tubules of the reticulum.

In summary, the different ways a hormone might enter into cell functions are a) to attach at a specific site on the membrane, b) to penetrate various layers of the double-layered membrane, c) to enter a pore, d) to enter the exterior opening of an endoplasmic reticulum or other tubule, e) to enter or send a membrane message through the protein lining of the edges of mosaics, f) to provide a special means, *i.e.*, specific carrier, or g) a combination of the above. Whatever the mode of entry, specificity of each target cell for a certain hormone is maintained, while the subsequent reaction series within the cell may be common to many types of target tissues. The resulting reaction (product) of the cell is preprogrammed by the previous differentiation of that cell.

Table 12.4. Effect of antigen on lymphocytes

1. Enhanced endocytosis.
2. Increased membrane phospholipid turnover.
3. Increased transport of adenosyl cyclase.
4. Cyclase activation.
5. Increased cAMP concentration.
6. Increased cAMP esterase activity.
7. Lysosomal alterations.
8. Nuclear changes, including histone acetylation, protein phosphorylation, and increased dye uptake by DNA.
9. Synthesis of new RNA, increased total RNA, and decreased ribosomal RNA degradation.
10. Protein synthesis and increased enzyme synthesis.
11. Increased enzyme activity, including RNA polymerase, purine kinases, and DNA polymerases.
12. Synthesis and/or elaboration of antibody and/or mediators of cellular immunity.
13. Increased cytotoxic activity by direct contact.
14. Redistribution of lysosomal enzymes.
15. Proliferation of Golgi apparatus, smooth endoplasmic reticulum, mitochondria, and lysosome.
16. Mitosis.
17. Division.
18. Increased number of cells producing specific antibody if antigen were present during the stimulation.

In antibody formation, the antigen acts as a signal, "hormone equivalent," for lymphocyte production. Actions noted upon lymphocyte activation by mitogens *in vitro* are much slower than those induced by thymic hormones and antigens *in vivo*. Events noted following stimulation have been listed by Wilson and Weissman (1971) and Cooper and Ginsburg (1971). Table 12.4 presents reactions noted.

Hypothetical thymic hormone actions

Rational speculation about the role of each compound isolated from the thymus and its place in the generalized hormone action leads to the following concepts. Starvation, irradiation, or other stress causes a decrease in total thymic size. The lymphocytes are the most labile cells within the thymus. The work of Comsa suggests that the hormone-producing cells are controlled in a pituitary feedback system. Excepting this and the increase in thymic hormones seen in lymphoma, there seems to be little effect of any external stimuli directly on the thymic parenchyma. The increment of thymus and thymic hormone is postnatal life and the eventual involution of the thymus must be major factors in controlling the quantity of thymic hormone produced. Effects from this change are seen clearly in newborn animals and indirectly in aged animals which have decreased immunologic competence. The thymic hormone rapidly confers to white cells immunologic competence which may last for their lifetime. Thus thymectomy of mature animals gives little detectable response for several weeks. This is atypical for hormones but not for cytocrines.

The molecular weights of LSH_r (80,000) and LSH_h (17,000) suggest that both of these compounds should meet with difficulty going through cell membranes. In a diagram of a classic cell membrane (Fig. 12.4), these compounds and probably thymosin would have an effect on the outer molecules of the membrane. If these and other thymic hormones act as classic hormones, the initiated cell reaction could continue with the activation of adenyl cyclase, production of cyclic AMP, and other secondary messengers. If each membrane mosiac unit must be affected, then each cell affected might be expected to utilize about 10^4 molecules.

However, the effect of thymic hormones upon lymphocytes is not expected to follow the classic hormone cell interaction; instead, there appears to be a permanent change effected in the cell by the first contact of the cell with the hormone. LSH increases lymph node and spleen cell populations as well as the development of individual lymphocyte types as judged by the increased L/P ratio. Lymphocytes touched by thymic hormones have a competence which they did not have before the hormones contacted them. The compounds cause differentiation. Presumably, this change is carried on through the clone of succeeding cells in peripheral lymphatic tissues. It is surprising that thymic hormones do not effectively penetrate bone marrow to activate bone marrow cells at their source. The major function of thymic hormones for lymphocytes appears to be the initiation of recognition for the next foreign protein. Thereafter, this specific antigen acts like a hormone for that particular cell; it becomes a specific signal for antibody synthesis. This concept will be pursued later.

Presumably, thymosin compounds could act comparably to those of the LSH series. They are active in establishing cell-mediated immunologic competence, while LSH compounds are active in conferring competence for antibody production. It may be anticipated that the two groups of compounds will be similar to each other when tested under comparable conditions.

The molecule of Tallberg and coworkers (1966, 1968) resembles LSH_r

in its physical characteristics. Although its biologic activities appear to be antagonistic, this cannot be assumed until the compounds have been tested under similar conditions. A small excess of LSH depresses antibody formation, is harmful to cells, and is toxic to mice.

HTH, with a molecular weight of approximately 2000, would be likely to pass into a cell. The carbohydrate and possible nucleic acid components would slow passage through the lipid layers. It may be attracted to the outer and/or the inner protein layers of the cell membrane or through the protein-coated edges of mosaics or pores. Since the thymus appears to have approximately 1000 times more HTH than LSH, it could be anticipated that HTH could act not only within the cell membrane but further down the chain of the hormone messenger complex. Using the cyclase system as a model of messenger enzyme cascade, one might anticipate that this molecule could act upon the esterase to inhibit cyclic AMP breakdown, upon a kinase, on messenger RNA, or within nuclear reactions. The fact that it is a small molecule and acts on the pituitary in a negative feedback system lends credence to the suggestion that it does indeed enter the cell and participate directly or indirectly in reactions concerned with protein synthesis at the levels of transcription or translation.

Thymosterin (Chapter 11) may penetrate and affect the multilayered portion of the cell membrane more readily, than the pores or mosaic edges. The physiologic relationships between prostaglandins and steroids is not yet clear. Prostaglandins A_1 and F_1 stimulate lymphocyte cyclase to increase intracellular cAMP (Franks, MacManus, and Whitefield, 1971). However, it could be anticipated that thymosterin will be associated with proteins and transported to the nucleus as are steroid hormones.

The small size of thymus humoral factor (THF) reported in Chapter 6 would allow penetration of cell walls. It is no greater in size than two cyclic nucleotides. Trainin's classic experiment shows that at least one of these compounds can be transferred to bone marrow cells *in vitro* to provide activation for recognition and to convey immunologic competence to these cells. Comparable effects have been reviewed for thymosin in cell-mediated immunity (Chapter 7). HTH has this capability in situations reviewed by Comsa in Chapter 4. One injection of nanogram quantities of LSH provides suckling mice with immune competence before natural competence is obtained (see Chapter 8). Therefore, all of the compounds examined thus far exhibit effects on one or more targets.

12.3 Thymic hormones in differentiation and cancer

Thymic hormones have all of the characteristics normally attributed to
most hormones; yet they do not entirely fit the criterion that a hormone is
essentially a signal which, when received by the cell, activates it to produce a given product until the message for that product has been utilized.
Classically, target cells are ready to respond a second time when a new
supply of hormone reaches them. This concept may fit the role of a thymic
hormone in its interaction with other endocrine glands. However, it does
not fit the role of the thymic compounds which affect immune competence.
Thymic hormones may activate a gene set for stem cell differentiation or
lymphocyte immune response equivalent to the action proposed for
juvenile hormone to control one gene set for pupation and another master
gene set for adulthood in insects (Williams, 1971). Resembling the sex
hormones or the juvenile hormone of insects, thymic hormones affect
cell development, differentiation, and maturation, while the role of
hormone or trigger is assumed by the antigen. Since the antigen is usually
from a different species, it represents the same general biologic class of
compounds as pheromones. In other words, it is an external molecule
which evokes a specific reaction from the host. This concept contributes
to later generalizations.

Thymic hormones resemble factors causing tissue differentiation, an
action expected within the close confines of a developing tissue. Thymic
hormones undoubtedly act on lymphocytes within the thymus and appear
to be exported to other tissues. Presumably the thymic hormones can
act on lymphocytes wherever the two occur in the same milieu, as
shown by the experiments of Trainin and coworkers in Chapter 6. Since
the spleen appears to have the second highest concentration of thymic
hormone in mammals, and nodes have the next highest concentration, it
is apparent that thymic hormone concentration correlates with the
mature lymphocyte population.

Maturation of stem cells and individual lymphocytes appear to be two
places where LSH functions as a differentiation factor. The changed L/P
ratios suggest this thymic hormone affects the development of stem cells
to provide a greater proportion of lymphocytes. Since LSH_r provides an
increase in total lymphocytes, a more basic cell type may also be affected;
however, this could reflect increased reproduction or decreased rate of
destruction of lymphocytes by physiologic levels of thymic hormone.

The direct action of some thymic compounds, notably thymosterin,
in tumor inhibition was noted. An indirect action is suggested for other

thymic hormones: surveillance as a means of cancer prevention. The well-known thymic involution with age is followed by immunologic senescence. Does this allow increased cancer with age? Walford and Yunis (1971) reported that antibody production was maximal in mice at 15 weeks of age and declined to 15% of this maximum response in 2 years. This decline was not related to a change in capabilities of bone marrow cells. They indicated that thymic-dependent immune responses decrease faster than does antibody production. When the ratio of time *in utero* to time of life was compared for a large variety of species (Luckey, 1965c), it was noted that the life expectancy of man and domestic animals was about twice that of wild species. This suggests that thymic activity is maintained throughout biologically determined life expectancy; a doubling of life expectancy in man allowed immunologic senescence to develop prior to our fourscore years. Thymus parenchyma waxes and wanes more by its innate time clock than does the tissue of other glands. Depressed hormone production would undoubtedly lead to a gradually decreased immune competence. The consequence of this decreased self-nonself discrimination could mean increased survival of new tumors. Thus, one genetic trait involved in cancer susceptibility is the involution pattern of the thymus with decreased production of thymic hormones and subsequent decline in immune competence. This part of cancer susceptibility could be determined by serum examination for the quantity of a circulating thymic hormone such as LSH_r. The potential for this cancer susceptibility test is presently being explored in our laboratory. A negative correlation would suggest a possible preventive therapy. Injection of thymic hormones into susceptible persons could conceivably enhance immune surveillance and prevent tumor establishment.

Thymic hormones induce recognition and antibody synthesis

It is clear that thymic hormones evoke immune competence in bone marrow cells. Without the thymus, B cells (naive lymphocytes) show no special response to certain particulate antigens. Following a pilgrimage to the thymus, reaction with a variety of injected thymic hormones, interaction with thymocytes, or a brief bath in thymic extract, B cells sequentially a) differentiate between self and nonself materials, b) respond to one, and usually only one, nonself macromolecule, c) produce a complement to that molecule, either the antibody or its cell membrane equivalent, and d) become passive to other antigenic molecules. Thymic hormones activate, in a receptive cell, a state of responsiveness which can be satisfied by any of a variety of antigens and not by those of the usual (self) environment. This general action may be important in differentiation during development and in other areas of biology, as discussed in the next sections. Some of the mechanisms suggested for this interaction were reviewed by Dutton *et al.* (1971). Although thymic hormone activation could be essential for the subsequent action of antigen in the cell or for the cell production of antibody, it first activates the cell to respond to the antigen by an initiation of recognition of nonself molecules in a manner distinctly different from a simple surface adsorption without this activation. Steward (1971) has shown that antigen is adsorbed to the surface of lymphocytes of thymectomized rats; no detectable antibody was made in the absence of the thymus. This allows much speculation.

The simplest place for the thymic hormone reaction to occur would be on the outer protein part of the membrane or in a combination of it with other parts. During formative stages, the cell was exposed to all elements of its surrounding (self) environment, and these molecules provided both the substance and milieu of the new cell. Large and small self-molecules reacted in a dynamic equilibrium with the cell membrane throughout its formation to form whatever unions were possible. These reactions must continue throughout the life of the cell as a permanent part of the cell membrane exchange with its pico environment. In the same manner, antigenic molecules enter into the membrane of cells; they attach and react according to their affinity and reactiveness with component parts of the membrane. To this extent they become a part of that membrane; this is usually described as adsorption by the cell. Steward (1971) showed that antigen adsorption occurred in measurable quantities in about one splenic lymphocyte per 10^4 cells with essentially no difference in adsorption whether or not the rats had been thymectomized. No specificity was shown. When a cell is activated by thymic hormone, a new receptiveness occurs. Now the next antigenic (usually macro-) molecule which contacts the cell is accepted into the inner functions of the cell; it is incorporated into the economy of the cell as a trigger or signal for the cellular production of its complement. The differentiated cell now a) assumes a stable membrane which will not usually react to other antigens, b) responds to a specific antigenic signal, c) produces a large amount of antibody which is complementary to that signal, d) either exports the antibody into the surrounding humors or incorporates it into significant areas of the cell membrane, and e) forms a clone which possesses this newly acquired complementarity and sensitivity to the subsequent presence of the antigen. This two-step reaction requires both thymic hormone activation and antigen attachment to or entry within the membrane. Antigen-RNA may represent antigen in these concepts.

Reasonable speculation on how this might occur can be made. Large molecules such as LSH_r must affect the outer protein coat of a cell membrane and probably become incorporated into it to change a relatively stable structure into one which has reactive sites having no special reactions with self molecules. Possibly this site is occupied by "native antibody," and LSH allows the attachment of the antigenic molecule. This attachment restabilizes the total membrane, and normally neither more hormone nor other antigenic molecules will reactivate this cell to other antigens. Thus, new cells must be available to react with other species of antigenic molecules.

The immunocompetent cell and its clone not only have new permanent recognition sites for the imprinted molecule, but that molecule has directed the protein-synthesizing system of the cell to make the complement of more of the same imprinting molecule. Concepts presented earlier in this chapter suggest that the antigen becomes the hormone or signal for the cellular production of its complement. Thus, the arrival of the antigen triggers the transmission of a signal, probably through cyclase (Table 12.3), for the production of antibody. Secondly, protein production directly or indirectly involves the specific antigen as template. Since the complement to the antigen is made, the antigen cannot provide the complete reversal of the protein synthesis dogma, *i.e.*, protein directs RNA synthesis which directs DNA synthesis and reverses to give the antibody molecule eventually because this could provide only more antigen. The antigen could send its complement from the membrane to activate RNA, but this entails making the complement *de novo* in or near the membrane. The antigen could also help derepress the specific DNA preprogrammed through phylogeny for each antigen; however, this complementarity would need translation (Fig. 12.5) by an antibody-RNA complex or its equivalent.

If the concept of preprogrammed antibody for each potential antigen (Aristotelian preformation) is correct, we would need a majority of our DNA committed to this function. If the recent hypothesis of Crick (1971) that the majority of DNA is involved in regulation and is not available for transcription is correct, then there is not enough genetic material to code for the great potential of antibodies possible and there is need for much epigenesis. Butler (1968) states that the number of genes would be insufficient to provide a separate gene for each antigen and suggests that combinations of a few thousand genes or protein chains would be ade-

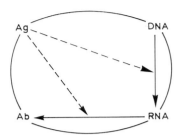

Fig. 12.5. Complementarity between immune structures.

quate. The increased overlapping found in antigen-antibody reactions suggests a simplification of read-out which may be based not upon 20 amino acids but upon common functional groups: a) free amino, b) free carboxyl, c) benzene ring, d) phenol, e) nonpolar chain, f) alcohol on side chain, g) sulfhydryl, h) methyl, i) histidyl, and j) indole.

Another solution to the genetic poverty problem may be a modified protein synthesis during m-RNA readout. Since peptides can form independently of m-RNA in certain peptide antibiotics, it is reasonable to suggest that bits of the variable portion of an antibody could be directed by a complementary protein, the antigen, with or without macrophage processing and RNA. Such a system, as Lipmann (1971) suggested, is intermediate between fatty acid synthesis and m-RNA-directed protein synthesis. In antibiotic synthesis, amino acid sequence is directed "by a protein template laid out on a polyenzyme system" (Lipmann, 1971). The major portion of the variable chains resembles the constant portion enough to suggest that a native antibody genome was interrupted during translation to give areas of variability which complement sites on the antigen. If the RNA-protein complex found in macrophages were found in antibody-producing plasma cells, such informosomes (Waddington, 1966) might conceivably allow the transition desired; the constant portion of antibody from the regular RNA template would be modified to give a variable portion from the antigen-complement template. This might involve obtaining antigen-m-RNA complex in the macrophage; it becomes more complex than protein-modified protein synthesis. Haurowitz (1970) suggested antigen-directed protein synthesis for the specific combining sites in antibody. When antigen is injected, several percent of the total lymphocytes in a lymph node appear to be activated to reproduce (the number doubles in less than 12 hr, Chapter 8), while only about one lymphocyte in a million produces antibodies specific to that antigen (Talmage, 1969). Antigens generally initiate reproduction in lymphocytes. Feldman (1970) indicated that replication is essential for both the primary and secondary responses in antibody production. Specific antibody production must come from a very few of the cells which replicate following antigen administration. This specificity indicates the small proportion of lymphocytes newly activated by thymic hormone in the primary immune response.

The hypothesis suggests that concepts of hormone action, second messengers, cascade amplification, and protein-directed protein synthesis may be useful to visualize the role of antigens in antibody formation.

Figure 12.5 suggests diagrammatically the interrelationships between antigen and antibody, antigen and RNA, and antigen and DNA, and the rough complementarity which exists in these four compounds. It is well established that constant-chain antibody is made in classic fashion: DNA → RNA → AB. Since antigen affects the production of a specific antibody, antigen may help derepress a preprogrammed gene and/or it may modify classic protein synthesis during the reading of the messenger RNA while an otherwise constant AB is being synthesized (Haurowitz, 1970). RNA-antigen from the macrophage or antigen itself may interrupt this reading to produce spots of antigen-active sites on the variable portions of antibody accomplished by a modification of the phylogenetic vestige of protein-directed protein synthesis seen in antibiotics (Lipmann, 1971). Both possibilities are indicated in the diagram, and both would have appropriate functions. Antigen-RNA complex could be effective in both.

The concept proposed is that one or a few genes of one class of lymphocytes are programmed for the peptide chains, constituting a complete "native antibody." During replication, these genes are unmasked and, to the extent of available molecules and energy, native (all constant chain) antibody is made until that gene is repressed. RNA attached to part of an antibody becomes a logical repressor; this would provide both the translation and complementarity which is otherwise missing for any antibody-gene interaction. Some native antibody is probably incorporated into the membrane. Feldman (1970) has shown specific antibody to be present in lymphocyte membranes.

Antigen from the environment specifically imprints itself upon the cell in several ways (Fig. 12.6): a) a discriminator is formed on the cell membrane; b) it signals the cell to activate protein production; c) it affects a component part of the protein-synthesizing apparatus of the cell; and

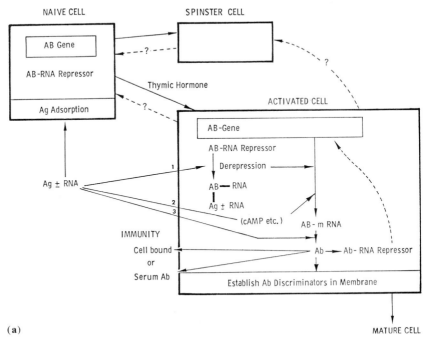

Fig. 12.6. Proposed antigen action on: a) naive and activated cells, and b) mature cells. Note that antigen and antibody may react at three places: a) at cell membranes in signal recognition; b) at the point of gene derepression; and c) at template perturbations during antibody synthesis when the general gene (AB) produces AB-mRNA which produces a specific, antibody (Ab). The complex may include RNA; *i.e.*, AB – RNA
$$\underset{\text{Ag} \pm \text{RNA}}{|}$$

d) it provides memory. Each could involve the antibody in the mature cell. This model for communication between environment and organism by way of molecular imprinting is most useful.

Signal recognition must be a function of the cell membrane and is specific for the one antigen which first becomes associated into that cell. The simplest concept would suggest that one main reaction provides the discriminator to the membrane-specific antibody and memory. The following is proposed (Fig. 12.6). a) Activation of lymphocyte by thymic hormone facilitates entrance of an antigen (and/or antigen fragment-RNA complex). This could be readily accomplished by thymic hormone reacting with a conjugated moiety to expose native antibody in the membrane. Antigen reacts with it. The Ag-AB complex (note the use of

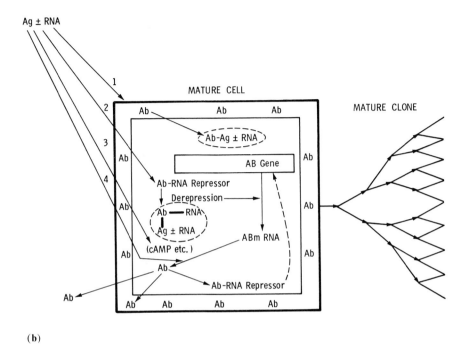

(b)

AB to indicate native antibody and Ab to indicate specific antibody)
allows more antigen to enter the cell. b) Antigen reacts with the AB-RNA
repressor of the immature cell, and the Ag-AB-RNA complex dere-
presses the AB gene and allows the production of AB-mRNA. c) The
production of AB is modified in a few places to produce variations in the
peptide chain; thus, native antibody (AB) is modified into specific antibody (Ab), as indicated previously. d) Antibody reacts with all the antigen
in the cell. e) Specific antibody incorporates into Ab-RNA repressor,
which now has specific affinity for the subsequent appearance of one
specific antigen (Ag). f) Specific antibody without the moiety reactive to
thymus hormone is incorporated into the cell membrane as discriminator
for the specific antigen. g) Antibody is exported into the serum by some
lymphocytes; others hold all antibody produced in the membrane for
cell-mediated immunity. Cell membrane native antibody (AB) could be
replaced by specific antibody (Ab) most readily during cell reproduction
in the presence of Ag when the cell is full of Ab. h) The clone is given

cytoplasmic Ab, Ab-RNA, and discriminator-Ab to provide specificity for a few subsequent generations. i) Subsequent appearance of the
specific antigen will neutralize the Ab discriminator to allow Ag into
the cell, where it will have high affinity for the Ab-RNA repressor and
renew the supply of antibody for each function. j) Activation of this
cell to reproduce in the absence of antigen may gradually decrease the
Ab supply. To this extent memory may be lost. Möller (1969) reviewed the
evidence for antibody repression of antibody production and the negative
feedback of antibody to restrict cell reproduction.

Antigens imprint memory. The lifetime immunity that follows various
infections suggests that an effective memory exists in certain lymphocytes.
What is the length of life of the memory cells, how is memory stored, and
how is memory passed to subsequent cell generations as a specific event?
One or more specific molecules must be involved. In order to find a
stable portion of the cell over a long period, the molecule might best
be stored intimately connected with the chromosome in a cell which
would be very slow in reproduction and remain quiescent until more
antigen appeared, as in the small lymphocyte. Ab-RNA repressor molecules provide specific memory molecules with compartmentalization to
protect them from many hydrolytic enzymes. When antigen triggers this
cell to respond, the specific antibody produced would replenish the Ab
supply, renew the membrane discriminator site, and adhere to the
chromosomal moiety following depression. This provides a teleologic
reason why usually only one antigen activates any given lymphocyte; if
more than one activated it, those antibodies not represented by antigen
during antibody synthesis would be lost. The mature cell uses specific
antibody as the memory molecule at the levels of both membrane discrimination and AB gene repression. Proposed multiple functions of
thymic hormone (LSH) and antigen in immunity are summarized in
Figure 12.7. This is a model for one type of molecular imprinting which
provides for both specific cell reaction and memory from a foreign
molecule.

12.4 Generalization: communication by molecular imprinting

Communication by molecular imprinting is the utilization by the cell
of one or more specific molecules in the organism-environment interchange. Molecular imprint communication suggests that memory systems
may be constituted of molecules and/or their arrangement to provide the
organism's interpretation of its environment and memory of previous

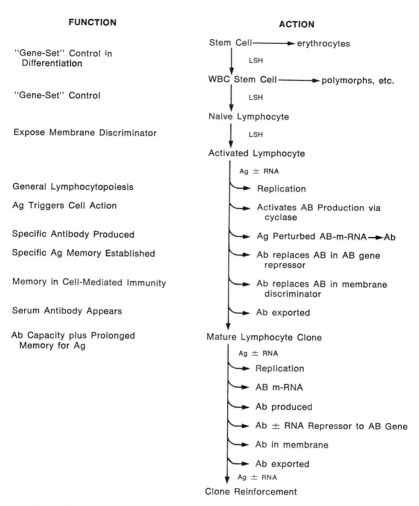

FUNCTION   **ACTION**

"Gene-Set" Control in
Differentiation

"Gene-Set" Control

Expose Membrane Discriminator

General Lymphocytopoiesis

Ag Triggers Cell Action

Specific Antibody Produced

Specific Ag Memory Established

Memory in Cell-Mediated Immunity

Serum Antibody Appears

Ab Capacity plus Prolonged
Memory for Ag

Stem Cell ⟶ erythrocytes
        LSH
WBC Stem Cell ⟶ polymorphs, etc.
        LSH
Naive Lymphocyte
        LSH
Activated Lymphocyte
    Ag ± RNA
    ⟶ Replication
    ⟶ Activates AB Production via
       cyclase
    ⟶ Ag Perturbed AB-m-RNA ⟶ Ab
    ⟶ Ab replaces AB in AB gene
       repressor
    ⟶ Ab replaces AB in membrane
       discriminator
    ⟶ Ab exported
Mature Lymphocyte Clone
    Ag ± RNA
    ⟶ Replication
    ⟶ AB m-RNA
    ⟶ Ab produced
    ⟶ Ab ± RNA Repressor to AB Gene
    ⟶ Ab in membrane
    ⟶ Ab exported
    Ag ± RNA
Clone Reinforcement

Fig. 12.7. Proposed functions of LSH and antigen in immunity. Note the use of *AB* for native, nonspecific antibody and *Ab* for specific antibody. Ab–Ag affinity must be much greater than AB−Ag affinity.

organism-environment interchange. The most primitive form of this communication system is chemotaxis and must include at least a part of differentiation. Most bacteria and plants which feed primarily by osmotic processes provide a well-defined cell wall to exclude nonself particles, macromolecules, and other cells. Once endocytosis becomes established in an organism, other defense mechanisms must develop to identify itself from nonself. This recognition of foreignness has been discussed by Burnet and Fenner (1949) and Nossal and Ada (1964). Understanding of this discrimination is immunology. Indistinct as immunologic mechanisms may be, they provide a useful model for a generalized consideration of how cells and organisms communicate with each other and their environment. The concept may be broadened, with adequate documented research, to be considered a general theory of biology.

Three distinct types of communication are evident. First is the direct communication in which a molecule or particle from the environment is taken into the organism and reacts directly with one or more cells; immune reactions and probably chemotaxis are the prototypes of this form. Modifications include the molecular interplay between cells within the same organism; hormones and differentiation inducers represent this modification. The first type is nonsensual; the second is sensual. The second type involves a molecular interpretation of the environment's message by intermediate cells. Environmental changes effect light, odor, or other sensing cells which send a message to information storage cells within the brain. This communication class is characterized by the variety of specialized cells working as one unit: the different kinds of sensory cells, message-carrying cells with their long axons, ganglia coordinator cells, brain storage cells, and many auxiliary types of cells. Memory storage cells provide the focus for later discussion. The third type of communication is cerebration. It ignores the environment and becomes cell-cell interaction within the brain. It is a modification of the second category in which direct involvement of the environment is excluded; indirectly it may be represented by memory. In all three types, molecules within a cell or on the cell membrane are affected, and memory can result.

In order to avoid using descriptive phrases, general terms useful for molecular imprint communication are suggested in Table 12.5. The prototype for this generalization is primarily immunology. *Xenogen* (from the Greek *xeno*, stranger) designates the nonself molecule which has entered the organism. *Xenospond* (the verb) comes from the above with the suffix from the Greek *sponde*, the plural for treaty. The xenogen includes antigens, odor and taste molecules, pheromones, and other *semiochemicals*. The xenogen enters the organism, and the xenosponse is the reaction of one or more molecules which incorporates some image of that xenogen. A molecule made or altered by the organism in response to the presence of the xenogen may be called a *homule* (a combination of the Greek,

Table 12.5. General terms useful for molecular imprint communication

Specific example	General term	General meaning
Antigen, pheromone	Xenogen	A nonself molecule inside the organism.
Antibody production	Xenosponse	The generalized response to a xenogen to produce a homule.
Antibody	Homule	A molecule made in response to the presence of the xenogen.
Hormone, choline esterase	Homogen	A molecule produced in the organism which acts equivalent to a xenogen.
Photophobin production	Karasponse	The response to a sensation by central nerve cells to produce a karule.
Memory molecule	Karule	A molecule made in response to a sensation or a set nervous expression.

homos, meaning self, with the suffix *ule*). A homule reflects the molecular and particulate input of the environment into the organism. Indirect communication, in which the environment is interpreted, starts with a sensing cell and subsequent transmission of the message leads to the production of a *karule* in the brain cell. A karule may be a molecule altered, as RNA may be altered in learning (Hyden and Lang, 1970), synthesized, as photophobin of Ungar and Fjerdingstad (1971), and/or numerically increased, as dendrites become more complex or synapses become "strengthened." The prefix *kara* is from the Greek, meaning head. The sensing cells must work through a transmission which limits the kinds of chemical and physical events transmitted to the brain from the nervous cell. Therefore, the memory molecule of the brain must be an interpretation system on a spatial arrangement of cells and/or compartmentalized dendrites. It is also possible that the karule will vary with the intensity of the nervous response and with the number of cells or dendrites affected in the immediate environment. *Karasponse* is the response to a sensation that results in the production of a karule.

Some general characteristics of molecular imprint communication can be discerned. The organism, cell, or cell compartment must acquire an activated state for fast imprinting. Activation may be a cell surface phenomenon brought about by differentiation inducers. The diagrams (Fig. 12.6 a and b) suggest immune concepts; general terms could have been used, and perhaps dendrite may be substituted for cell to contemplate cerebral functions. The cell is unreactive before contact with the differentiating factor. The time that a cell membrane can remain in the activated state has not been determined. This time must be relatively short; the cell probably becomes a spinster cell if it does not respond while activated. This information could readily be obtained in immunology; the short time is noted in psychologic imprinting. Second, the first xenogen (Ag ± RNA) to enter the pico environs is accepted as a discrimination model for the cell and subsequently becomes the signal for cell production to begin, probably via the second messenger routine (Table 12.3). The xenogen stimulates formation of a memory system which can be transmitted to a clone. This xenosponse indicates that a permanent specific receptiveness is established between the cell and the xenogen. Attachment of the xenogen stabilized the cell surface with recognition sites which now react only to that specific xenogen or closely related molecules. The xenogen next induces the cell to form a permanent production of a homule, an antibody, or some less directly complementary molecule. The major product will be preprogrammed. Molecular interpretation of the environmental message may be made by an intermediate cell. This indirect molecular imprinting usually involves a chemical simplification of the signal. This role is played by the macrophage in some immune reactions to provide Ag-RNA complex; this role is of prime importance in sensual communication. Significant development may have occurred with the increased specialization for communication by brain neurons. Predictably, these specialized cells with thousands of individual dendrites could provide intracellular compartmentalization and communication which could represent a sizeable savings in numbers of cells involved in recording complex sensations. Each synapse compartment could produce a peptide or other molecule as multiple components of a tremendously increased total cell versatility; each could be equivalent to a single less-specialized cell in other systems, as in the immune response.

12.5 Biologic implications of molecular imprint communication

Biologic implications of molecular imprint communication will be considered in three categories previously considered from a functional viewpoint: a) nonsensual or direct; b) sensual or indirect; and c) cerebral. Communication with the environment is one of the characteristics of life and is a major function of all organisms. Some involve a large proportion of their body for this activity, *i.e.*, the nervous system plus the special sensing cells plus lymphocytes. Many communication systems must exist, some have been delineated, and a few have components which are well studied. Each has a physical-chemical basis recorded as new or modified molecules in cells and reflects a change in the environment. Information about one may be useful in understanding others and a possible common phylogenetic basis.

Immunology

Molecular imprinting as a means of nonsensual communication between organism and environment rests upon known immunologic facts. The role of macrophage as a nonspecific sometime helper (Nossal and Ada, 1971) suggests the phylogenetic origin of indirect systems. When immunologic memory was compared with induced enzyme synthesis, Talmage (1969) noted that immunologic memory had an almost infinite variety, was much longer lasting, and could be either positive or negative. Hirschborn (1966) suggests that lymphocyte stimulation and reaction to one antigen is representative of other cellular events, such as fertilization of sea urchin eggs. The enhancement of antibody formation by added cyclic AMP suggested to Ishizuka *et al.* (1970) the similarity between immunologic and hormonal events. The function of thymic hormones to induce a state of activation in the continuously renewed lymphocyte population could be a general concept for the induction of recognition. Implications of this concept for other biologic phenomena provide new understandings of the full implications of immunology and return immunology to the mainstream of biology.

Endocrinology

Endocrine glands react to one specific molecule among thousands in their immediate environment. Molecular imprinting following the induction of recognition supplies one answer to the question of how such a cell is capable of responding to one specific signal. By analogy a differentiation factor, such as thymic hormone, could induce recognition of the homogen (hormone in this case) by activating the virgin target cell to react to new molecules in its environment. The homogen is imprinted into the cell and subsequently is the signal for that cell to produce. Once the specificity is established, subsequent transmission and amplification of the signal seems to involve a few common systems; *i.e.*, cyclase → cAMP → active kinases → RNA → protein → "everything else."

In endocrinology, target cells must be introduced to "their" hormone at an appropriate state of each newly differentiated cell. This induction of recognition may be brought about by differentiation factors equivalent to thymic hormones as previously outlined. During ontogeny of an endocrine gland, the supply of new cells would provide a relatively broad "time window" to encompass the time that the homogen (the hormone) first appeared in its milieu. Although this hormone is made by the organism, its first appearance provides the conditions needed to make it become the specific signal for those cells recently activated. These cells have products different from those of lymphocytes or muscle cells because their developmental background is different. Thus a single hormone signals the production of different specific compounds from cells of different tissues. Clones from the differentiated cells would be expected to respond to the same hormone as did the parent cell. Both membrane recognition site and repressor may involve a complement (antibody-like) molecule.

Differentiation

The proposed action of thymic hormones to initiate a state of receptiveness in naive cells may be one explanation for the development of immune competence in lymphocytes and for the initiation of hormone response in target cells. This is differentiation. Comparable phenomena could occur for cells of any developing organism; when an activated state is induced in cells, they incorporate a new portion of the changing molecular environment into their structure to provide the trigger for functional capability. This change may provide the new milieu needed for the next activated cell to react to a different stimulus and to produce different products. Such a sequential cascade of new products provides the changing molecular basis for continuous differentiation of a developing tissue or organism. These cell products are not species-specific (Moscona, 1971). The acceptance of each imprinted molecule provides a new orientation for cells in the ontogeny of the individual. Some compounds which induce differentiation appear to be proteins (Tiedemann, 1967). These cause one-way development in cell-cell interactions.

Molecular imprinting in parasitology

Molecular imprinting may explain the choosing by a freely moving parasite of a particular host for feeding or egg laying. Hypothetically, a xenogen from the host would be imprinted into the parasite at hatch. Although literature search revealed no evidence for this mechanism, such induction of recognition would be simple to study. Read (1970) noted animal parasites which infect only one of two closely related species in nature; when both were fed the same food in the laboratory, both were readily infected. He stated, "a symbiont can always live in more species of hosts than the number in which it is found in nature."

Molecular imprinting by pheromones

Most of the comments about molecular imprinting by antigens could be made about pheromones and other semiochemicals. Different organisms provide the xenogens. Since pheromones are usually small molecules, they might combine with a protein for their specific action on cells. The simple lipid structure of many pheromones suggests that they might function as primitive prostaglandin moieties. The imprinting of sex attractants may be equivalent to what affects the parasitic host for egg laying (*i.e.*, wasps in specific spider species); insects were previously imprinted from compounds of the respective parent or host egg. Immunologic paralysis suggests why mature female insects are not attracted to their own sex pheromones. The review by Law and Regnier (1971) suggests that pheromones and other semiochemicals usually provide olfactory or gustatory sensations. Thus, they act through indirect imprinting. A broad view of the chemicals, allelochemics, used for interactions between species is reviewed by Whittaker and Feeny (1971).

Molecular imprinting in homing instincts

Homing instincts, as seen in fish, may be explained by molecular imprinting. The extensive development in fish of taste for food and of smell for social functions has been examined by Todd (1971). Fish with hundreds of thousands of taste buds through the epidermis are provided guidance by remarkably few molecules from the environment. Since both this and the tremendously specialized olfactory sense in bullheads have a central nervous component, these functions must be related to molecular imprinting of memory, considered later. Gurim and Carr (1971) found 10^{-10} molar concentration of a glycoprotein was stimulatory for chemoreception in marine snails. They noted the analogy between hormone binding to target organs and the binding specificity of xenogens to receptor membranes.

Differences exist between molecular imprinting in parasitology and homing. Homing requires a sequence of molecules involved as the young

travel, whereas parasitology and possibly pheromones and other semiochemicals would require primarily a single source imprinting. This impact
imprinting resembles psychologic imprinting.

Psychologic imprinting

The psychologic attachment of young ducks and other mobile neonatal
animals to any well-impressed (by movement and sound) object suggests
this phenomenon has an indirect molecular imprinting component. Hess
(1959) found that neontal imprinting reaches a peak 12 hr following
birth or hatch and that it recedes to zero in the 1-day-old animal. The
term "puppy love" applied to youth suggests that psychologic imprinting
is unique to neither birds nor canines. It suggests that there are special
receptive occasions when psychologic or emotional attachments may be
readily made; love at first sight suggests such an imprinting. This state of
special receptiveness resembles the initiation of recognition clearly seen
in the activation of lymphocytes when immune competence was conferred.

Young ducks probably begin "sound imprinting" prior to hatch, according to Hess (1972), who also noted the importance of activation: "the
parental behavior of the female mallard is primed by certain neuro-
endocrine mechanisms" in response to the sounds of the hatching duck-
ling.

Emotional-psychologic imprinting in certain species climaxes rapidly
when a mother goat or sheep establishes her attachment to neonatally
mobile offspring shortly after parturition. Mother love is imprinted in
5 min in goats. Klopfer (1971) proposed that the appearance of oxytoxin
or a hormonal imbalance at parturition activates a sensory (odor) basis
for recognition of young in the goat. This imprinting window has a half-
life of less than 30 min postpartum. If no contact with the kid is made
during the first hour following parturition, few mothers will accept young.
This evidence was used to formulate that part of the general thesis which
suggested that the activated state was short-lived.

Is activation for psychologic imprinting triggered by unusual excite-
ment or stress when a given event is "burned into memory"?

Cortical imprinting and memory

"How and where does the brain store its memories? This a great mystery"
(Ladik and Greguss, 1971). The finding that new RNA (presumably
messenger) or specific peptides in animals with learned responses can be

transferred (Golub *et al.*, 1971; Ungar and Fjerdingstad, 1971) suggests that sensations can evoke the production and/or storage of specific compounds in brain cells which are specific to the concept learned. Since this might include intellectual activity, the concept of outside influence may be extended to a self-feeding system within the brain. This is similar to imprinting in endocrinology and differentiation. Other concepts of memory molecules (karules) of considerable complexity and/or spatial arrangement in, on, and/or between telodendron membranes were reviewed by Schmitt, Samson, and Irwin (1970). These include mucopolysaccharides (Adey, 1969), mosaics in the membrane and intercellular space, specific glycoproteins (Barondes, 1968, 1970) with the secreted carbohydrate moiety responsible for specificity of message for any given neuron, and glycoprotein-ganglioside complexes (Bogoch, 1969). Emphasis upon an intercellular matrix finds support from the need to add gangliosides to provide maximum *in vitro* responsiveness to cerebral cortex slices and isolated neurons (Hillman and Hyden, 1965). This extension of membrane into the intercellular space, the synaptosomes, was studied by radioglucosamine incorporation into synaptosome protein (Barondes, 1968). Anatomical concepts of the cells of the central nervous system suggest a multifunctional cell; each synapse may be a separate mosaic of the cell membrane and may be compartmentalized so that each provides the equivalent communication of a whole cell in less highly developed tissue. An analogy is seen in reticular cells which trap antigen in dendritic processes (Mitchell and Abbott, 1965; McDevitt *et al.*, 1966). Rasmussen (1970) indicated common modalities in hormonal and nervous message transmission between cells; both involve small molecule release and uptake.

In memory, no external molecule directly contacts the brain cell; thus the stored molecule, the karule, was made in response to a set of nerve impulses. The placement of these within different areas of brain, the immediate reactions of the cells about them, and the number of single cell synapses in synchronous action could give a great variety of conditions for the synthesis of different compounds or of similar compounds in different loci. The reaction of the target-sensing organ may be outlined as indicated in Table 12.3. Since the brain has the body's highest concentration of adenyl cyclase, Greengaard and Costa (1970) suggest that synaptic transmissions are facilitated by cAMP. Miller, Gorman, and Bitensky (1971) have found both cyclase and phosphodiesterase in the outer segments of retinal photoreceptor cells. Inactivation of the cyclase produces effects equivalent to bleaching of the rhodopsin, and application of cAMP plus methylxanthine minimizes the effects of illumination in *Limulus* photoreceptor cells.

Since brain cells are not continually renewed as are lymphocytes, the memory stored could last long in cell compartments storing each karule. Since new cells are not continuously available for induction of the activated state, brain cells may be open to recognition at all times. This would be facilitated by the fact that xenules are not involved. However, the variety of impulses must act as different xenules. Thus learning supplies the equivalent of a xenule and produces a response of homules in groups of cells or dendrites involved (possibly depending upon the complexity and intensity of the perception). If the signal for recall is required to resupply homules, it must come from the common denominator of new impulses.

12.6 Summary

In summation, the mammalian thymus produces a variety of stimulatory and inhibitory compounds which are important in differentiation, immunology, endocrinology, calcium regulation, cell growth, and metabolism. Those compounds studied disappear from serum, spleen, lymph nodes, and urine within a few days following thymectomy. Other tissues examined contain zero to 1% as much activity as the thymus.

Thymosterin is a steroid derivative which inhibits tumor growth *in vitro* and *in vivo* and plays a protective role in X-radiation. Lipid extract with high quantities of thymosterin stimulates antibody formation and lymphocytopoiesis. HTH, the homeostatic hormone of Comsa, contains amino sugars and amino acids and possibly a nucleotide within a structure of 2,000 molecular weight. It replaces thymus for many functions and can best be understood endocrinologically as a permissive factor in endocrine functions, particularly in the negative feedback control to the hypo-thyalmic-pituitary complex from other endocrines. It is antagonistic to glucocorticoids and thyroxine and enhances some pituitary hormone activity, *i.e.*, growth hormone. Preliminary experiments indicate that it is active immunologically. THF, the thymic humoral factor being isolated by Trainin, Small, and Kimhi, is less than 1,000 in molecular weight and is active in lymphocytopoiesis and cell-mediated immunity. It evokes immune competence in bone marrow cells bathed in solutions for 1 to

2 hr. It was not found in spleen or lymph nodes. The most purified thymosin preparations appear to contain three proteins of 10,000 to 70,000 in molecular weight. This material is active in cell-mediated immunity. LSH, a lymphocyte-stimulating hormone, appears to be a complex of several compounds with overlapping activity. LSH_h is a heat-labile protein of about 17,000 molecular weight. LSH_r appears to be a conjugated protein four times larger than LSH_h; both compounds increase the lymphocyte to polymorph ratio and, when injected into neonatal mice, confer the capability for antibody synthesis.

Thymic hormone appears to induce a state of active recognition in lymphocytes. Previously ignored surface-absorbed antigens are incorporated into antibody formation, possibly as derepressors and site templates. It was proposed that specific antibody is incorporated into structures which depend upon specificity of molecule identification in immunity. This is possible in a membrane discriminator or an antibody component of a gene repressor and could include a cell reproduction inhibitor. Each would be neutralized by the next entry of specific antigen. Thymic hormone induces differentiation and maturation in lymphocytes; thereafter antigen acts as an external signal to a particular group of cells to produce antibody.

This immunologic concept was generalized to provide a communication theory between an organism and its environment. The general mechanism is molecular imprinting in certain host cells. In direct imprinting, molecules, particles, or cells from the environment enter the organism to form a permanent response pattern within activated cells. The prime example is the immune response. Indirect imprinting involves the interaction of a third cell to interpret the signal from the environment. The macrophage may be a component of this system. Examples of indirect imprinting which involve activated cells include the pheromones which are well studied in insects, mechanisms of parasite choice of host, and the homing instinct of fish which may operate through olfactory sensing of waterways.

Neonatal imprinting and mother love imprinting are activated through sight and odor, respectively. These provide impact memory at special times in the life of the organism. Environmental stimuli are translated by sensor cells which send chemical messages to the brain. Synapses within brain cells form molecules which become the imprinted memory. In learning from thinking, both stimuli and response come from within the brain; this is comparable to the molecular imprinting of a target cell by the hormone during the formative period of the target tissue. Such is the course of differentiation. The collation of these concepts gives immunology a broad impact on biology. Elucidation of the generalized concept of molecular imprint communication promises another exciting decade of research.

Literature Cited

Abderhalden, E. 1926. Uber das Wesen der Wirkung der Verfutterung von Thymusgewebe auf Washstum und Entwicklung von Froschlarven. Pfluegers Arch. 211:324–332.

Abelous, J. E., and Billard, A. 1896. Recherches sur les fonctions du thymus. Arch. Physiol. Norm. Path. 28:898–907.

Abraham, A. D. 1971. Evidence of steroid biosynthesis in the thymus of white rat using (1^{-14}C) acetate and 4^{-14}C) cholesterol as precursors. Rev. Roum. Endoc. (Symposium sur le Thymus, Cluj., Roumanie, 1969).

Abramoff, A., and LaVia, M. 1970. Biology of the immune response. McGraw-Hill, New York.

Ackerman, G. A. 1967. Developmental relationship between the appearance of lymphocytes and lymphopoietic activity in the thymus and lymph nodes of the fetal cat. Anat. Rec. 158:387–399.

Adey, W. R. 1969. Neural information processing; windows without and the citadel within, pp. 1–33. In L. D. Proctor (ed.), Biocybernetics of the central nervous system. Little Brown, Boston.

Adinolfi, M., and Humphrey, J. 1969. Immunology and development. William Heinemann, Medical Books, Ltd., London.

Adler, H. 1937. Thymus und Myasthenie. Arch. Klin. Chir. 189:529–532.

Adler, H. 1938. Thymusfunktion und Nebenniesen. Dtsch. Z. Chir. 252: 241- 247.

Adler, H. 1938. Hypofunktion des Thymus als Visache von Myotonic und Darmin-vagination. Dtsch. Z. Chir. 252:658–663.

Adner, M. M., Sherman, J. D., and Dameshek, W. 1965. The normal development of the lymphoid mass in the golden hamster and its relationship to the effect of thymectomy. Blood 25:511–521.

Agnew, H. D. 1967. Immunologic restoration of neonatally thymectomized rats with thoracic duct lymphocytes. Proc. Soc. Exp. Biol. Med. 125: 132–142.

Aisenberg, A. C. 1962. Studies on delayed hypersensitivity in Hodgkin's disease. J. Clin. Invest. 41:1964–1970.

Aisenberg, A. C. 1966. Manifestations of immunologic unresponsiveness in Hodgkin's disease. Cancer Res. 26:1152–1160.

Aisenberg, A. C. and Davies, C. 1968. The thymus and recovery of the sheep erythrocyte response in irradiated mice. J. Exp. Med. 128:1327–1338.

Aisenberg, A. C. and Wilkes, B. 1965. Partial immunological restoration of neonatally thymectomized rats with thymus-containing diffusion chambers. Nature 205:716–717.

Aisenberg, A. C., Wilkes, B., and Waksman, B. H. 1962. The production of runt disease in rats thymectomized at birth. J. Exp. Med. 116:759–772.

Aldrich, R. A., Steinberg, A. C., and Campbell, D. C. 1954. Pedigree demonstarting sex-linked recessive condition characterized by draining ears, eczematoid dermatitis and bloody diarrhea. Pediatrics 13:133–139.

Allen, R. J. L. 1940. The estimation of phosphorus. Biochem. J. 34:858–865.

Allibone, E. O., Goldie, W., and Marmion, B. P. 1964. Pneumocystis carinii pneumonia and progressive vaccinia in siblings. Arch. Dis. Child. 39: 26–34.

Allison, A. C., and Taylor, R. B. 1967. Observations on thymectomy and carcinogenesis. Cancer Res. 27:703–707.

Ambrose, C. T. 1964. The requirement for hydrocortisone in antibody-forming tissue cultivated in serum-free medium. J. Exp. Med. 119:1027-1049.

Amos, B. 1971. Progress in immunology. Academic Press, New York. 1554 p.

Anderson, D. H. 1932. Studies on the physiology of reproduction. I. The effect of thymectomy and of season on the age and weight at puberty in the female rat. J. Physiol. 74:49–64.

Anigstein, L., Anigstein, D. M., Rennels, E. G., and O'Steen W. K. 1966. Induced alternation of resistance to transplantable mammary adenocarcinoma in mice neonatally inoculated with rat thymus antiserum. Cancer Res. 26:1867–1971.

Archer, O.K. and Pierce, J. C. 1961. Role of the thymus in development of the immune response. Fed. Proc. 20:26.

Arnason, B. G., deVaux St. Cyr, C., and Grabar, P. 1963. Immunoglobulin abnormalities of the thymectomized rat. Nature 199:1199–1200.

Arnason, B. G., de Vaux St. Cyr, C., and Relyveld, H. E. 1964. Role of the thymus in immune reactions in rats. Arch. Allergy Appl. Immunol. 25: 206.

Arnason, B. G., de Vaux St. Cry, C., and Shaffner, J. B. 1964. A comparison of immunoglobulins and antibody production in the normal and thymectomized mouse. J. Immunol. 93:915–925.

Arnason, B. G., Jankovic, B. D., and Waksman, B. H. 1964. The role of the thymus in immune reactions in rats, pp. 492–501. In R. A. Good and A. E. Gabrielsen (eds.), The thymus in immunobiology: Structure, function and role in disease. Hoeber-Harper, New York.

Arnason, B. G., Jankovic, B. D., Waksman, B. H., and Wennersten, C. 1962. Role of the thymus in immune reactions in rats. II. Suppressive effect of thymectomy at birth on reactions of delayed (cellular) hypersensitivity and the circulating small lymphocyte. J. Exp. Med. 116:177–186.

Arvin, G. C., and Allen, H. E. 1928. Variations in weight of thymus glands following administration of ovarian hormone and anterior hypophysis. Anat. Rec. 38:39.

Asanuma, Y., Goldstein, A. L., and White, A. 1970. Reduction in the incidence of wasting disease in neonatally thymectomized CBA/W mice by the injection of thymosin. Endocrinology 86:600–610.

Asher, D. 1933. Weitere Isolierung des Wachstumsfordernden Thymocrescins. Biochem. Z. 257:209–212.

Asher, L. and Landolt, E. 1934. Die Wirkung der Thymusexstripation auf das Wachstum bei vitaminarmer Nahrung. Pfluegers Arch. 234:605–613.

Asher, L., and Scheinfinkel, N. 1929. Untersuchungen uber den Einfluss eines gereinigten Thymus praparates auf die Muskelermudung. Endokrinologie 4:241–248.

Askonas, B. A., and White, R. G. 1956. Site of antibody production in the guinea pig. The relation between *in vitro* synthesis of anti-ovalbumin and γ-globulin and distribution of antibody-containing plasma cells. Brit. J. Exp. Pathol. 37:61–74.

Aspinall, R. L., Meyer, R. K., Graetzer, M. A., and Wolfe, H. R. 1963. Effect of thymectomy and bursectomy on the survival of skin homografts in chickens. J. Immunol. 90:872–877.

Auerbach, R. 1960. Morphogenetic interactions in the development of the mouse thymus gland. Dev. Biol. 2:27–84.

Auerbach, R. 1961. Experimental analysis of the origin of cell types in the development of the mouse thymus. Dev. Biol. 3:336–354.

Auerbach, R., and Globerson, A. 1966. *In vitro* induction of the graft-*versus*-host reaction. Exp. Cell Res. 42:31–41.

August, C. S., Levey, R. H., Berkel, A. I., Rosen, F. S., and Kay, H. E. M. 1970. Establishment of immunological competence in a child with congenital thymic aplasia by a graft of fetal thymus. Lancet 1:1080–1083.

August, C. S., Rosen, F. S., Filler, R. M., Janeway, C. A., Markowski, B., and Kay, H. E. M. 1968. Implantation of a fetal thymus, restoring immunological competence in a patient with thymic aplasia (DiGeorge's Syndrome). Lancet 2:1210–1211.

Azar, H. A. 1964. Bacterial infection and wasting in neonatally thymectomized rats. Proc. Soc. Exp. Biol. Med. 116:817–823.

Azar, H. A., Williams, J., and Takatsuki, K. 1964. Development of plasma cells and immunoglobins in neonatally thymectomized rats, pp. 75–87. *In* V. Defendi and D. Metcalf (eds.), The thymus. The Wistar Institute, Philadelphia.

Babes, V. T., Badescu, D., Mreana, G., Petrescu, A., and Potop, I. 1971. L'Effet stimulateur des extraits thymiques (B et TP) sur les cellules de la rate, anti-corps-formatrices. Rev. Roum. Endocr. (in press).

Babes, V. T., Rutter, G., Badescu, D., Babes, B. A., and Potop, I. 1970. Studiul raspunsului imunitar in gripa experimentala sub influenta unor extracte de timus. I. Studiul anticorpilor serici HAI la hamsteri. Stud. Cercet. Inframicr. 21:3–6.

Bach, J. F., Dardenne, M., Goldstein, A. L., Guha, A., and White, A., 1971. Appearance of T-cell markers in bone marrow rosette-forming cells after incubation with thymosin, a thymic hormone. Proc. Natl. Acad. Sci. U.S.A. 68:2734–2738.

Bachmann, H. 1934. Fortgesetzte Untersuchungen uber die Wirkungsweise des Thymocrescins. Biochem. Z. 268:272–284.

Bachmann, R. 1965. Studies on the serum γ-A-globulin level. III. The frequency of A-γ-A-globulinemia. Scand. J. Clin. Lab. Invest. 17:316–320.

Bachra, B. N., Dauer, A., and Sobel, A. E. 1958. The complexometric titration of micro and ultramicro quantities of calcium in blood serum, urine and inorganic salt solutions. Clin. Chem. 4:107–119.

Ball, W. D., and Auerbach, R. 1960. *In vitro* formation of lymphocytes from embryonic thymus. Exp. Cell Res. 20:245–247.

Balner, H. 1970. Immunosuppression and neoplasia. Rev. Europ. Etudes Clin. Biol. 15:599–602.

Balner, H., and Dersjant, H. 1966. Neonatal thymectomy and tumor induction with methylcholanthrene in mice. J. Natl. Cancer Inst. 36:513–521.

Barclay, T. J. 1964. Discussion of thymic function, pp. 117–119. *In* V. Defendi and D. Metcalf (eds.), The thymus. The Wistar Institute, Philadelphia.

Barondes, S. H. 1968. Incorporation of radioactive glucosamine into macromolecules at nerve endings. J. Neurochem. 15:699–706.

Barondes, S. H. 1970. Two sites of synthesis of macromolecules in neurons. *In* S. H. Barondes (ed.), Cellular dynamics of the neuron, Vol. 8. International Society Cellular Biology, Academic Press, New York. 383 p.

Basch, K. 1906. Beitrage zur Physiologie und Pathologie der thymus. Jahrb Kinderheilk 64:285–335.

Basch, R. S. 1966. Immunologic competence after thymectomy. Int. Arch. Allergy Appl. Immunol. 30:105–119.

Beauvieux, Y. J. 1963a. Apports experimentaux a la physiologie du thymus. Presse Med. 71:1367–1370.

Beauvieux, Y. J. 1963b. Donnees experimentales sur l'un des aspects de la physiologie du thymus. C. R. Acad. Sci. (Paris) 256:2914–2917.

Bedo, K., Horvath, M., Losonczi, V. L., Laszlo, J., Szollosi, A., and Balint, E. 1971. Stimulating and inhibiting effects of the borine thymus extracts. Rev. Rom. d'Endocrin. 8:89–90.

Benedict, E. B., Putnam, T. J., and Teel, H. M. 1930. Early changes produced in dogs by injections of sterile active extract from anterior lobe of hypophysis. Am. J. Med. Sci. 179:489–497.

Berek, L., Bános, Z., Szeri, I., Anderlik, P. and Aszodi, K. 1968. Osseal changes in mice following neonatal thymectomy. Experientia 24:721–723.

Bernardi, G., and Comsa, J. 1965. Purification chromatographique d'une preparation de thymus douée d'activité hormonale. Experientia 21:416–417.

Bethenod, M., Nivelon, J. L., Gilly, J., and Pouillaude, J. M. 1966. Un nouveau cas d'aplaisie lympho-plasmocytaire avec agammaglobulinémie et pneumonie à "Pneumocystis Carinii." Echec d'une greffe de thymus. Pediatrie 21:87–94.

Beutner, E. H;, Chorzelski, T. P., Hale, W. L., and Hausmanowa-Petrusewicz,

I. 1968. Autoimmunity in concurrent myasthenia gravis and pemphigus erythematosus. J. Am. Med. Assn. 203:845–849.

Bezssonoff, N. A., and Comsa, J. 1958. Preparation d'un extrait purifie de thymus, application a l'urine humaine. Ann. Endocr. 19:222–227.

Bickis, I. J., Henderson, I. W. D., and Quastel, J. H. 1966. Biochemical studies of human tumor. II. *In vitro* estimation of individual tumor sensitivity to anticancer agents. Cancer 19:103–113.

Bierring, F. 1960. CIBA Foundation Symposium, Hemopoiesis: cell production and its regulation, G. E. W. Wolstenholme and M. O'Connor (eds.) Little Brown, Boston. 490 p.

Billingham, R. E., and Brent, L. 1958. Quantitative studies on tissue transplantation immunity. IV. Induction of tolerance in newborn mice and studies on the phenomenon of runt disease. Phil. Trans. Roy. Soc. B. 242:439–477. Biomet, 1895, Quoted in Hammar (1936).

Birch, C. A., Cooke, K. B., Drew, C. E., London, D. R., MacKenzie, D. H., and Milne, M. D. 1964. Hyperglobulinaemic purpura due to a thymic tumour. Lancet 1:693–697.

Bjorneboe, M., Gormsen, H., and Lundqvist, F. R. 1947. Further experimental studies on the role of the plasma cells as antibody producers. J. Immunol. 55:121–129.

Blalock, A. 1944. Thymectomy in the treatment of myasthenia gravis. Report of twenty cases. J. Thoracic Surg. 13:316–339.

Blalock, A., Harvey, A. M., Ford, F. R., and Lilienthan, J. L., Jr. 1941. The treatment of myasthenia gravis by removal of the thymus gland. Preliminary report. J. Am. Med. Assn. 117:1529–1533.

Blalock, A., Mason, M. F., Morgan, H. J., and Riven, S. S. 1939. Myasthenia gravis and tumours of the thymic region. Report of a case in which the tumour was removed. Ann. Surg. 110:544–561.

Blecher, T. E., Soothill J. F., Voyce, M. A., and Walker, H. C. 1968. Antibody deficiency syndrome: A case with normal immunoglobulin levels. Clin. Exper. Immunol. 3:47–56.

Block, M. 1964. The blood-forming tissues and blood of the newborn oppossum (*Didelphys virainiana*) Ergel. Anat, Entwicklungsgesch 37:237–366.

Block, R., Durrum, E., and Zweig, G. 1958. Manual of paper chromatography and paper electrophoresis, 2nd ed. Academic Press, New York. 710 p.

Bloom, W. 1948. Histopathology of irradiation from external and internal sources. McGraw-Hill, New York. 808 p.

Boder, E., and Segwick, R. P. 1958. Ataxia-telangiectasia. Pediatrics 21:526–554.

Boeru, V., and Potop, I. 1971. Influenta timectomiei asupra dezvoltarii tumorale la sobolanul nou nascut. Stud. Cercet. Endocr. (in press).

Bogoch, S. 1969. On recognition molecules in brain circuitry: pigeon brain mucoids in training, learning and memory, pp. 104–113. *In* S. Bogoch (ed.), Future of the brain sciences. Plenum Press, New York.

Bomskov, C. 1940. Der thymus als inner sekretorisches Organ. Dtsch. Med. Wochenschr. 66:589–594.

Bomskov, C., and Holscher, B. 1942. Die thymektomie und ihr Erscheinungsbild. Pfluegers Arch. Ges. Physiol. Menschen Tiere. 245:455–482.

Bomskov, C., Kaulla, K. N., and Maurath, I. 1941. Uber die Wirkung von Sterinderivaten auf Stoffwechsel; uber die Wirkung des Digitalissubstanzen auf Leber-Herz-und Muskelgykogen. Archiv. Exp. Pathol. Pharmakol. 198: 232–244.

Bomskov, C., and Kucker, G. 1940. Uber die Wirkung Thymushormones an Kaltbluterlarven. Pfluegers Arch. Gesamte Physiol. Menschen Tiere. 244:246–340.

Bower, T. G. R. 1971. The object in the world of the infant. Amer. Sci. 225:30–38.

Boyd, E. 1932. The weight of the thymus gland in health and in disease. Am. J. Dis. Child. 43:1162–1214.

Braun, H. 1968. On the action of radiation protection substances on thymus cells. Experimentia 24: 1145–1146.

Braun, W., Ishizuka, M., Winchurch, R., and Webb, D. 1971. On the role of cycle AMP in immune response. Cyclic AMP and Cell Function, Ann. N. Y. Acad. Sci. 185:417–422.

Brown, H. D. (ed.). 1971. Chemistry of the cell interface. Vol. I:338, Vol. II:327. Academic Press, New York.

Buadze, S. 1938. Zum Pronlem der Hormonalen Beeinflussung des Kreatin-Stoffwechsels. Zschr. Exper. Med. 96:763.

Brumby, M. and Metcalf, D. 1967 Migration of cells to the thymus demonstrated by parabiosis. Proc. Soc. Exptl Biol, Med. 124:99–103.

Buckley, R. H., and Sidbury, J. B., Jr. 1968. Hereditary alterations in the immune response: coexistence of "agammaglobulinemia," acquired hypogamma-globulinemia and selective immunoglobulin deficiency in a sibship. Pediat. Res. 2:72–84.

Bull, D. M., and Tomasi, T. B. 1968. Deficiency of immunoglobulin A in intestinal disease. Gastroenterology 54:313-320.

Burnet, F. M., and Fenner, R. 1949. The production of antibodies. MacMillan and Co., Melbourne.

Burnet, F. M., and Holmes, M. C. 1964. Thymic changes in the mouse strain NZB in relation to the auto-immune state. J. Path. Bact. 88:229–241.

Burnet, M. 1959. Auto-immune disease. I. Modern immunological concepts. Brit. Med. J. 2:645–650.

Burnet, M 1962. Role of the thymus and related organs in immunity. Brit. Med. J. 2:807–811.

Bush, I. E. 1952. Methods of paper chromatography of steroids applicable to the study of steroids in mammalian blood and tissues. Biochem. J. 50:370–378.

Butcher, E. O., and Persike, E. C. 1938. The effect of Antuitrin-S on the thymus of the young albino rat. Endocrinology 23:501–506.

Butler, J. A. V. 1968. Gene control in the living cell. Basic Books, Inc., New York. 164 p.

Bystryn, J. C., Graf, M. U., and Uhr, J. W. 1970. Regulation of antibody formation by serum antibody. II. Removal of specific antibody by means of exchange transfusion. J. Exptl. Med. 132:1279–1287.

Bystryn, J. C. 1970. Regulation of antibody formation by serum antibody. II. Removal of specific antibody by means of exchange transfusion.

Caffrey, R. W., Rieke, W. O., and Everett, N. B. 1962. Radioautographic studies of small lymphocytes in the thoracic duct of the rat. Acta. Haematol. 28:145–154.

Calzolari, A. 1898–1899. Recherches experimentales sur un rapport probable entre la fonction du thymus et celle des testicules. Arch. Ital. Biol. (Turin) 30:71–77.

Cameron, A. H. 1965. Malformations of the thymus and the cardiovascular system. Arch. Dis. Child. 40:334.

Capocaccia, J., and Cicchini, T. 1955. Azione del timo in conigli inoculation streptococci piogeni e salmonelle tifose. Arch. Ital. Sci. Med. Tropic. 34:565–568.

Caridroit, F. 1924. Effects de la thymectomie sur le rat alimente au riz pali. C. R. Soc. Biol. 90:1330–1331.

Carriere, G., Morel, J., and Gineste, P. J. 1938. Influence de l'extrait de lobe anterieur d'hypophyse sur la morphologie du thymus chez le rat thyreoprive. C. R. Soc. Biol. 128:1151–1153.

Carter, R. O., and Hall, J. L. 1940. The physical chemical investigation of certain nucleoproteins. I. Prepartion and general properties. J. Am. Chem. Soc. 62:1194–1196.

Casazza, A. R., Duvall, C. P., and Carbone, P. O. 1966. Summary of infectious complications occurring in patients with Hodgkin's disease. Cancer Res. 26:1290–1296.

Caster, P., Garner, R., and Luckey, T. D. 1966. Antigen-induced morphological changes in germfree mice. Nature 209:1202–1204.

Castleman, B., and Norris, E. H. 1949. The pathology of the thymus in myasthenia gravis. A study of 35 cases. Medicine 28:27–58.

Cazal, P. 1969. Les fonctions du thymus. Pathologie du thymus chez l'adulte, par A. Bernadou. Congres français de medecine, 37th. Masson, P., Paris.

Ceglowski, W. S., Freedman, H., Robey, W. G., and Luckey, T. D. 1972. Thymus protein mediated enhancement of immunologic competence in neonatal mice. Abstract 8th National Reticuloendothelial Society Meeting, J. Ret. Soc. 1972. 4:412–413.

Ceglowski, W. S., Hand, T. L., and Friedman, H. 1970. Alterations in immunologic responsiveness of neonatal mice by calf thymus extracts. Bact. Proc. 1970:92 (Abstr.).

Cesarini, J. P., Benkoel, L. and Bonneau, H. 1969. Ultrastructure comparee du thymus chez le hamster jeune et adulte. C. R. Soc. Biol. 162:1975–1979.

Chamblin, J. G., and Bridges, J. B. 1964. Effects of cell-free extracts of thymus in leucopenic rats. Transplantation 2:785–787.

Chiodi, H. 1939. Action de la castration des adultes sur le poids du thymus. C. R. Soc. Biol. 130:457–458.

Claman, H. N., Chaperon, E. A., and Selmer, J. 1968. Thymus-marrow immuno-competence. III. The requirement for living thymus cells. Proc. Soc. Exp. Biol. Med. 127:462–466.

Claman, H. N., Chaperon, E. A., and Triplett, R. F. 1966a. Immuno-competence of transferred thymus-marrow cell combinations. J. Immunol. 97:828–832.

Claman, H. N., Chaperon, E. A., and Triplett, R. F. 1966b. Thymus-marrow cell combinations. Synergism in antibody production. Proc. Soc. Exp. Biol. Med. 122:1167–1171.

Clark, E. P., and Collip, J. B. 1925. A study of the Tisdall method for the determination of blood serum calcium with a suggested modification. J. Biol. Chem. 63:461–464.

Clark, I., and Stoerk, H. C. 1956. Uptake of P^{32} by nucleic acids of lymphoid tissue undergoing atrophy. J. Biol. Chem. 222:285–292.

Clem, L. W., and Leslie, G. A. 1969. Phylogeny of immune structure and function, pp. 62–88. *In* M. Adinolphi and J. Humphrey (eds.), Immunology and development. Heineman Medical Books, Ltd., London.

Cleveland, W. W., Fogel, B. J., Brown, W. T., and Kay, H. E. M. 1968. Foetal thymic transplant in a case of DiGeorge's syndrome. Lancet 2:1211–1214.

Cohn, R. B., Toll. G. D., and Castleman, B. 1960. Bronchial adenomas in Cushing's syndrome: Their relation to thymomas and oat cell carcinomas associated with hyperadrenocorticism. Cancer 13:812.

Comings, D. E. 1965. Congenital hypogammaglobulinemia. Arch. Intern. Med. 115:79–87.

Comsa, J. 1938. Consequences de la thymectomie totale chez le cobaye male. C. R. Soc. Biol. 27:903–905.

Comsa, J. 1940. Action de l'extrait de thymus sur le cobaye thymiprive. C. R. Soc. Biol. 133:24.

Comsa, J. 1944, Effets de la thymectomie totale sur creation urinaire du cobaye. C. R. Soc. Biol. 138:773–74.

Comsa, J. 1945. Role de la thyroide dans la genese de la creatinurie thymiprive chez le cobaye. C. R. Acad. Sci. 220:227–228.

Comsa, J. 1947. Nouvelles recherches sur la creatinurie de castration chez le cobaye. C. R. Soc. Biol. 141:413–415.

Comsa, J. 1950. Recherches sur le mechanisme determinant de l'afflux des lymphocytes vers le thymus. C. R. Acad. Sci. 230:2337–2339.

Comsa, J. 1951a. Action sur l'ovaire du cobaye d'un extrait thymique hautement purifie. Ann. Endocr. 12:91–92.

Comsa, J. 1951b. Influence des gonades sur l'activite thyreotrope de l'urine du cobaye thymiprive. Ann. Endocr. 12:565–568.

Comsa, J. 1951c. Action de l'extrait de thymus sur l'elimination du facteur thyreotrope chez le cobaye thymiprive. Ann. Endocr. 12:562–564.

Comsa, J. 1951d. Activation de la thyroide du jeune cobaye par des injections d'urine de cobaye thymiprive. C. R. Acad. Sci. 232:1245–47.

Comsa, J. 1952a. Activation thyreotrope des urines du cobaye par la rupture de l'equilibre thymus-thyroide-gonades. Experientia 8:196–197.

Comsa, J. 1952b. Modification de l'action anti-thyroidienne de l'extrait de thymus chez la cobaye irradie aux rayons X. Experientia 8:267–268.

Comsa, J. 1952c. Activation thyreotrope des urines du cobaye traite aux rayons X. Ann. Endocr. 13:931–934.

Comsa, J. 1952d. Role de la thyroide dans le determinism des lesions du thymus chez le cobaye irradie. Ann. Endocr. 13:935–937.

Comsa, J. 1952e. Utilization of antithyroid action test for bioassay of thymus hormone. Am. J. Physiol. 166:550–554.

Comsa, J. 1952f. Renal excretion of a substance closely related to thymus hormone in man. Am. J. Physiol. 170:528–531.

Comsa, J. 1953a. Nouvelles recherches sur les connexions physiologiques entre le thymus et les hormones sexuelles et le thymus chez le cobaye. Physiol. Comp. Oecol. 3:128–134.

Comsa, J. 1953b. Nouvelles recherches sur l'incidence du thymus dans l'interaction thyroxine-testosterone chez le cobaye. J. Physiol. 45:377–384.

Comsa, J. 1953c. Nouvelles recherches sur l'incidence du thymus dans l'interaction entre la thyroxine et oestradiol chez le cobaye. J. Physiol. 45:385–392.

Comsa, J. 1954. Nouvelles recherches sur l'interaction thymus-thyroide-gonades chez le cobaye. J. Physiol. 46:577–583.

Comsa, J. 1956a. Influence d'un extrait hautement purifie de thymus sur les consequences de l'irradiation aux rayons X sur les glandes endocrines du cobaye. Ann. Endocr. 17:777–84.

Comsa, J. 1956b. Effect of the thymus upon throxin metabolism in guinea pigs. Acta Endocr. 21:396–402.

Comsa, J. 1956c. Influence d'un extrait purifie de thymus sur les organes hematopoietiques chez le cobaye irradie. C. R. Soc. Biol. 150:516–518.

Comsa, J. 1957a. Action d'un extrait hautement purifie de thymus sur la croissance du cobaye. Physiol. Comp. Oecol. 4:270–276.

Comsa, J. 1957b. Influence de la castration sur la stimulation thymiprive de la corticosurrenale chez le cobaye. Ann. Endocr. 18:764–766.

Comsa, J. 1957c. Consequences of thymectomy upon leucopoiesis in guinea pigs. Acta Endocr. 26:361–365.

Comsa, J. 1957d. Effect of thymectomy upon the functional condition of the adrenal cortex in guinea pigs. Nature 179:872–873.

Comsa, J. 1957e. Wirkung des Thymusextraktes von Bezssonoff and Comsa beim thyreopriven Meerschweinchen. Pfluegers Arch. Ges. Physiol. Menschen Tiere. 264:383–385.

Comsa, J. 1958a. Influence du thymus sur l'action gonadotrope de l'hypophyse chez le rat. Ann. Endocr. 19:1042–1045.

Comsa, J. 1958b. Role of the thymus in the effect of thyroxin on leucopoiesis in guinea pigs. Acta Endocr. 27:455–463.

Comsa, J. 1958c. Nouveau procede de mesure de l'activite anti-thyroidienne du thymus. J. Physiol. 50:825–830.

Comsa, J. 1958d. Influence of the thymus on the reaction of the adrenal to adrenocorticotropic hormone in the rat. Nature 182:57–58.

Comsa, J. 1958e. Influence of the thymus upon the reaction of the rat to anterior pituitary growth hormone. Nature 182:728.

Comsa, J. 1959a. Physiologie et physiopathologie du thymus. Doin, Paris. 152 p.

Comsa, J. 1959b. Influence de l'hypophyse sur la teneur du thymus en principe actif. Ann. Endocr. 20:795–798.

Comsa, J. 1959c. Effect of adrenalectomy on the hormone content of the thymus in the rat. Nature 184:279.

Comsa, J. 1959d. Einflub der Wechselbeziehung zwischen Schilddruse und Gonaden auf den Funktionszustand des Thymus. Pfluegers Arch. Ges. Physiol. Menschen Tiere. 269:361–365.

Comsa, J. 1963. Allgemein-somatische Aspekte der Sexualitat. Z. Naturwiss-Med. Grundlagenforsch 1:201.

Comsa, J. 1964. Die endokirnen Drusen im experimentellen Strahlensyndrom. Strahlentherapie 126:366–385; 541–564.

Comsa, J. 1965a. Les mecanismes possibles de l'influence du thymus sur les lymphocytes. Pathol. Biol. 13:665–669.

Comsa, J. 1965b. Action de l'hormone thymique sur la consommation de glucose du diaphragm du rat. Ann. Endocr. 26:472–475.

Comsa, J. 1965c. Influence de l'hormone thymique purifie sur le choc au blanc d'oeuf chez le rat. Ann. Endocr. 26:476–478.

Comsa, J. 1965d. Influence de l'hormone thymique sur l'action des hormones hypophysaires. Ann. Endocr. 26:525–534.

Comsa, J. 1965e. Die endokrinen Drusen im experimentellen Strahlensyndrom. Strahlentherapie 126:541–564.

Comsa, J. 1965f. Action of the purified thymus hormone in thymectomized guinea pigs. Am. J. Med. Sci. 250:79–85.

Comsa, J. 1971. Physiology of the thymus. Rev. Roum. Endocr. (Symposium sur le thymus, Cluj. Roumanie,) 3:1–22.

Comsa, J., and Bezssonoff, M. A. 1958. Preparation and bioassay of a purified thymic extract. Acta Endocr. 29:257–266.

Comsa, J., and Bezssonoff, M. A. 1959. Origin of the supposed thymus hormone. Acta Endocr. 30:621–624.

Comsa, J., and Filipe, G. 1966. Influence de l'hormone thymique sur la production d'anticorps chez le cobaye thymiprive. Ann. Instit. Pasteur 110:365–372.

Comsa, J., and Gros, C. M. 1956. Wirkung eines hochgereinigten Thymus praparetes auf rontgenbestrahlten Meerschweinchen. Fortschr. Ront. 85:274–281.

Comsa, J., and Leroux, H. 1955. Influence of a highly purified thymus extract upon the adrenals in guinea pigs. J. Endocr. 13:7–10.

Comsa, J., and Leroux, H. 1956. Role de la thyroide dans l'action du thymus sur la surrenale chez le cobaye. Ann. Endocr. 17:785–788.

Comsa, J. and Philipp, E. M. 1971. Essai de demonstration de la secretion de l'hormone thymique. J. Physiol. (Paris) 63:193a.

Cone, L., and Uhr, J. W. 1964. Immunological deficiency disorders associated with chronic lymphocytic leukemia and multiple myeloma. J. Clin. Invest. 43:2241–2248.

Constant, G., Porter, E. L., Andronis, A., and Rider, J. A. 1949. Effect of thymic extracts on neuromuscular response. Texas Rep. Biol. Med. 7:350–354.

Constant, G. A., Porter, E. L., Seybold, H. M., and Andronis, A. 1949. Effect of thymic extracts on neuro-muscular response. Am. J. Physiol. 159:565.

Cooper, H. L., and Ginsberg, H. 1971. Lymphocyte activation I, pp. 1147–1150. In B. Amos (ed.), Progress in immunology. Academic Press, New York.

Cooper, M. D., Chase, H. P., Lowman, J. T., Krivit, W., and Good, R. A. 1968. Immunologic defects in patients with Wiskott-Aldrich Syndrome. Birth Defects 4:378.

Cooper, M. D., Gabrielson, A. E., Peterson, R. D. A., and Good, R. A. 1967. Ontogenetic development of the germinal centers and their function— relationship to the bursa of Fabricius, pp. 28–33. In Cottier, H., Odart-chenko, N., Schindler, R. and Congdon, C. C. (eds.), Germinal centers in immune responses. Springer, New York.

Cooper, M. D., Peterson, R. D. A., and Good, R. A. 1965. Delineation of the thymic and bursal lymphoid systems in the chicken. Nature 205:143–146.

Cooper, M. D., Peterson, R. D. A., South, M. A., and Good, R. A. 1966. The functions of the thymus system and the bursa system in the chicken. J. Exp. Med. 123:75–102.

Courrier, R. 1928. Action de l'ingestion de corps thyroide sur le thymus, sur le testicule et sur la thyroide. Contribution a l'histophysiologie throidienne. Rev. Endocr. 6:10–48.

Crabbe, P. A., and Heremans, J. F. 1967. Selective IgA deficiency with stea-torrhea: a new syndrome. Amer. J. Med. 42:319–326.

Crede, R. H., and Moon, H. D. 1940. Effect of adrenocorticotropic hormone on thymus of rats. Proc. Soc. Exp. Biol. Med. 43:44–46.

Crick, R. 1971. General model for the chromosomes of higher organisms. Nature 234:25–27.

Crieder, Q. E., Alampovic, P., Hillsbery, J., Yen, C. and Bradford, R. H. 1964. Separation of lipids by silica-gel G column chromatography. J. Lipid Res. 5:3, 479–481.

Cristofalo, V. J., Kabakjian. R. J., and Kritchevsky, D. 1967. Enzyme activities of some cultural human cells. Proc. Soc. Exp. Biol. Med. 126:273–276.

Cross, A. M., Leuchars, E., and Miller, J. F. A. P. 1964. Studies on the recovery of the immune response in irradiated mice thymectomized in adult life. J. Exp. Med. 119:837–850.

Dalmasso, A. P., Martinez, C., Archer, O. K., Pierce, J. C., and Papermaster, B. W. 1962. The role of the thymus in development of immunologic capacity in rabbits and mice. J. Exp. Med. 116:773–795.

Dalmasso, A. P., Martinez, C., and Good, R. A. 1962a. Further studies of suppression of the homograft reaction by thymectomy in the mouse. Proc. Soc. Exp. Biol. Med. 111:143–146.

Dalmasso, A. P., Martinez, C., and Good, R. A. 1962b. Failure of spleen cells from thymectomized mice to induce graft vs host reactions. Proc. Soc. Exp. Biol. Med. 110:205–208.

Dalmasso, A. P., Martinez, C., Sjodin, K., and Good, R. A. 1963. Studies on the role of the thymus in immunobiology. Reconstitution of immunologic capacity in mice thymectomized at birth. J. Exp. Med. 118:1089–1109.

Dameshek, W. 1966. The significance of auto-immune disease. In The thymus: Experimental and clinical studies, Ciba Foundation Symposium, ed. by G. E. Wolsternholme and R. Porter. Churchill, London. 538 p.

Dameshek, W., and Sherman, J. D. 1963. Wasting disease following thymectomy in the hamster. Nature (London) 197:469–471.

Davies, A. J. S. 1969a. The thymus humoral factor under scrutiny. Agents and Action 1(1):1–7.

Davies, A. J. S. 1969b. The thymus and the cellular basis of immunity. Transplant. Rev. 1:43–91.

Davies, A. J. S., Leuchars, E., Wallis, V., and Koller, P. C. 1966. The mitotic response of thymus-derived cells to antigenic stimulus. Transplantation 4:438–451.

Davis, S. D., Ching, Y. C., Shaller, J., Shurtleff, D. B., Hecht, F., and Wedgwood, R. J. 1967. The congenital agammaglobulinemias. A heterogeneous group of immune defects. Amer. J. Dis. Child. 113:186–194.

Davis, W., Jr., and Cole, L. 1969. Retarded immunological recovery in sub-lethally X-irradiated mice by additional thymic exposure. Reversal with injected marrow cells. NRLD-TR-68-119. U. S. Naval Radiol. Def. Lab. 1–14, Oct. 24, 1968. Cit. No. 4075474.

Davis, W. E., Jr., Tyan, M. L., and Cole, L. J. 1964. Homografts in thymectomized irradiated mice: Responses to primary and secondary skin grafts. Science 145:394–395.

Dean G. O., Earle, A. M., and Reilly, W. A. 1951. Failure of thymectomy in lymphatic leukemia. Surgery 63:695.

Deane, H. W., and Shaw, J. H. 1947. Cytochemical study of responses of the adrenal cortex of the rat of thiamine, riboflavin and pyridoxine deficiences. J. Nutr. 34:1–15.

Defendi, V., and Metcalf, D. (eds.). 1964. The thymus. The Wistar Institute. Philadelphia. 145 p.

De Koning, J., Dooren L. J., van Bekkum, D. W., van Rood, J. J., Dicke, K. A. and Rádl, J. 1969. Transplantation of bone-marrow cells and fetal thymus in an infant with lymphopenic immunological deficiency. Lancet 1:1223–1227.

Delbrez, M., and Hoat, J. 1968. Greffes de cellules medullaries associes a des cellules lymphoides ou thymiques chez le souris irradiee a dose lethale. C. R. Soc. Biol. 162:2038–2041.

DeSomer, P., Denys, P., Jr., and Leyten, R. 1963. Activity of a non-cellular calf thymus extract in normal and thymectomized mice. Life Sci. 11:810–819.

DeVaal, O. M., and Seynhaeve, V. 1959. Reticular dysgenesia. Lancet 2:1123–1125.

DeVries, M. J., Van Putten, L. M., Balner, H., and Van Bekkum, D. W. 1964. Lesions suggerant une reactivite auto-immune chez des souris. Atteintes de la "Runt Disease" apres thymectomie neonatale. Etud. Clin. Biol. 9:381–397.

Dieter, M. P. 1971. Further studies on the relationship between vitamin C and thymic humoral factor. Proc. Soc. Exp. Biol. Med. 136:316–322.

Di George, A. M., Lischner, H. W., Dacou, C., and Arey, J. B. 1967. Absence of the thymus. Lancet 1:1387–1388.

Diomede-Fresa, V., Fumarola, D., and de Rinaldis, P. 1959. Influenza degli estratti timici sugli anticorpi serici. Acad. Pugl. Sci. Atti 2:561–564.

Dische, M. R. 1968. Lymphoid tissue and associated congenital malformations in thymic agenesis. Findings in one infant and two severely malformed stillborns. Arch. Path. 86:312–316.

Dischler, W., and Rudali, G. 1961. La thymectomie totale chez le souriceau nouveau-ne. Rev. Fr. Etud. Clin. Biol. 6:88–92.

Dixon, F. J., Weigle, W. O., and Roberts, J. C. 1957. Comparison of antibody responses associated with the transfer of rabbit lymph node, peritoneal exudate and thymus cells. J. Immunol. 78:56–62.

Doak, P. B., Montgomerie, J. Z., North, J. D. K., and Smith, F. 1968. Reticulum cell sarcoma after renal homotransplantation and azathioprine and prednisone therapy. Brit. Med. J. 4:746–748.

Doenhoff, M. J., Davies, A. J. S., Leuchars, E., and Wallis, J. 1970. The thymus and circulating lymphocytes of mice. Proc. Roy. Soc. B 176:69–85.

Doniach, D., and Roitt, I. M. 1962. Auto-antibodies in disease. Ann. Rev. Med. 13:213–240.

Doniach, I. 1957. Lack of effect of thymectomy on thyroid function in weanling rats. J. Endocr. 16:294–297.

Dooren, L. J., de Vries, M. J., van Bekkum, D. W., Cleton, F. J., and de Koning, J. 1968. Sex-linked thymic epithelial hypoplasia in two siblings. Attempt at treatment by transplantation with fetal thymus and adult bone marrow. J. Pediat. 72:51–62.

Dougherty, T. F. 1952. Effects of hormones on lymphatic tissue. Physiol. Rev. 32:339–340.

Dufour, D., and Rochette, A. 1961. Etude de l'influence des acides nucleiques du thymus sur la reponse nonspecifique a l'agression. Annal. Endocr. 22:9–13.

Dunn, T. B., Trainin, N., and Levey, R. H. 1964. Studies of thymic function, pp. 105–117. In V. Defendi and D. Metcalf (eds.), The thymus. The Wistar Institue, Philadelphia.

Dustin, A. P. 1963. Thymocytes et lymphocytes, demonstration experimentale de leurs differences de potentialite. Rev. Fr. Endocr. Clin. 1:332–345.

Dutton, R. W. 1967. *In vitro* studies of immunological responses of lymphoid cells. Adv. Immunol. 6:253–336.

Dutton, R. W., Falkoff, R., Hirst, J. A., Hoffmann, Kapplor, J. W., Kettman, J. R., Lesley, J. F., and Vann, D. 1971. Is there evidence for a non-antigen specific diffusable chemical mediator from the thymus derived cell in the initiation of the immune response? pp. 355–368. *In* B. Amos (ed.). Progress in immunology. Academic Press, New York.

Earle, A. M., Reilly, W. A., and Dean, G. O. 1951. Thymectomy and ACTH in lymphatic leucemia. J. Pediat. 38:63–68.

East, J., and Parrott, D. M. V. 1964. Prevention of wasting in mice thymectomized at birth and their subsequent rejection of allogeneic leukemic cells. J. Natl. Cancer Inst. 33:673–685.

Eaton, L. M. 1942. Myasthenia gravis: Its treatment and relation to thymus. Proc. Staff Meet., Mayo Clinic 17:81–87.

Eaton, L. M., and Clagett, O. T. 1950. Thymectomy in the treatment of myasthenia gravis; Results in seventy-two cases compared with one hundred and forty-two control cases. J. Am. Med. Assn. 142:963–967.

Eaton, L. M., and Clagett, O. T. 1955. Present status of thymectomy in treatment of myasthenia gravis. Am. J. Med. 19:703–717.

Eaton, L. M., Clagett, O. T., and Bastron, J. A. 1953. The thymus and its relationship to diseases of the nervous system: Study of 374 cases of myasthenia gravis and comparison of 87 patients undergoing thymectomy with 225 controls. Proc. Assn. Res. Nerv. Ment. Dis. (Research Publication) 32:107.

Eilber, F. R., and Morton, D. L. 1970. Impaired immunologic reactivity and recurrence following cancer surgery. Cancer 25:362–367.

Ellinger, F. 1947. Some effects of desoxycorticosterone acetate on mice irradiated with X-rays. Proc. Soc. Exp. Biol. Med. 64:31–35.

Eskelund, V., and Plum, C. M. 1953. Experimental investigations into the healing of fractures: Influence of extract of thymus and other tissues. Acta Endocr. 12:171–178.

Evans, H. M., and Simpson, M. E. 1934. Reduction of thymus of gonadotropic hormone. Anat. Rec. 60:423–435.

Fahey, J. L., Barth, W. F., and Law, L. W. 1965. Normal immunoglobulins and antibody response in neonatally thymectomized mice. J. Natl. Cancer Inst. 35:663–675.

Feldman, J. D. 1950. The *in vitro* reaction of cells to adrenal cortical steroids with special reference to lymphocytes. Endocrinology 46:552–562.

Feldman, M. 1970. Critical periods in development. *In* Environmental Influences on Genetic Expression. Kretchmer, N., and Walcher, D. N. (eds.). Academic Press, New York. pp. 7–15.

Ferguson, F. R. 1962. A critical review of the clinical features of myasthenia gravis. Proc. Roy. Soc. Med. 55.49–52.

Ferguson, F. R., Hutchinson, E. C., and Liversedge, L. A. 1955. Myasthenia gravis, results of medical management. Lancet 2:636–639.

Fiaccavento, W. 1952. Variazioni del'attivita fosfatasica del tessuto osseo in seguito alla timectomia. Ormonologia 12:260–261.

Ficchera, G. 1933. I fattori interni nello sviluppo dei tumori a gli odierni saggi di terapia biologica. Milano, U. Hoepil. 213 p.

Fish, L. A., Pollara, B., and Good, R. A. 1966. Characterization of an immuno-globulin from the paddlefish (*Polyodon spathula*). *In* Phylogency of Immunity, Smith, R. T., Miescher, P. A., and Good, R. A. (eds). University of Florida Press, Gainesville, Fla. pp. 99–104.

Fisher, B., Fisher, E. R., Lee, S., and Sakai, A. 1965. Renal homotransplantation in neonatal thymectomized puppies. Transplantation 3:49–53.

Fisher, E. R., and Fisher, B. 1965. Role of the thymus in skin and tumor transplantation in the rat. Lab. Invest. 14:546–555.

Fiske, C. H., and Subbarow, Y. 1925. The colorimetric determination of phosphorus. J. Biol. Chem. 66:375–400.

Franks, D. J., MacMus, J. P., and Whitfield, J. F. 1971. The effect of prostaglandins on cyclic AMP production and cell proliferation in thymus lymphocytes. Biochem. Biophys. Res. Commun. 44:1177–1183.

Fudenberg, H. H. 1966. Immunologic deficiency, autoimmune disease and lymphoma: Observations, implications and speculations. Arthritis Rheum. 9:464–472.

Fudenberg, H., German, J. L., and Kunkel, H. G. 1962. The occurrence of rheumatoid factor and other abnormalities in families of patients with agammaglobulinemia. Arthritis Rheum. 5:565–588.

Funk, C., and Douglas, M. 1913. Studies on beriberi. VIII. The relationship of beriberi to glands of internal secretion. J. Physiol. 47:471–478.

Gabrielsen, A. E., Cooper, M. D., Peterson, R. D. A., and Good, R. A. 1969. The primary immunologic deficiency diseases. *In* Textbook of immunopathology. Meischer, P. A., and Muller-Eberhard, H. J. (eds.) Grune and Stratton. New York. p. 385.

Gaburro, D., and Volpato, S. 1955. Aspetti metabolici della sindrome timoprivi sperimentale. Minerva Pediatr. 18:9–445.

Galante, L., Gudmundsson, T. V., Matthews, E. W., Tse, A., Williams, E. D., Woodhouse, N. J. Y., and MacIntyre, I. 1968. Thymic and parathyroid origin of calcitonin in man. Lancet 2:537–538.

Gaugas, J. M., Chesterman, F. C., Hirsch, M. S., Rees, R. J. W., Harvey, J. J., and Gilchrist, C. 1969. Unexpected high incidence of tumours in thymectomized mice treated with anti-lymphatic globulin and *Myocobacterium leprae*. Nature 221:1033–1036.

Gebele, V. 1929. Uber Thymus und Schilddruse. Dtsch. Z. Chir. 215: 186–195.

Giedion, V. A., and Scheidegger, J. J. 1957. Kongenital Immunoparese bei Fehlen spezifisher β_2-Globuline und quantitativ normalen γ-Globulinen. Helv. Paediat. Acta 12:241–259.

Gilbert, C., and Hong, R. 1964. Qualitative and quantitative immunoglobulin deficiency. Amer. J. Med. 37:602–609.

Gill, G. N., and Garren, L. D. 1971. Role of the receptor in the mechanism of action of adenosine 3':5'-cyclic monophosphate. Proc. Nat. Acad. Sci. 68:786–790.

Gitlin, D., and Craig, J. M. 1963. The thymus and other lymphoid tissues in congenital agammaglobulinemia. I. Thymic alymphoplasia and lymphocytic hypoplasia and their relation to infection. Pediatrics 32:517–530.

Gitlin, D., Vawter, G., and Craig, J. M. 1964. Thymic alymphoplasia and congenital aleukocytosis. Pediatrics 33:184–192.

Glanzmann, E. 1923. Die rolle der akzessorischen Washstumfaktoren (Vitamine A und B) bei der Biochemie des Wachstums. Msch. f. Kinderhk. 25: 178–200.

Glanzmann, E., and Riniker, P. 1950. Essentielle Lymphocytophthise. Ein nues Krankheits bild aus der Sauglingspathologie. Ann. Paediat. 175:1–32.

Glaser, M. 1926. Thyroxinversuche an weizen Mausen. Z. Anat. Entwicklungsgesch. 80:704–725.

Glimstedt, G. 1932. Das Leben ohen Bakterien. Sterile Aufziehung von Meerschweinchen. Verhandl. Anat. Ges. Jena 41:79–89.

Glimstedt, G. 1933. Nagra nya ron baserade pa jamforelser mellan steriltuppfodda djur och kontrolldjur. Med. Foren. Tdschkr. 11:271–277.

Glimstedt, G. 1936. Bakterienfreie Meerschweinchen, Aufzucht, Lebensfahigkeit und Wachstum, nebst Untersuchungen uber das lymphatische Gewebe. Acta Pathol. Microbiol. Scand. (Suppl.) 30:1–295.

Goedbloed, J. R., and Vos, O. 1965. The capacity for skin rejection in mice thymectomized neonatally or in adult life. Transplantation 3:368–379.

Goldman, A. S., Ritzmann, S. E., Houston, E. W., Sidwell, S., Bratcher, R., and Levin, W. C. 1967. Dysgammaglobulinemic antibody deficiency syndrome. J. Pediat. 70:16–27.

Goldstein, A. L. 1971. Thymus-hormones workshop. Proceedings of the First International Congress of Immunology. Unpublished Report.

Goldstein, A. L., Asanuma, Y., Battisto, J. R., Hardy, M. A., Quint, J., and White, A. 1970. Influence of thymosin on cell-mediated and humoral immune responses in normal and immunologically deficient mice. J. Immunol. 104:359–366.

Goldstein, A. L., Asanuma, Y., and White, A. 1970. The thymus as an endocrine gland: Properties of thymosin, a new thymus hormone. Recent Progr. Horm. Res. 26:505–538.

Goldstein, A. L., Banerjee, S., Schneebele, G. L., Dougherty, T. F., and White, A. 1970. Acceleration of lymphoid tissue regeneration in X-irradiated CBA-W mice by injection of thymosin. Radiat. Res. 41:579–593.

Goldstein, A. L., Banerjee, S., and White, A. 1967. Preparation and properites of thymostatin, a new thymic inhibitor of DNA and RNA synthesis. Proc. Natl. Acad. Sci. U.S.A. 57:821–828.

Goldstein, A. L., Guha, A., Howe, M. L., and White, A. 1971. Ontogenesis of cell-mediated immunity in murine thymocytes and spleen cells and its acceleration by thymosin, a thymic hormone. J. Immunol. 106:773–780.

Goldstein, A. L., Guha, A., Zatz, M. M., Hardy, M. A. and White, A., 1972. Purification and biological activity of thymosin, a hormone of the thymus gland. Proc. Natl. Acad. Sci. U.S.A. 69:1800–1803.

Goldstein, A. L., Guha, A., Zatz, M. M., and White, A. 1972. Biological properties of thymosin, a thymic hormone. Fed. Proc. 31:418.

Goldstein, A. L., Slater, F. D., and White, A. 1966. Preparation, assay and partial purification of a thymus lymphocyotpoietic factor. Proc. Natl. Acad. Sci., U.S.A. 56:1010–1017.

Goldstein, A. L., and White, A. 1970a. The thymus as an endocrine gland: Hormones and their actions. In Biochemical actions of hormones, I. Litwach, G. (ed.). Academic Press, New York. pp. 465–502.

Goldstein, A. L., and White, A. 1970b. Current Topics in Experimental Endocrinology, James, V. H. T., and Martini, L. (eds.). Academic Press, New York, vol. 1.

Goldstein, A. L., and White, A. 1971. The thymus gland: Experimental and clinical studies of its role in the development and expression of immune functions. Adv. Metab. Disord. 5:149–182.

Goldstein, G. 1966a. Plasma cells in the human thymus. Aust. J. Exp. Biol. Med. Sci. 44:695–699.

Goldstein, G. 1966b. Thymitis and myasthenia gravis. Lancet 2:1164–1167.

Goldstein, G. 1968. The thymus and neuromuscular function. A substance in thymus which causes myositis and myasthenic neuromuscular block in guinea pigs. Lancet 2:119–123.

Goldstein, G. 1970. The thymus, thymosin and antithymosin. Vox Sang. 19:97–104.

Goldstein, G., and Hoffmann, W. W. 1968. Electrophysiological changes similar to those of myasthenia gravis in rats with experimental autoimmune thymitis. J. Neurol. Neurosurg. Psychiat. 31:453–459.

Goldstein, G., and Hofmann, W. W. 1969. Endocrine function of the thymus affecting neuromuscular transmission. Clin. Exp. Immun. 4:181–189.

Goldstein, G., and Mackay, I. R. 1965. Contrasting abnormalities in the thymus in systemic lupus erythematosus and myasthenia gravis: A quantitative histological study. Aust. J. Exp. Biol. Med. Sci. 43:381–390.

Goldstein, G., and Mackay, I. R. 1967. The thymus in systemic lupus erythematosus: A quantitative histopathological analysis and comparison with stress involution. Brit. Med. J. 2:475–478.

Golub, A. M., Maslarz, F. R., Villars, T., and McConnell, J. V. 1971. Incubation effects upon transfer of training in rats. In Biology of memory, Adam, G. (ed.). Plenum Press, New York.

Good, R. A., Copper, M. D., Peterson, R. D., Kellum, M. J., Sutherland, E. R., and Gabrielsen, A. E. 1966. The role of the thymus in immune process. Ann. N.Y. Acad. Sci. 135:451–478.

Good, R. A., Dalmasso, A. P., Martinez, C., Archer, O. K., Pierce, J. C., and

Papermaster, B. W. 1962. The role of the thymus in development of immunological capacity in rabbits and mice. J. Exp. Med. 116:773–796.

Good, R. A., and Fisher, D. W. (eds.). 1971. Immunology. Sinauer Associates, Inc., Stamford, Conn., 305 p.

Good, R. A., and Gabrielsen, A. E. 1964. The thymus in immunobiology; Structure, function and role in disease. Hoeber Medical Division, Harper and Row, New York. 778 p.

Good, R. A., Gatti, R. A., Hong, R., and Meuwissen, H. J. 1969. Graft treatment of immunological deficiency. Lancet 1:1162.

Good R. A., Gatti, A., Hong, R., and Meuwissen, H. J. 1969. Successful marrow transplantation for correction of immunologic deficit in lymphopenic agammaglobulinemia and treatment of immunologically induced pancytopenia. Exper. Hemat. 19:4–5.

Good, R. A., Peterson, R. D., and Martinez, C. 1965. The thymus in immunobiology: With special references to auto-immune disease. Ann N.Y. Acad. Sci. 124:73–94.

Goodman, J. W. 1971. Cellular interaction between thymocytes and transplanted marrow stem cells. Transplantation Proc. 3:430–433.

Goodman, J. W., and Grubs, C. G. 1970. The relationship of the thymus to erythropoiesis. In Hemopoietic cellular proliferation. Stohlman, F., Jr. (ed.). Grune and Stratton, New York. p. 26–35.

Goslar, H. G. 1958. Uber die Wirkung eines standardisierten Thymusextraktes auf die Hautungsvorgange und auf einige Orange von Natrix. L. Arch. Exp. Path. 233:201–25.

Gotoff, S. P. 1968. Lymphocytes in congenital immunological deficiency diseases. Clin. Exp. Immun. 3:343–356.

Gowans, J. L., and McGregor, D. O. 1965. The immunological activities of lymphocytes. Progr. Allergy. 9:1–78.

Gowans, J. S., and Knight, E. J. 1964. The route of re-circulation of lymphocytes in the rat. Proc. Roy. Soc. Biol. 159:257–282.

Goya, N., Fujimoto, T., and Sumiyoshi, A. 1967. Congenital immunologic deficiency diseases. Acta Haemat. Jap. 30:11–23.

Goya, N., Kodate, S., Kuroki, Y., and Sumiyoshi, A. 1968. Influence of transplantation of thymus and spleen cells on patients with ataxia teleangiectasia. XII. International Kongress Pediatrie, Mexico.

Graetzer, M. A., Wolfe, H. R., Aspinall, R. L., and Meyer, R. K. 1963. Effect of thymectomy and bursectomy on precipitin and natural hemagglutinin production in the chicken. J. Immunol. 90:878–887.

Grant, G. A., and Miller, J. F. A. P. 1962. Effect of neonatal thymectomy on the induction of sarcoma in C57BL mice. Nature 205:1124–1125.

Greengard, P., and Costa, E. (eds.). 1970. Role of cyclic AMP in cell function. Adv. Biochem. Psychopharm., III. Raven Press, New York. 383 p.

Gregoire, C. 1935. Recherches sur la symbiose lymphoepitheliale au niveau du thymus de mammifere. Arch. Biol. 46:717–720.

Gregoire, C. and Duchateau, G. 1956. A study on lymphoepithelial symbiosis in thymus. Arch. Biol. Liege 67:269–296.

Gross, L. 1959. Effect of thymectomy on development of leukemia in C3H mice inoculated with leukemic passage virus. Proc. Soc. Exp. Biol. Med. 100:325–328.

Gudernatsch, J. F. 1912. Feeding experiments on tadpoles. Arch. Entwcklngsmechn. Organ. Leipz. 35:457–483.

Guha, A., Goldstein, A. L. and White, A. 1972 Thymosin, a thymic hormone: purification and chemical properties, Fed. Proc. 31:418.

Gunn, A., Michie, W., and Irvine, W. J. 1964. The thymus in thyroid disease. Lancet 2:776–777.

Gurim, S., and Carr, W. E. 1971. Chemoreception in *Nassarius obsoletus*: The role of specific stimulatory proteins. Sci. 174:293–295.

Gyllensten, L. 1953. Influence of thymus and thyroid on the postnatal growth of the lymphatic tissue in guinea pigs. Acta Anat. Suppl. 18–1:1–163.

Gyorgy, P., and Goldblatt, H. 1940. Choline as a member of the vitamin B_2 complex. J. Exp. Med. 72:1–9.

Hammar, J. A. 1921. The new views as to the morphology of the thymus gland and their bearing on the problem of the function of the thymus. Endocrinology 5:543–573, 731–760.

Hammar, J. A. 1936. Die Normal-morpholgische Thymus-furschung im Letzten Vierteljahrhundert; Analyse und Synthese, nebst einigen Worten su der Funkionsfrage. Barth, Leipzig. 453 p.

Hammett, F. S. 1926. Studies of the thyroid apparatus. XXXVII. The role of the thyroid apparatus in the growth of the thymus. Endocrinology 10:370–384.

Hand, T., Caster, P., and Luckey, T. D. 1967. Isolation of a thymus hormone, LSH. Biochem. Biophys. Res. Commun. 26:18–23.

Hand, T. L., Ceglowski, W. S., Damrongsak, D., and Friedman, H. 1970. Development of antibody forming cells in neonatal mice: Stimulation and inhibition by calf thymus fractions. J. Immunol. 105:442–450.

Hand, T. L., Ceglowski, W. S., and Friedman, H. 1970. Calf thymus fractions: Enhancement and suppression of immunocompetent cells. Experientia 26:653–655.

Hannig, K., and Comsa, J. 1963. Factionnement electrophoretique de l'extrait de thymus. C. R. Acad. Sci. [D] 256:1855–1957.

Harboe, M., Pande, H., Brandtzaeg, P. Tveter, K. Y., and Hjort, P. E. 1966. Synthesis of donor type gamma-G-globulin following thymus transplantation in hypo-gamma-globulinemia with severe lymphopenia. Scand. J. Haemat. 3:351–374.

Hardy, M. A., Quint, J., Franco, D. J., and Monaco, A. P. 1969a. Modification of immunosuppressive effects of antilymphocyte serum by a thymic humoral factor, thymosin. Brit. J. Surg. 56:616.

Hardy, M. A., Quint, J., Goldstein, A. L., State, D., and White, A. 1968. Effect of thymosin and an antithymosin serum on allograft survival in mice. Proc. Natl. Acad. Sci. U.S.A. 61:875–882.

Hardy, M. A., Quint, J., Goldstein, A. L., White, A., State, D., and Battisto, J. R. 1969b. Effects of an antiserum to calf thymosin on lymphoid cells *in vitro*. Proc. Soc. Exp. Biol. Med. 130:214–219.

Hardy, M. A., Quint, J., and State, D. 1969. Prolongation of skin allograft survivals in mice by an antiserum to calf thymosin. Transplantation 7:223–725.

Harms, J. W. 1952a. Exstirpation mit anschliebender Transplantation des Thymus bei *Xenopus laevis*. Daubin Z. Naturforsch [B] 7:622–630.

Harms, J. W. 1952b. Experimentell-morphologische Untersuchungen uber den Thymus von *Xenopus laevis*. Daudin Gegenbaurs Morphol. Jahrb. 92:256–338.

Harris, J. E., and Ford, L. E. 1964. Cellular traffic of the thymus: Experiments with chromosome markers. Evidence that the thymus plays an instructional part. Nature 201:884–885.

Harvey, A. M. 1948. Some preliminary observations on clinical course of myasthenia gravis before and after thymectomy. Bull. N.Y. Acad. Med. 24:505–522.

Harvey, A. M., Lilienthal, J. L., Jr., and Talbot, S. A. 1942. Observations on the nature of myasthenia gravis. The effect of thymectomy on neuromuscular transmission. J. Clin. Invest. 21:579–588.

Haskill, J. S., Byrt, P., and Marbrook, J. 1970. *In vitro* and *in vivo* studies of the immune response to sheep erythrocytes using partially purified cell preparations. J. Exp. Med. 131:57–76.

Hathaway, W. E., Brangle, R. W., Nelson, T. L., and Roeckel, I. E. 1966. Aplastic anemia and alymphocytosis in an infant with hypogammaglobulinemia: Graft-*versus*-host reaction? J. Pediat. 68:713–722.

Hathaway, W. E., Fulginiti, V. A., Pierce, C. W., Githens, J. H., Pearlman, D. S., Muschenheim, F., and Kempe, C. H. 1967. Graft-*vs*-host reaction following a single blood transfusion. J.A.M.A. 201:1015–1020.

Hathaway, W. E., Githens, J. H., Blackburn, W. R., Fulginiti, V., and Kempe, C. H. 1965. Aplastic anemia, histiocytosis and erythrodermia in immunologically deficient children. Probable human runt disease. New Engl. J. Med. 273:953–958.

Haurowitz, F. 1970. Molecular basis of immunity. *In* Developmental aspects of antibody formation and structure, II. Sterzl, J. and Riha, I. (eds.). Academic Press, New York. pp. 91–917.

Hays, E. F. 1967. The effects of allografts of thymic epithelial reticular cells on the lymphoid tissue of neonatally thymectomized mice. Blood 29:29–40.

Hellman, T. and White, G, 1930. Das Verhatten des lymphatischen Gewebes während eines Immunisierungsprozesses. Virchows Arch, 278:221–257.

Hermans, P. E., Huizenga, K. A., Hoffman, H. N., Brown, A. L., and Markowitz, H. 1966. Dysgammaglobulinemia associated with nodular lymphoid hyperplasia of the small intestine. Amer. J. Med. 40:78–89.

Hess, E. H. 1959. Imprinting. Science 130:133–134.

Hess, E. H. 1972. "Imprinting" in a natural laboratory. Sci. Am. 227:24–31.

Hess, M. W. 1968. Experimental thymectomy, possibilities and limitations. Springer, Berlin. 107 p.

Hess, M. W., Cottier, H., and Stoner, R. D. 1963. Primary and secondary antitoxin responses in thymectomized mice. J. Immunol. 91:425–430.

Hess, M. W., and Stoner, R. D. 1966. Further studies on tetanus antitoxin responses in neonatally thymectomized mice. Int. Arch. Allergy Appl. Immunol. 30:37–47.

Hillman, H., and Hyden, H. 1965. Membrane potentials in isolated neurones *in vitro* from Dieters' nucleus of rabbit. J. Physiol. 177:398–410.

Hirabagashi, R. N., and Lindsay, S. 1965. The relation of thyroid carcinoma and chronic thyroiditis. Surg. Gynec. Obstet. 121:243–252.

Hirota, O. 1938. Relations between thymus and vitamins. (Japanese, summary in German), Fol. Endocr. Jap. 15:73–76.

Hirschborn, K. 1966. Lymphocyte activation. *In* Mediators of cellular immunity, Lawrence, H. S., and Landy, M. (eds.) Academic Press, New York.

Hirst, E. and Robertson, T. I. 1967, The syndrome of thymoma and erythroblastopenic anemia, Med. 46:225.

Hitzig, W. H. 1960. Praktische und theoretische Ergebnisse neuerer Bluteiweiss-Untersuchungen. Schweiz. Med. Wchnschr. 90:1449–1458.

Hitzig, W. H., Barandun, S., and Cottier, H. 1968. Die schweizerische Form der Agammaglobulinämie. Ergebn. Inn. Med. Kinderh. 27:79–154.

Hitzig, W. H., Biro, Z., Bosch, H., and Huser, H. J. 1958. Agammaglobulinamie und Alymphocytose mit Schwund des lymphatischer Gewebes. Helv. Paediat. Acta 13:551.

Hitzig, W. H., Kay, H. E. M., and Cottier, H. 1965. Familial lymphopenia with agammaglobulinaemia. An attempt at treatment by implantation of foetal thymus. Lancet 2:151–154.

Hnilica, L. S. 1971. The structure and biological function of histones. C. R. C. Press, Cleveland. 200 p.

Hobbs, J. R., Milner, R. D. G., and Watt, P. J. 1967. Gamma-M-deficiency predisposing to meningococcal septicaemia. Brit. Med. J. 4:583–586.

Hoene, R., Rindani, T. H., and Heuser, G. 1954. Influence of somato-trophic hormone and hydrocortisone acetate on the production of hemolytic antibodies in the rat. Am. J. Physiol. 177:19–26.

Hohn, E. 1959. Lack of effect of thymectomy on inguinal lymph gland weight and thyroid function in weanling rats. J. Biochem. 37:1453–1455.

Hohorst, H., Reim, M., and Barthel, H. 1962. Studies of the creatine kinase equilibrium in muscle and significance of ATP and ADP level. Biochem. Biophys. Res. Commun. 7:142–146.

Hong, R., Gatti, R. A., and Good, R. A. 1968. Hazards and potential benefits of blood-transfusion in immunological deficiency. Lancet 2:388–389.

Hong, R., Kay, H. E. M., Cooper, M. D., Meuwissen, H., Allan, M. J. G., and Good, R. A. 1968. Immunological restitution in lymphopenic immunological deficiency syndrome. Lancet 1:503–506.

Horacek, J., and Cernikova, M. 1959. Examination of lipids in human serum by disk chromatography. Biochem. J. 71:417–419.

Hoshino, T., Takada, M., Abe, K., and Ito, T. 1969. Early development of thymic lymphocytes in mice, studied by light and electron microscopy. Anat. Rec. 164:47–65.

Houssay, B. A., Houssay, A. B., Cardeza, A. F., and Pinto, R. M. 1955. Tumeurs surrenales oestrogeniques et tumeurs hypophysaires chez les animaux castres. Schweiz. Med. Wochenschr. 85:291–296.

Howe, M. L., Goldstein, A. L., and Battisto, J. R. 1970. Isogeneic lymphocyte interaction: Recognition of self antigens by cells of the neonatal thymus. Proc. Natl. Acad. Sci. U.S.A. 67:613.

Hudson, A., and Luckey, T. D. 1964. Bacteria-induced morphologic changes. Proc. Soc. Exp. Biol. Med. 116:628–631.

Huff, C. G. 1940. Immunity in invertebrates. Physiol. Rev. 20:68–88.

Humphrey, J. H., Parrott, D. M. V., and East, J. 1964. Studies on globulin and antibody production in mice thymectomized at birth. Immunology 7:419–439.

Hyden, H. and Lang, P. W. 1970 Brain cell protein synthesis specifically related to learning, Proc. Nat. Acad, Sci. 65:898–904.

Ingle, D. J. 1938. The effects of administering large amounts of cortin on the adrenal cortices of normal and hypophysectomized rats. Am. J. Physiol. 124:369–371.

Irvine, W. J., Stewart, A. G., and Scarth, L. 1967. A. clinical and immunological study of adrenocortical insufficiency (Addison's disease). Clin. Exp. Immun. 2:31–70.

Irvine, W. J., and Sumerling, M. D. 1965. Radiological assessment of the thymus in thyroid and other diseases. Lancet 1:996–999.

Isakovic, K., and Jankovic, B. D. 1964. Role of the thymus and the bursa of Fabricius in immune reactions in chickens. Int. Arch. Allergy Appl. Immunol. 24:296–310.

Ishizuka, M., Gafni, M., and Braun, W. 1970. Cyclic AMP effects on antibody formation and their similarities to hormone-mediated events. Proc. Soc. Exp. Biol. Med. 134:963–967.

Ito, Y., and Mizutani, A. 1952a. Salivary gland hormones. XIV. Isolation of crystalline parotin by fractional precipitation with ammonium sulfate. J. Pharm. Soc. Jap. 72:244–248.

Ito, Y., and Mizutani, A. 1952b. Salivary gland hormones. XVII. Comparison of properties of parotin and organ extracts acting like parotin on serum calcium level. J. Pharm. Soc. Jap. 72:1468–1471.

Jaffe, H. L. 1924a. The influence of the suprarenal gland on the thymus. Re-generation of the thymus following double suprarenalectomy in the rat. J. Exp. Med. 40:325–342.

Jaffe, H. L. 1924b. The influence of the suprarenal gland on the thymus. II. Direct evidence of regeneration of the involuted thymus following double supra-renalectomy. J. Exp. Med. 40:619–625.

Jailer, J. W. 1941. Effect of testosterone propionate on creatinuria of experi-mental hyperthyroidism in male and female monkeys. Endocrinology 29:89–92.

Jankovic, B. D., and Isakovic, K. 1964. Role of the thymus and bursa of Fabricius in immune reactions in chickens. Int. Arch. Allergy Appl. Immunol. 24:278–295.

Jankovic, B. D., Isvaneski, M., Milosvic, D., and Popeskovic, L. 1963. Delayed hypersensitive reactions in bursectomized chickens. Nature 198:298–299.

Jankovic, B. D., Waksman, B. H., and Arnason, B. G. 1962. Role of the thymus in immune reactions in rats. I. Immunologic response to bovine serum albumin (antibody formation, Arthus reactivity, and delayed hypersensitiv-ity) in rats thymectomized or splenectomized after birth. J. Exp. Med 116:159–175.

Janower, M. L., and Miettinen, O. S. 1971. Neoplasms after childhood irradiation of the thymus gland. J. Am. Med. Assn. 215:753–756.

Jeejeebhoy, J. F. 1965. Effects of rabbit anti-rat-lymphocyte plasma on immune response of rats thymectomised in adult life. Lancet 2:106–107.

Jehn, U. W., and Karlin, L. 1971. Independent action of thymus and bone marrow cells during the secondary responses of direct plaque-forming cells. J. Immunol. 106:946–950.

Joel, D. D., Hess, M. W., and Cottier, H. 1971. Thymic lymphocytes in develop-ing Peyer's patches of newborn mice. Nature (New Biol.) 231:24–25.

Jolley, W. B., and Hinshaw, D. B. 1965. Basic peptides isolated from the thymus gland and blood and their possible role in homograft reaction. Surg. Forum 16:211–213.

Jolly, J., and Levin, S. 1911. Sur les modifications de poids des organes lymphoids a la suite des jeune. C. R. Soc. Biol. 71:320–323.

Jones, R. N., and Herling, F. 1956. The infrared spectra of acetoxysteroids below 1350 Cm^{-1}. J. Am. Chem. Soc. 78:1152–1161.

Jones, R. N., Herling, F., and Katzenellbogen, E. 1955. The infrared spectra of ketosteroids below 1350 Cm^{-1}. J. Am. Chem. Soc. 77:651–661.

Jonson, A. 1909. Die accidentelle thymusinvolution im Hunger. Arch. Mikrosk. Anat. Entwicklungsmech. 73:390–443.

Joske, R. A. 1958. The effects of thymectomy on the lymphocyte count in patients with myasthenia gravis. Med. J. Aust. 45:859–861.

Kampschmidt, R. F., and McCoy, T. A. 1960. Effect of tumor cell fractions upon plasma iron, liver catalyase, and organ weights of rats. Proc. Soc. Exp. Biol. Med. 103:869–871.

Kaplan, H. S. 1947. Observations on radiation-induced lymphoid tumors of mice. Cancer Res. 7:141–147.

Kaplan, H. S. 1954. On the etiology and pathogeny of leukemia—A review. Cancer Res. 14:535–548.

Kaplan, H. S. 1966. Interaction of occult leukaemogenic viruses with ionzing radiation and other external leukaemogenic agents in the induction of thymic lymphosarcoma in the mouse. In The thymus: Experimental and clinical studies, Wolstenholme, G. E. W., and Porter, R. (eds.), Ciba Found. Symp. Churchill, London. p. 310.

Kaplan, H. S., Brown, M. B., and Paul, J. 1953. Influence of postirradiation thymectomy and of thymic implants on lymphoid tumor incidence in C-57BL mice. Cancer Res. 13:677–680.

Kaplan, H. S., Marder, S. N., and Brown, M. B. 1951. Adrenal cortical function and lymphoid tumors of mice. Cancer Res. 11:629–633.

Karaklis, A., Valaes, T., Pantelakis, S. N., and Doxiadis, S. A. Thymectomy in an infant with autoimmune haemolytic anaemia. Lancet 2:778–780, 1964.

Kellum, M. J., Sutherland, D. E. R., Eckert, E., Good, R. A., and Peterson, R. D. A. 1965. Wasting disease Coombs-positivity and amyloidosis in rabbits subjected to central lymphoid tissue extirpation and irradiation. Int. Arch. Allergy Appl. Immunol. 27:6–26.

Kelly, W. D. 1963. The thymus and lymphoid morphogenesis in the dog. Fed. Proc. 22:600.

Kersey, J. H., Meuweissen, J. J., and Good, R. A. Allogeneic hematopoietic cells. 1971. Human Pathol. 2:389–392.

Keynes, G. 1946. Surgery of thymus gland. Brit. J. Surg. 33:201–214.

Keynes, G. 1949. The results of thymectomy in myasthenia gravis. Brit. Med. J. 2:611–616.

Keynes, G. 1954a. The physiology of the thymus gland. Brit. Med. J. 2:659–663.

Keynes, G. 1954b. Surgery of the thymus gland. Second (and third) thoughts. Lancet 1:1197–1202.

Keynes, G. 1955. Investigations into thymic disease and tumour formation. Brit. J. Surg. 42:449–462.

Kirk, B. W., and Freedman, S. O. 1967. Hypogammaglobulinemia, thymoma, and ulcerative colitis. Canad. M. A. J. 96:1272–1277.

Kirkpatrick, C. H., Waxman, D., Smith, D. O., and Schimke, R. N. 1968. Hypogammaglobulinemia with nodular lymphoid hyperplasia of the small bowel. Arch. Int. Med. 121:273–277.

Klein, J. J., Goldstein, A. L., and White, A. 1965. Enhancement of in vivo incorporation of labeled precursors into DNA and total protein of mouse lymph nodes after administration of thymic extracts. Proc. Natl. Acad. Sci. U.S.A. 53:812–817.

Klein, J. J., Goldstein, A. L., and White, A. 1966. Effect of the thymus lymphocytepoietic factor. Ann. N.Y. Acad. Sci. 135:485–495.

Klein, J. J., Gottleib, A. J., Mones, R. J., Appel, S. H., and Osserman, K. E. 1964. Thymoma and polymyositis: Onset of myasthenia gravis after thymectomy: Report of two cases. Arch. Int. Med. 113:142.

Kliwanskaia-Kroll, E. 1938. Zur morphologie des experimentellen Hyperthyroid-ismus. Das inkretorische System des in Wachstum begriffenen Organisms bei systematischer Futterung mit Schilddruensubstanz. Virchows Arch. Pathol. Anat. Physiol. 268:374–394.

Klopfer, P. H. 1971. Mother love: What turns it on? Am. Scientist 59:404–447.

Klose, H. 1914. Thymusdruse und rachitis. Zentralbl. Allg. Pathol. 25:1–7.

Klose, H. and Vogt, H. 1910. Klinik und Biologie der Thymusdruse. Bietr. klin. Chim, 69:1–200.

Kmieciak, M. 1971. Effects of calf thymus extract on human peripheral blood lymphocytes growing *in vitro*. Folia Morphol. 30:301–309.

Knoll, W. 1929. Z. Undersuchungen uber embryonale Blutbildung bieun Hens-chen. Z. Mikrosk. Anat. Forsch. 18:199–232.

Kornberg, J. A., Daft, F. S., and Sebrell, W. H. 1954. In The Vitamins, Sebrell, W. H., and Harris, R. S. Ed. Academic Press, New York.

Kough, R. H., and Barnes, W. T. 1964. Thymoma associated with erythroid aplasia, bullous skin eruption and the lupus erythematosus cell phenomenon. Ann. Int. Med. 61:308–315.

Kreel, I., Genkins, G., Osserman, K. E., Jacobsen, E., and Baronofsky, I. D. 1960. Studies in myasthenia gravis and improved techniques in thymectomy. Arch. Surg. 81:251–258.

Kreel, I., Osserman, K. E., Genkins, G., and Kark, A. E. 1967. Role of thym-ectomy in the management of myasthenia gravis. Ann. Surg. 165:111–117.

Kretschmer, R., Jeannet, J., Mereu, T. R., Kretschmer, K., Winn, H., and Rosen, F. S. 1969. Hereditary thymic dysplasia: A graft-*versus*-host reaction induced by bone marrow cells with a partial 4a series histoincompatibility. Pediat. Res. 3:34–40.

Krizenecky, J. 1926. Einflub der Schilddreuse und des Thymus auf die Entwick-lung des Gefieders. Roux' Arch. 107:583–585.

Kruger, J., and Gershon, R. K. 1971. Immune response to hemocyanin in normal thymus-deprived and reconstituted mice. J. Immunol. 106:1065–1073.

Kruger, J., Goldstein, A. L., and Waksmann, B. 1970. Immunologic and anatomic consequences of calf thymosin injection in rats. Cell. Immunol. 1:51–61.

Kun, H., and Peczennik, O. 1936. Geschlechtsspezifische Wirkung der Sexual-hormone auf den Kreatinstoffwechsel. Pfluegers Arch. 236:471–480.

Kushner, D. S., Dubin, A., Donlon, W. P., and Bronsky, D., 1960. Familial hypogammaglobulinemia, splenomegaly, and leukopenia with a review of the etiological factors of the hypogamma globulinemias. Amer. J. Med. 29:33–42.

Lacassagne, A., and Gricouroff, G. 1941. Action des radiations sur les tissus. Masson, Paris. 170 p.

Ladik, J., and Greguss, P. 1971. Possible molecular mechanisms of information storage in the long term memory. Biology of Memory, ed. Adam, G. Plenum Press, New York. 343 p.

Larsson, O. 1963. Thymoma and systemic lupus erythematosus in the same patient. Lancet 2:665–666.

Lattes, R. 1962. Thymoma and other tumors of the thymus. An analysis of 107 cases. Cancer 15:1224–1260.

Law, J. H., and Regnier, F. E. 1971. Pheromones. Ann. Rev. Biochem. 40:533–548.

Law, L. W. 1947. Effect of gonadectomy and adrenalectomy on the appearance and incidence of spontaneous lymphoid leukemia in C58 mice. J. Natl. Cancer Inst. 8:157–159.

Law, L. W. 1965. Neoplasmas in thymectomized mice following room infection with polyoma virus. Nature 205:672–673.

Law, L. W. 1966. Studies of thymic function with emphasis on the role of the thymus in oncogenesis. Cancer Res. 26:551–574.

Law, L. W., and Agnew, H. D. 1968. Effect of thymic extracts on restoration of immunologic competence in thymectomized mice. Proc. Soc. Exp. Biol. Med. 127:953–956.

Law, L. W., Goldstein, A. L., and White, A. 1968. Influence of thymosin on immunological competence of lymphoid cells from thymectomized mice. Nature 219:1391–1392.

Law, L. W., and Miller, J. H. 1950a. Observations on the effect of thymectomy on spontaneous leukemias in mice of the high-leukemic strains, RIL and C58. J. Natl. Cancer Inst. 11:253–262.

Law, L. W., and Miller, J. H. 1950b. The effect of thymectomy on the incidence, latent period and type of leukemia in high leukemia strains of mice. Cancer Res. 10:230 p.

Law, L. W., and Miller, J. H. 1950c. The influence of thymectomy on the incidence of carcinogen-induced leukemia in strain DBA mice. J. Natl. Cancer Inst. 11:425–437.

Law, L. W., Trainin, N., Levey, R. H., and Barth, W. F. 1964. Humoral thymic factor in mice: Further evidence. Science 143:1049.

Lazar, A. 1966. Transplantation and function of a histo-incompatible tumor in thymectomized rats. Nature 210:1380–1381.

Leblond, C. P., and Segal, G. 1942. Differentiation between direct and indirect effects of roentgen rays upon organs of normal and adrenalectomized rats. Am. J. Roetgenol. Rad. Ther. Nucl. Med. 47:302–306.

Leduc, E. H., Coons, A. H., and Connelly, J. M. 1955. Studies on antibody production. II. The primary and secondary responses in the popliteal lymph node. J. Exp. Med. 102:61–72.

Leriche, J. 1948. Cancerologie; facteurs etiologiques, etats cancereux, precancereux, diagnostique biolgique, les glandes endocrines et autres organes et les cancers, les corps chimiques et les cancers, le traitement chimio-glandu-laire. Librairie Maloine, Paris, 989 p.

Leuchars, E., Cross, A. M., and Dukov, P. 1965. The restoration of immuno-logical function by thymus grafting in thymectomized irradiated mice. Transplantation 3:28–38.

Levey, R. H., Trainin, N., and Law, L. W. 1963. Evidence for function of thymic tissue in diffusion chambers implanted in neonatally thymectomized mice. Preliminary Report. J. Natl. Cancer Inst. 31:199–217.

Levey, R. H., Trainin, N., Law, L. W., Black, P. H., and Rowe, W. P. 1963. Lymphocytic choriomeningitis infection in neonatally thymectomized mice bearing diffusion chambers containing thymus. Science 142:483–485.

Levinthal, J. D., and Buffett, R. F. 1961. Thymectomy and thymic grafts in mouse viral leukemia. Proc. Soc. Exp. Biol. Med. 106:426–432.

Levy, R. L., Huang, S., Bach, M. L. Bach, F. H., Hong, R., Ammann, A. J., Bortin, M., and Kay, H. E. M. 1971. Thymic transplanation in a case of chronic mucocutaneous candidasis. Lancet 7730:898–903.

Li, C. P., Prescott, B., Chi, L. L., and Martino, E. 1963. Antiviral and anti-bacterial activity of thymus extracts. Proc. Soc. Exp. Biol. Med. 114:504–509.

Lipmann, F. 1971. Attempts to map a process evolution of peptide biosynthesis. Science 173:875–884.

Lishner, H. W., and Di George, A. M. 1969. Role of the thymus in humoral im-munity. Lancet 2:1044–1046.

Litwac, G. 1970. Biochemical actions of hormones. Academic Press, New York.

Loiseleur, J. 1954. Techniques de laboratoire, 2nd ed., Toma, I. (ed.). Masson, Paris.

Lopez-Lomba, J. 1923a. Modifications ponderales des organes chez le pigeon au cours de l'avitaminose B. C. R. Acad. Sci. (D) 176:1417–1421.

Lopez-Lomba, J. 1923b. Modifications ponderales des organes chez le cobaye au cours de l'avitaminose C. C. R. Acad. Sci. (D) 176:1752–1754.

Louis-Bar, M. 1941. Sur un syndrome progressif comprenant des telangiectasies capillaires cutanees et conjonctivales symmetriques a des positions naevoide et des troubles cerebelleux. Confin. Neurol. 4:32–42.

Lowry, O., Rosebrough, N., Farr, A., and Randall, R. 1951. Protein measure-ment with the Folin phenol reagent. J. Biol. Chem. 193:265–275.

Luca, R. de, Santangelo, G., and Cotadini, V. 1966. Indagini sul ricambio gluci-dico a livello epatico in ratti distimizzati. Minerva Pediatr. 18:492–495.

Lucien, M., and Parisot, J. 1910. Contribution a l'etude des fonctions du thymus. Arch. Med. Exp. Anat. Path. 22:98–137.

Lucien, M., Parisot, J., and Richard, G. 1925. Traite d'endocrinologie. Le parathyroides et le thymus. Doin, Paris.

Luckey, T. D. 1959. Antibiotics in nutrition. Antibiotics, their chemistry and non-medical uses, Goldberg, H. S. (ed.). D. Van Nostrand, Princeton: pp. 174–321.

Luckey, T. D. 1963. Germfree life and gnotobiology. Academic Press, New York. 490 p.

Luckey, T. D. 1965. Gnotobiology and aerospace systems. Advances in germfree research and gnotobiology, Miyakawa. M., and Luckey, T. D. (eds.). C. R. C. Press, Cleveland. pp. 317–353.

Luckey, T. D. 1965b. Gnotobiologic evidence for functions of the microflora. Ernahrungs Forschung. 10:192–250.

Luckey, T. D. 1965c. Effects of microbes on germfree animals. Adv. Appl. Microbiol. 7:169–223.

Luckey, T. D. 1971. Thymic hormones. Recorded at workshop fifty-five of the First International Congress of Immunology, Washington.

Lykke, A. W. J., Willoughby, D. A., and Kosche, E. R. 1967. Thymic permeability factor: Its relationship to lymph-node permeability factor and its antagonism by pyridinol carbamate (Anginin) and other anti-inflammatory agents. J. Pathol. Bacteriol. 94:381–388.

Mackay, I. R. 1966. Histopathology of the human thymus. In the thymus: Experimental and clinical studies, Ciba Found. Symp. Wolstenholme, G. E., and Porter, R. (ed.). Churchill, London. p. 449–475.

Mackay, I. R., Goldstein, G., and McConchie, I. H. 1963. Thymectomy in systemic lupus erythematosus. Brit. Med. J. 2:792–793.

Mackay, I. R., and Smalley, M. 1966. Results of thymectomy in systemic lupus erythematosus: Observations on clinical course and serological reactions. Clin. Exp. Immun. 1:129–138.

Maisin, J. H. F. 1963. Le role du thymus et des antigenes specifiques dans la cancerisation par le 20-methycholantrene. C. R. Soc. Biol. 157:1519–1522.

Maisin, J. H. F; 1964. L'immunoprophylaxie du cancer experimental. Brux. Med. 44:323–335.

Mandel, P. 1963. Nekotirie aspecta reguleatii biosinteza nucleinovih kislot v normalnih i racovih tkaniah. Vopr. Onkol. 9:7–24.

Marabini, B., and Natali, G. 1952. Dati sperimentali sull' antagonismo tra estratto timico e ACTH. Rass. Neurol. Veg. 9:341–363.

Marine, D., Manley, O. T., and Bauman, E. J. 1924. The influence of thyroidectomy, gonadectomy, suprarenalectomy, and splenectomy on the thymus gland of rabbits. J. Exp. Med. 40:429–443.

Masson, E. E., Chin, T., Li, Y. W., and Ziffrin, S. E. 1960. Cancer and human liver catalase. Cancer Res. 20:1474–1481.

Matti, H. 1911. Untersuchungen uber die Wirkung experimenteller Ausschaltung der Thymusdruse; un Beitrag zur Physiologie und Pathologie der Thymus. Mitteil. Grenzgeb. Med. 24:664–821.

Maximow, A. 1901. Untersuchungen uber Blut und Bindegewebe. II. Uber die Histogenese des thymus Beisaugetieren. Arch. Mikroskop. Anat. Entwicklungsmech. 74:525–621.

McDivitt, H. O., Askonas, B. A., Humphrey, J. H., Schechter, I. and Sela, M. 1966. The localization of antigen in relation to specific antibody-producing cells. I. Use of a synthetic polypeptide labelled with iodine-125. Immunol. 11:337–351.

McEndy, D. P., Boon, M. C;, and Furth, J. 1944. On the role of thymus, spleen, and gonads in the development of leukemia in a high-leukemia stock of mice. Cancer Res. 4:377–383.

McGregor, D. 1968. Bone marrow origin of immunologically competent lymphocytes in the rat. J. Exp. Med. 127:953–966.

McIntire, K. R., Sell, S., and Miller, J. F. A. P. 1964. Pathogenesis of the postneonatal thymectomy wasting syndrome. Nature 204:151–155.

McQueeney, A. J., Ashburn, L. L., Daft, F. S., and Faulkner, R. 1947. Tissue changes and sodium balance in pantothenic acid-deficient rats. Endocrinology 41:441–450.

Metcalf, D. 1956a. A lymphocytosis stimulating factor in the plasma of chronic lymphatic leukemic patients. Brit. J. Cancer 10:169–178.

Metcalf, D. 1956b. Further studies on the plasma lymphocytosis stimulating factor in chronic lymphatic leukemia and some other disease states. Brit. J. Cancer 10:431–441.

Metcalf, D. 1956c. The thymic origin of the plasma lymphocytosis-stimulating factor. Brit. J. Cancer 10:442–457.

Metcalf, D. 1958. The thymic lymphocytosis-stimulating factor. Ann. N.Y. Acad. Sci. 73:113–119.

Metcalf, D. 1959. The thymic lymphocytosis stimulating factor and its relation to lymphatic leukemia. In Becq. R. W. Proceedings Third Canadian Cancer Conference, Academic Press, N.Y. pp. 351–366.

Metcalf, D. 1960. The effect of thymectomy on the lymphoid tissues of the mouse. Brit. J. Haematol. 6:324–333.

Metcalf, D. 1964. Functional interactions between the thymus and other organs. In The Thymus, Defendi, V. and Metcalf, P. (eds.). The Wistar Institute Press, Philadelphia, pp. 53–72.

Metcalf, D. 1965. Delayed effect of thymectomy in adult life on immunological competence. Nature 208:1336.

Metcalf, D. 1966a. Recent results in cancer research. Springer-Verlag, Inc., New York:

Metcalf, D. 1966b. The thymus; Its role in immune responses, leukemia development and carcinogenesis. Springer-Verlag, Inc., New York.

Metcalf, D., and Buffet, R. F. 1957. Lymphocytosis response in mice and its relation to thymus and adrenal. Proc. Soc. Exp. Biol. Med. 95:576–579.

Metcalf, D., and Wakonig-Vaartaja, R. 1964. Stem cell replacement in normal thymus grafts. Proc. Soc. Exp. Biol. Med. 115:731–735.

Meuwissen, H. J., Bach, F. H., Hong, R., and Good, R. A. Lymphocyte studies in congenital thymic dysplasia: The one-way stimulation test. J. Pediat. 72:177–185.

Micklem, H. S., Ford, C. E., Evans, E. P., and Gray, J. 1966. Interrelationships of myeloid and lymphoid cells. Studies with chromosome-marked cells transfused into lethally irradiated mice. Proc. Roy. Soc. Biol. 165:78–102.

Milcu, S. M., Babes, A., Istrati, F., and Petrea, I. 1954. Contributiuni la studiul histofisilogiei timusului. Stud. Cercet. Endocr., 5, 115.

Milcu, S. M., and Lupulescu, A. 1952a. Inhibitia cirozei estradiolice prin extract protidic de timus. Com. Acad. RPR 2:9–10.

Milcu, S. M., and Lupulescu. A. 1952b. Actinuea inhibitorie a extractului protidic de timus asupra tumorilor estradiolice. Stud. Cercet. Endocr. 3, 1:220.

Milcu, S. M., and Pitis, M. 1943a. Contibutinui la studiul corelatiilor dintre epifiza si timus. Acta Endocrinol. 9:38.

Milcu, S. M., and Pitis, M. 1943b. Contributions a l'etude de la corrélation thymoepiphisaire. Acta Endocr. 9:2–73.

Milcu, S. M., and Potop, I. 1955. Actinunea timusului asupra variatiilor continutului in apa si lipide totale al unor segmente dintesutul cerebral. Bul. St. Sect. St. Med. Acad. RPR 7:1182.

Milcu, S. M., and Potop, I. 1966. Influence du thymus sur le matabolism des acides nucleiques chez les rats normaux et ceux porteurs de tumeurs. Rev. Roum. Biochim. 3:183.

Milcu, S. M., and Potop. I. 1970. Farmacodinamia substantelor hormonal asemanatoare din timus. Edit. Acad. RPR., Bucharest.

Milcu, S. M., and Potop, I. 1971. Isolation of an antiblastic factor from the bovine thymus. Rev. Roum. Endocr. 8:1–73.

Milcu, S. M., Potop, I., Ciocirdia, S., Neacsu, C., and Simionescu, N. 1963. L'influence de l'administration du thymus et de l'athymie experimentale sur les proteins seriques chez le lapin. Acta Biol. Med. Germ. 11:371–377.

Milcu, S. M., Potop, I., Felix, E., and Costin, E. 1951a. Contributinui experimentale la studiul relatiilor dintre timus si crestere. Com. Acad. RPR 1, 2:201.

Milcu, S. M., Potop, I., Felix, E., and Costin, E. 1951b. Continutul oaselor in Ca, K, P, si Na in hiper si hipotimia experimentala. Com. Acad. RPR 1, 6:483.

Milcu, S. M., Potop, I., Hobvan, R., Mreana, G., and Boeru, V. 1965. Actinuea unor extracte timica asupra proliferarii cellulelor cultivate in vitro. Stud. Cercet. Endocr. 16:129–36.

Milcu, S. M., Potop, I., Holban-Petresco, R., Boeru, V., Ghinea, E., and Tasca, C. 1969. Effects of some fractions isolated from a lipid thymus extract (extract II B) on tumor cell proliferation in vitro. Neoplasma 16:473–484.

Milcu, S. M., Potop, I., Holban-Petresco, R., and Ghinea, E. 1966. Effet d'un extrait lipidique de thymus (fraction "II B") sur la proliferation des cultures des cellules tumorales KB in vitro. C. R. Soc. Biol. 160:1326–1364.

Milcu, S. M., Potop, I., Holban-Petresco, R., Ghinea, E., Boeru, V., and Mreana, G. 1966. Action de certains extraits isoles du thymus sur proliferation des cellules cultives in vitro. Acta Biol. Med. Ger. 16:606–616.

Milcu, S. M., Potop, I., and Mreana, G. 1963. Date referitorare la influenta estimizarii si administrarii de extracte timice asupra ATP-ului din muschi. Com. Acad. RPR 13, 10:909.

Milcu, S. M., and Simionescu, N. 1953. Rolul sistemului nerves central in desfasurarea hipertrofiei de compensatie a glandei suprarenale le animalele tratate cu extract de timus. Stud. Cercet. Endocr. 6, 3–4:535.

Milcu, S. M., and Simionescu, N. 1960. Influenta timectomiei asupra hipertrofiei de compensatie a glandei suprarenal. Stud. Cercet. Endocr. 11 (1):128.

Milcu, S. M., Stanescu, V., Florea, I., Juvina, E., and Ionescu, V. 1960. Efectele timectomiei si ale administrarii de cortizon asupra nucleoproteinelor sanghine. Stud. Cercet. Endocr. 11:203–207.

Miller, J. F. A. P. 1960. Recovery of leukaemogenic agent from non-leukaemic tissues of thymectomized mice. Nature 187:703 p.

Miller, J. F. A. P. 1961a. Immunological function of the thymus. Lancet 2:748–749.

Miller, J. F. A. P. 1961b. Analysis of the thymus influence in leukaemogenesis. Nature 191:248–249.

Miller, J. F. A. P. 1961c. Etiology and parthogenesis of mouse leukemia. Adv. Cancer Res. 6:291–368.

Miller, J. F. A. P. 1962a. The role of the lymphoid system in homotransplantation reactions. I. Role of the thymus in transplantation immunity. Ann. N. Y. Acad. Sci. 99:340–354.

Miller, J. F. A. P. 1962b. Effect of neonatal thymectomy on the immunological responsiveness of the mouse. Proc. Roy. Soc. Biol. 156:415–428.

Miller, J. F. A. P. 1962c. Immunological significance of the thymus of the adult mouse. Nature 195:1318–1319.

Miller, J. F. A. P. 1963a. Tolerance in the thymectomized animal. Tolerance aquise et tolerance naturelle a l'egard du substances antigeniques definies. Colloque du Centre National de la Recherche Scientifique, Paris p. 47–75.

Miller, J. F. A. P. 1963b. Role of the thymus in immunity. Brit. Med. J. 2:459–464.

Miller J. F. A. P. 1964a. Recovery of immunological responsiveness in thymectomized animals by thymus grafting. In The thymus, Defendi, V., and Metcalf, D. (eds.). The Wistar Press, Philadelphia. pp. 99–101.

Miller, J. F. A. P. 1964b. The thymus and development of immunologic responsiveness. Science 144:1544–1550.

Miller, J. F. A. P. 1964c. Effect of thymic ablation and replacement. In The thymus in immunobiology; Structure, function and role in disease, Good, R. A., and Gabrielson, A. E. (eds.). Hoeber-Harper, New York. pp. 436–464.

Miller, J. F. A. P. 1964d. Influence of thymectomy on tumor induction of polyoma virus in C57BL mice. Proc. Soc. Exp. Biol. Med. 116:323–327.

Miller, J. F. A. P. 1965a. Influence of the thymus on the development of the immune system. Series Haematol. 8:41.

Miller, J. F. A. P. 1965b. The thymus and transplantation immunity. Brit. Med. Bull. 21:111–117.

Miller, J. F. A. P. 1965c. Effect of thymectomy in adult mice on immunological responsiveness. Nature 208:1337–1338.

Miller, J. F. A. P. 1966. The thymus in relation to the development of immunological capacity. The CIBA Found. Symp. Thymus: Experimental and clinical studies, Wolstenholme, G. E. W., and Porter, R. (eds.). Churchill, London. pp. 153–174.

Miller, J. F. A. P. 1967. The thymus, yesterday, today, tomorrow. Lancet 2:1299–1302.

Miller, J. F. A. P., Block, M., Rowlands, D. T., Jr., and Kind, P. 1965. Effect of thymectomy on hematopoietic organs of the opossum "embryo." Proc. Soc. Exp. Biol. Med. 118:916–921.

Miller, J. F. A. P., Doak, S. M. A., and Cross, A. M. 1963. Role of the thymus in recovery of the immune mechanism in the irradiated adult mouse. Proc. Soc. Exp. Biol. Med. 112:785–792.

Miller, J. F. A. P., Grant, G. A., and Roe, F. J. C. 1963. Effect of thymectomy on the induction of skin tumors by 3,4-benzopyrene. Nature 199:920–922.

Miller, J. F. A. P., and Howard, J. G. 1964. Some similarities between the neonatal thymectomy syndrome and graft-versus-host disease. J. Reticuloend. Soc. 1:369–392.

Miller, J. F. A. P., Marshall, A. H. E., and White, R. G. 1962. The immunological significance of the thymus. Adv. Immunol. 2:111–162.

Miller, J. F. A. P., and Mitchell, G. F. 1967. The thymus and the precursors of antigen reactive cells. Nature 216:659–663.

Miller, J. F. A. P., and Mitchell, G. F. 1968. Cell to cell interaction in the immune response. J. Exp. Med. 128:801–820.

Miller, J. F. A. P., and Mitchell, G. F. 1969. Thymus and antigen-reactive cells. Transplant. Rev. 1:3–42.

Miller, J. F. A. P., Mitchell, G. F., and Weiss, N. S. 1967. Cellular basis of the immunological defects in thymectomized mice. Nature 214:992–997.

Miller, J. F. A. P., and Osoba, D. 1964. The lymphoid tissues and immune responses of neonatally thymectomized mice bearing thymus tissue in millipore diffusion chambers. J. Exp. Med. 119:177–194.

Miller, J. F. A. P., and Osoba, D. 1967. Current concepts of the immunological function of the thymus. Physiol. Rev. 47:437–520.

Miller, M. E. 1967. Thymic dysplasia ("Swiss agammaglobulinemia") I. Graft versus host reaction following bone-marrow transfusion. J. Pediat. 70:730–736.

Miller, W. H., Gorman, R. E., and Bitensky, M. W. 1967. Cyclic adenosine monephosphate: Function in photoreceptors. Science 295:295–297.

Milne, J. A., Anderson, J. R., Macsween, R. N., Fraser, R., Short, I., Stevens, J., Shaw, G. B., and Tankley, H. I. 1967. Thymectomy in acute systemic lupus erythematosus and rheumatoid arthritis. Brit. Med. J. 1:461.

Mitchell, G. F., and Miller, J. F. A. P. 1968. Cell to cell interaction in the immune response. II. The source of hemolysin-forming cells in irradiated mice given bone marrow and thymus or thoracic duct lymphocytes. J. Exp. Med. 128:821–837.

Mitchell, J., and Abbot, A. 1965. Ultrastructure of the antigen-retaining reticulum of lymph node follicles as shown by high resolution autoradiography. Nature 208:500–502.

Mizutani, A., Saito, Y., Sato, H., and Saito, M. 1970. The search for a hypocalcemic factor in the thymus gland. I. Separation of fractions producing hypocalcemia in rabbits from bovine thymus gland by precipitation with calcium chloride. J. Pharm. Soc. Jap. 90:445–451.

Mizutani, A., Terada, M., Toda, Y., and Yamamoto, K. 1969. A search for hypocalcemic factor in the thymus gland. III. Fundamental experiment for an improved method of the extraction of substance producing hypocalcemia in rabbits. Ann. Rept. Pharm. Nagoya City Univ. 17:16–19.

Mizutani, A., Yamamoto, K., Kawaguchi, H., and Mizutani, M. 1968. Staining method of differential counting of lymphocytes and polymorphonuclear leucocytes in rabbit blood. Ann. Rept. Pharm. Nagoya City Univ. 16:22–23.

Mizutani, A., Yamamoto, K., Sato, H., Saito, Y., Kitsugawa, H., and Yamamoto, H. 1971. A search for a hypocalcemic factor in the thymus gland. II. Improved method for the purification of the substance producing hypocalcemia in rabbits. J. Pharm. Soc. Jap. 91:297–302.

Molnar, P., and Kovacs, K. 1953. Wirkung eines Thymusextraktes auf das Brown-Pearce-Karzinom des Kaninchens. Archiv. Geschwulstforsch. 5:47–53.

Möller, G. 1969. Regulatory mechanisms in antibody synthesis. In Homeostatic Regulators, Wolstenholme, G. E. W., and Knight, J. (eds.). J. and A. Churchill, Ltd., London. pp. 197–221.

Monaco, A. P., Wood, M. L., and Russell, P. S. 1965. Adult thymectomy: Effect on recovery from immunologic depression in mice. Science 149:432.

Monnerot-Dumaine, 1965. Influence de la thymectomie sur la carcinogenesis chez le rat. Presse Med. 73:3157.

Moscona, A. A. 1971. How do cells know their place. Nature (New Biology) 234:131.

Mosier, D. E., Fitch, F. W., Rowley, D. A., and Davies, A. J. S. 1970. Cellular deficit in thymectomized mice. Nature 225:276–277.

Nagareda, C. S., and Kaplan, H. S. 1959. Effect of hypothyroidism and thyroid grafts on lymphoid tumors in irradiated C57BL mice. Cancer Res. 19:292–296.

Nakamoto, O. 1957a. Influence of thymus on blood picture especially on lymphocytes. II. Influence of thymic extract on peripheral blood lymphocytes. Acta Haematol. Jap. 20:187–199.

Nakamoto, O. 1957b. Influence of thymus on blood picture especially on lymphocytes. I. Effects of thymectomy on the peripheral blood and lymph nodes. Acta Haematol. Jap. 20:179–187.

Neogy, R. K., and Bose, S. 1965. RNA and DNA metabolism in liver cells of normal and cancer bearing mice. Experientia 19:575–577.

Nettesheim, P., Williams, M. L., and Hammons, A. S. 1969. Regenerative potential of immunocompetent cells. III. Recovery of primary antibody-forming potential from X-irradiation. The role of the thymus. J. Immunol. 103:505–518.

Nezelof, C., Jammey, M. L., Lortholary, S., Labrune, B., and Lamy, M. 1964. l'hypoplaisie hereditaire du thymus. Sa place et sa responsibilite dans une observation d'aplaisie lymphocytaire normoplasmocytaire, et normoglobulinemique du nourisson. Arch. Franc. Pediat. 21:897–920.

Nitschke, A. 1928a. Darstellung und Wirkung eines aktiven Thymusdrusen-extraktes. Klin. Wochenschr. 7:2080.

Nitschke, A. 1928b. Darstellung und Wirkung eines aktiven Thymusdrusen-extraktes. Monatsschr. Kinderheikd. 41:128–134.

Nitschke, A. 1929a. Darstellung einer den Calciumgehalt unde einer den Phosphatgehalt des Serum senkenden Substantz. Nachweis in Milz und Lymphknoten. Z. Ges. Exp. Med. 65:651–654.

Nitschke, A., 1929b. Darstellung sweier wirksamer und spezifischer Thymussubstanzen, ihr Einflup auf Kalk und Phosphatgehalt des Kaninchenserums. Z. Ges. Exp. Med. 65:637–650.

Nitzescu, I. I., and Benetato, G. 1932. Sur la physiologie du thymus. Action des extracts thymiques sur le calcium et le phosphore du sang. Antagonisme entre ces extraits et la parathormone. C. R. Soc. Biol. 111:339–341.

Nossal, G. J. V. 1964. Studies on the rate of seeding of lymphocytes from the intact guinea pig thymus. Ann. N. Y. Acad. Sci. 120:171–181.

Nossal, G. J. V., and Ada, F. L. 1964. Recognition of foreignness in immune and tolerant animals. Nature 201:580–582.

Nossal, G. J. V., and Ada, G. L. 1971. Antigens, lymphoid cells, and the immune response. Academic Press, New York. 324 p.

Nowinski, W. W. 1930. Beitrage zu Physiologie der Drusen; Fortgesetzte Beitrage zur Funktion der thymus. Die wirkung des Thymocrescins auf das Wachstum. Biochem. Z. 226:415–428.

Nowinski, W. W. 1933. Die Beziehung zwischen Thymocrescin und Thyroxin beim Wachstum der tiere. Biochem. Z. 259:182—190.

O'Connell, E. J., Enriquez, P., Linman, J. W., Gleich, G. J., and McDuffie, F. C. 1966. Swiss-type agammaglobulinemia associated with an abnormality of the inflammatory response. 36th Ann. Meet. Soc. Ped. Research, Atlantic City, N.J.

Ogato, A., and Ito, Y. 1944. Studies on salivary gland hormones. V. Bioassay method based on the hypocalcemic activity in rabbits. J. Pharm. Soc. Jap. 64:332–337.

Ogier, R., Bastide, P., and Dastigue, G. 1966. L'equipement enzymatique du thymus. Pathol. Biol. 14:83–107.

Osgood, E. E. 1954. Number and distribution of human hemic cells. Blood 9:1141–1154.

Osoba, D. 1965a. The effects of thymus and other lymphoid organs enclosed in millipore diffusion chambers in neonatally thymectomized mice. J. Exp. Med. 122:633–650

Osoba, D. 1965b. Immune reactivity in mice thymectomized soon after birth: Normal response after pregnancy. Science 147:298–299.

Osoba, D. 1968. Thymic control of cellular differentiation in the immunological system. Proc. Soc. Exp. Biol. Med. 127:418–420.

Osoba, D. 1970. Some physical and radiobiological properties of immunologically reactive mouse spleen cells. J. Exp. Med. 132:368–383.

Osoba, D., and Miller, J. F. A. P. 1963. Evidence of a humeral thymus factor responsible for the maturation of immunological faculty. Nature 199:653–654.

Osoba, D., and Miller, J. F. A. P. 1964. The lymphoid tissues and immune responses of neonatally thymectomized mice bearing thymus tissues in millipore diffusion chambers. J. Exp. Med. 119:177–194.

Osserman, K. E. (ed.) 1966. Myasthenia gravis. Ann. N. Y. Acad. Sci. 135:312–327.

Pansky, B., House, E. L., and Cone, L. A. 1965. An insulin-like thymic factor: A preliminary report. Diabetes 14:325–332.

Paoletti, M. C. 1955. Le metabolisme du fer. J. Med. Bordeaux, Sud-ouest 5:498–512.

Papermaster, R. W., Dalmasso, A. P., Martinez, C., and Good, R. A. 1962. Suppression of antibody forming capacity with thymectomy in the mouse. Proc. Soc. Exp. Biol. Med. 111:41–43.

Papermaster, R. W., and Good, R. A. 1962. Relative contributions of the thymus and the bursa of Fabricius to the maturation of the lymphoreticular system and immunological potential in the chicken. Nature 196:838–840.

Pappenheimer, A. M. 1914a. The effects of early extirpation of the thymus in albino rats. J. Exp. Med. 19:319–338.

Pappenheimer, A. M. 1914b. Further experiments upon the effects of exterpation of the thymus in rats, with special reference to the alleged production of rachitic lesions. J. Exp. Med. 20:477–498.

Parhon, C. I. 1937. Apercu general sur le thymus au point de vue endocrinologique. Bull. Men. Sec. Endocr. 7:181.

Parhon, C. I. 1959. Endocrinologie generala, Glands tiroida, glandele paratiroida si timusu. Bucharesti: Academici Republicii Populare, Romine, Opere alese.

Parhon, C. I., and Apostol, N. 1954. Procesul enzimatic al respiratiei tesuturilor si actiunea unor hidrolizate proteice glandulare folosite in terapia hormonala. Bull. St. Sect. St. Med. Acad. RPR 6:687.

Parhon, C. I., and Cahane, M. 1931. Recherches experimentales concernant l'action du traitement thymique sur la croissance. C. R. Soc. Biol. 106:756–758.

Parhon, C. I., and Cahane, M. 1939. Recherches sur la calcemie et la kalimie des oiseaux ethymisees ou ethymises et hyperthyroidises. Bull. Mem. Soc. Endocr. 5:36–37.

Parhon, C. I., Cahane, M., and Marza, V. 1927. Sur la teneur en eau du sang, du tissu musculaire et de certains organs chez les animaux hyperthymises. C. R. Soc. Biol. 96:1177–1179.

Parhon, C. I., and Costin, E. 1953. Date biochimice asupra timectomiei la bobolanul tinar. Stud. Cercet. Endocr. 4:145.

Parhon, C. I., Kaplan-Banu, E., Flechner, I., and Biner, J. 1950. Actinunea unui extract de timus asupra continutului in acid, timus si ribonucleic in facat, creier si muschi la sobolanul alb. Bull. St. Sert. St. Med. Acad. RPR 2:151.

Parhon, C. I., Kaplan-Banu, E., Flechner, I., and Vaduva, M. 1950. Citeva contributiuni asupra compozitiei in lipide, fosfolipide si colesterol a creierului, ficatului si muschiului la bocaii batrini. Actinunea unui lizattimic asupra acestor componente. Bull. St. Sert. St. Med. Acad. RPR 2:691.

Parhon, C. I., Potop, I., Babes, A. Petrea, I., Felix, E., and Juvina, E. 1955a. Scaderea malignitatii tumorilor produse prin meticolantren la sobolanul alb in urma tratamentului cu timus (mezenchimom). Bull. St. Sect. St. Med. 7:863.

Parhon, C. I., Potop, I., Babes, A., Petrea, I., Juvina, E., and Felix, E. 1956. Cercetari morfologiee si biochimice asupra cancerului experimental la sobolanii etimizat. Bull. St. Sect. St. Med. 8:449. Proceedings of the international conference, Paris, 1957. Pergamon Press, UNESCO. pp. 30–33.

Parhon, C. I., Potop, I., Babes, A., Petrea, I., Juvina, E., Felix, E., and Boeru, V. 1955b. Actinunea timusului si a unor substante neurotrope in cancerul experimental. Bucharesti: Academici Republicii Populare, Romine, pp. 146–147.

Parhon, C. I., Potop, I., Boeru, V., Felix, E., and Petrea, I. 1952. Citeva date preliminare asupra rolului protector al extractului de timus in dezvoltarea cancerului experimental. Stud. Cercet. Endocr. 3:443.

Parhon, C. I., Potop, I., Boeru, V., Felix, E., and Petrea, I. 1954. Quelques donnees preliminaires sur le role protecteur de l'extrait thymique sur le development du cancer experimental. Rev. Sci. Med. 2:5.

Parhon, C. I., Potop, I., Felix, E., Neacsu, C., and Lupulescu, A. 1958a. L'influence du thymus sur l'incorporation du ^{32}P au cours de la cancerisation. Conf. Radioisot. Geneve. pp. 229–230.

Parhon, C. I., Potop, I., Juvina, E., Felix, E.. and Ciocirdià, C. 1958b. Actinunea timusului si influenta regimului alimentar proteic in cancerul experimental. Stud. Cercet. Endocr. 2:161.

Parhon, C. I., Potop, I., and Nicolescu-Zinca, D. 1957. Contributions a l'etude biochimique des processus tumoraux. L'influence du thymus sur l'incorporation du ^{32}P. *In* Radioisotopes in scientific research. Proc. Int. Cong. Paris, UNESCO Pergamon Press, pp. 30–33.

Park, B. H., Good, R. A., Beck, N. P., and Davis, B. B. 1971. Concentration of cyclic adenosine 3',5'-monophosphate in human leucocytes during phagocytosis. Nature (New Biology) 229:27–28.

Parkes, A. S. 1945. The adrenal-gonad relationship. Physiol. Rev. 25:203–254.

Parkes, J. D., and McKinna, J. A. 1967. Effect of thymic extract on the neuro muscular junction. Nature 214:1116–1117.

Parrott, D. M. V. 1962. Strain variation in mortality and runt disease in mice thymectomized at birth. Transplant. Bull. 29:474–476.

Parrott, D. M. V., and East, J. 1962. Role of the thymus in neonatal life. Nature 195:347–348.

Parrott, D. M. V., and East, J. 1964a. The thymus and immunity. The immunological status of thymectomized animals; A survey. Proc. Roy. Soc. Med. 57:147–151.

Parrott, D. M. V., and East, J. 1964b. Studies on a fatal wasting syndrome in mice thymectomized at birth. *In* The thymus in immunobiology: Structure, function and role in disease, Good, R. A., and Gabrielsen, A. E. (eds.). Hoeber-Harper, New York. pp. 523–541.

Parrott, D. M. V., de Sousa, M. A. B., and East, J. 1966. Thymus-dependent areas in the lymphoid organs of neonatally thymectomized mice. J. Exp. Med. 123:191–204.

Pastan, I., and Perlman, R. L. 1971. Cyclic AMP in metabolism. Nature (New Biology) 229:5–7.

Patey, D. H. 1963. A contribution to the study of Hodgkin's disease. Brit. J. Surg. 50:389–392.

Patten, B. N. 1948. Embryology of the pig, 3rd ed. McGraw Hill Book Co., New York.

Pelletier, M., Huron, M., and Delaunay, A. 1960. Substances antibacterien nes d'origine tissulaire. IV. Action d'un polypeptide extrait du thymus et de corps diverses dur le metabolisme respiratoire de quelques bacteries. Pathol. Biol. 8:715–720.

Perlmann, P., Hammarstrom, S., Lagercrantz, R., and Gustafsson, B. E. 1965. Antigen from colon of germfree rats and antibodies in human ulcerative colitis. Ann. N.Y. Acad. Sci. 124:377–394.

Perlo, V. P. 1960. The lymphocyte count in myasthenia gravis. *In* Myasthenia gravis: The Second International Symposium. Proceedings, H. R. Viets (ed). Charles C Thomas, Springfield, Ill. pp. 505–516.

Perlo, V. P., Poskanzer, D. C., Schwab, R. S., Viets, H. R., Osserman, K. E., and Genkins, G. 1966. Myasthenia gravis: Evaluation of treatment in 1,355 patients. Neurology 16:431–439.

Perri, G. C., Faulk, M., Shapiro, E., Mellors, J., and Money, W. L. 1963. Function of the thymus and growth of tumour homograft. Nature 200:1294–1296.

Peterson, R. D. A., Cooper, M. D., and Good, R. A. 1965. The pathogenesis of immunologic deficiency diseases. Am. J. Med. 38:579–604.

Peterson, R. D. A., Kelley, W. D., and Good, R. A. 1964. Ataxia telangiectasia, its association with defective thymus immunological deficiency disease and malignancy. Lancet 1:1189–1193.

Pierpaoli, W., and Sorkin, E. 1968. Hormones and immunologic capacity. I. Effect of heterologous anti-growth hormones (ASTH) antiserum on thymus and peripheral lymphatic tissue in mice. Induction of a wasting syndrome. J. Immunol. 101:1035–1043.

Pierpaoli, W., and Sorkin, E. 1969. Relationship between the developmental thymus hormones and immunological capacity. *In* Lymphatic tissue and germinal center in immune response. Plenum Press, New York. pp. 397–401.

Pierre, St. R. L., and Ackerman, G. A. 1965. Bursa of Fabricius in chickens: Possible humoral factor. Science 147:1307–1308.

Pifer, J. W., Hempelmann, L. H., Dodge, H. J., and Hodges, F. J., 1968. II. Neoplasma in the Ann Arbor series of thymus-irradiated children; A second survey. Am. J. Roent. Rad. Ther. Nucl. Med. 103:13–18.

Pinnas, J. L., and Fitch, F. W. 1966. Immunological competence of thymectomized rats to several soluble and particulate antigens. Int. Arch. Allergy Appl. Immunol. 30:217–230.

Plagge, J. C. 1940. Effect of thymectomy at birth on spermatogenesis in the albino rat. Proc. Soc. Exp. Biol. Med. 44:57–60.

Pora, E., and Toma, V. V. 1960a. Rolul timusului in repartitia ^{32}P la sobolanii albii. Stud. Cercet. Biol. 10:243.

Pora, E., and Toma, V. V. 1960b. Action des extraits de thymus sur le gastrocnemieɲ de grenouille intoxique aux acides lactique ou monoiodoacetique ou par la fatigue. Stud. Cercet. Biol. 12:285.

Pora, E., Toma, V. V., and Madar, I. 1962. L'utilisation du glucose et la synthese du glycogen par le diaphragme des rats ethymises. J. Physiol. 54:401.

Pora, E., Toma, V. V., and Oros, J. 1962. Incorporation du ^{32}P dans certains os du rat éthymise. J. Physiol. (Paris) 54:400–404.

Pora, E., Toma, V. V., Wittenberger, C., and Rusdea, D. 1961. Efectele etimizarii sogolanilor albi asupra activitatii colinestera zei, respiratiei tisulare si cronaxiei musculare. Studii, Univ. Babes-Bolyai, Biologie, Seria II, 2:202.

Potop, I. 1959. Contributiuni la studiul biochimic si morfologic in cancerologia experimentala. Stud. Cercet. Endocr. 10:7.

Potop, I. 1963. Contributinui la studiul biochimic al timusului. Stud. Cercet. Endocr. 14:697–702.

Potop, I. 1966a. Donnees concernant l'influence du thymus sur le cancer experimental. RRE. 3:185.

Potop, I. 1966b. Contributinui la studiul actinunii timusului asupra dezvoltarii tumorilor experimentala. "Omagu lui, C. I. Parhon," Burchuresti, Ed. Acad. RSR 415.

Potop, I. 1970. La fonction immunologique du thymus dans le development des neoplasies. Rev. Roum. Endocr. 7:305.

Potop, I., Beiner, J., Balaceanu, M., and Lupulescu, A. 191. Action de certaines fractions isolees, du thymus sur l'embryogenese et sur le developpement des greffes tumorales dans l'oeuf. V. Congr. Biochim. Moscova. MacMillan Co. New York. p. 308.

Potop, I., Beiner, J., Balaceanu, M., and Lupulescu, A. 1962. Action de certaines fractions isolees du thymus sur l'embryogenese et sur le developpement des greffes tumorales dan l'oeuf. Neoplasma 9:563–78.

Potop, I., Beiner, J., and Lupulescu, A. 1960. Modificari biochimice si morfologice in facatul sobolanilor tratati cu dieta cancertigena si extract timic. Stud. Cercet. Endocr. 11:217.

Potop, I., Beiner, J., Lupulescu, A., and Mreana, G. 1961. Action de certaines fractions isolees du thymus sur le developpement des tumeurs Guerin chez le rat albino. Neoplasma 8:157–164.

Potop, I., Beiner, J., and Mreana, G. 1965. Date referitoare la actinuea unui extract de timus embrionar de cal asupra dezvoltarii tumorilor ascito-genegene elrohich la soarece. Stud. Cercet. Endocr. 16:449–453.

Potop, I., and Boeru, V. 1951. Modificarile morfologice ale singelui in hipo-si himpertomia experimentala. Com. Acad. RPR 1:641.

Potop, I., Boeru, V., Babes, V., Juvina, E., Mreana, G., Stoian, M., and Badescu, D. 1970. L'action d'un extrait thymique liposoluble "B" sur le poids relatif, le contenu en sau et la phosphatase alcaline dans le thymus, l'hemoglobine et les leucocytes du sang. Rev. Roum. Endocr. 7:331.

Potop, I., Boeru, V., Juvina, E., Mreana, G., and Petrea, I. 1969. Influence d'un extrait lipidique isole du thymus sur le developpement des tumeurs Guerin. Arch. Geschwultstforsch. 33:233–243.

Potop, I., Boeru, V., and Mreana, G. 1966. The effect of thymus extracts on phosphorus compounds in muscle and serum, and on serum calcium. Biochem. J. 101:454–459.

Potop, I., Boeru, V., Mreana, G., and Juvina, E. 1969. Actiunea extractelor timice lipidice (B si fractiunea II B) asupra dezvoltarii carcinosarcomului Walker la sobolanul intact si timectomizat. Stud. Cercet. Endocr., 20:127–135.

Potop, I., Ciocirdia, C., Juvina, E., Lupulescu, A., Beiner, J., and Mreana, G. 1960. L'action de certaines fractions isolees du thymus sur le developpement des tumeurs experimentales. Acta Biol. Med. Ger. 5:205–220.

Potop, I., Felix, E., and Ciocirdia, C. 1959. K. Voprosu o Biochimii vilco-civoigeleza. Biokhimiia 24:388.

Potop, I., Halban-Petrescu, R., Boeru, V., Ghinea, E., and Mreana, G. 1971. Action de l'extrait thymique liposoluble "II B" sure le cancer thyroidien humain in vitro. Rev. Roum. Endocr. 8:2.

Potop, I., Halban-Petrescu, R., Mreana, G., Ghinea, E., and Juvina, E. 1971. Date asupra unor factori de variabilitate in activitates antitumorala a extractelor timice. Stud. Cercet. Endocr. (in press).

Potop, I., and Juvina, E. 1966. Influenta unor fractii timice asupra fierului plasmatic si a activitatii catalizei hepatice la sobolanii purtatori de tumori waslker. Stud. Cercet. Endocr. 17:349–353.

Potop, I., and Juvina, E. 1967. Influence de l'athymie experimentala et de l'administration d'un extrait proteique du thymus sur le Fe plasmatique, sur l'activite de la catalase hepatique et sur l'hemoglobin chez le rat. RPR Biol. Ser. Zool. 12:53.

Potop, I., Juvina, E., Beiner, J., and Mreana, G. 1967. Actiunea unor extracte timice asupra acizilor nucleici in ficat si a betaglucuronidazei in timusul soarecelui iradiat. Stud. Cercet. Endocr., 18:411–416.

Potop, I., Juvina, E., Cirocirdia, C., Lupulescu, A., and Mreana, G. 1961. Action protectrice de certaines fractions isolees du thymus sur le cancer experimental. V. Congr. Biochem. Pergamon Press, Moscova. 438 p.

Potop, I., Juvina, E., and Lupulescu, A. 1961. Vliv nekterych frakci extraku thymus na vyrag experimental nich malignich nadoru. Casopis, Lek. Cesk. 100:720–724.

Potop, I., Juvina, E., and Mreana, G. 1963. Citeva date asupra unor fractii lipidice active izolate din timus. Com. Acad. RPR 12:915.

Potop, I., Juvina, E., and Mreana, G. 1970. Action de l'extrait thymique "B" sur l'activite de glucose-6-phosphatase et de l'acide lactique. Rev. Roum. Endocr. 7:49.

Potop, I., Juvina, E., Mreana, G., and Beiner, J. 1966. L'action de certains extraits lipidiques prepares du thymus sur le developpement des tumeurs ascitogenes d'Ehrlich. Rev. Roum. Endocr. 3:55–62.

Potop, I., Juvina, E., Mreana, G., and Boeru, V. 1967a. Sur la presence dans le thymus de deux fractions a l'action antagoniste sur le developpement tumoral. Arch. Geschwulstforsch. 30:190–198.

Potop, I., Juvina, E., Mreana, G., and Boeru, V. 1967b. Actiunea inhibitorie a extractelor lipidice die timus asupra carcinomului Ehrlich. Stud. Cercet. Endocr. 18:139–145.

Potop, I., Juvina, E., Mreana, G., and Ispas, I. 1969. Effet d'un extrait thymique de nature lipidique (B) sur le developpement des tumeurs Guerin chez le rat irradie. Rev. Roum. Endocr. 6:133–140.

Potop, I., Juvina, E., Zimel, H., Mreana, G., and Macrineanu, A. 1967. Influence du thymus sur le developpement des tumeurs experimentales. Rev. Roum. Endocr. 4:295.

Potop, I., Lupulescu, A., and Beiner, J. 1961. Modifications morphologiques et biochimiques dans le foie des rats apres administration de diete cancerigene et de l'extrait thymique. Acta Biol. Med. Ger. 8:230–237.

Potop, I., Manitescu, F., Mreana, G., and Catargi, I. 1971. Influenta unor aspecte morfologice in singele soarecelui. Stud. Cercet. Endocr. (in press).

Potop, I., and Milcu, S. M. 1970. Isolation of an antiblastic factor from the bovine thymus. Rev. Roum. Endocr. 7:253.

Potop, I., Mreana, G., Holban-Petrescu, R., and Ghinea, E. 1971. Efectul anti proliferative al unor extracte preparate din timusul uman asupra culturilor de celule de carcinom uman. Stud. Cercet. Endocr. (in press).

Potop, I., Mreana, G., and Juvina, E. 1969. Influenta extractului lipidic "B" izolat din timus asupra dezvoltarii sarcomului Crocker 180 la soarece. Stud. Cercet. Endocr. 20:327–331.

Potop, I., Mreana, G., and Neacsu, C. 1963. L'influence de quelques hormones et extraits hormonaux sur l'incorporation du ³²P dans le cerveau du point de vue phylogentique. Res. Sci. Med. Acad. RPR 8:164.

Potop, I., Mreana, G., and Neacsu, C. 1967. Variations de la phosphrylation oxydative chez certaines classes de vertebres sous l'influence de la thyroxine, de l'hydrocortisone et d'un extrait lipidique prepare du thymus. RPR Biol. Ser. Zool. 12:263.

Potop, I., Sterescu, V., Boeru, V., Peloni, R., Petrescu, E., and Ghinea, E. 1970. Effect of an "S" purified thymus factor (isolated from and II B₃ thymus fraction) on the *in vitro* proliferation of tumor cells. Neoplasma 17:655–662.

Potts, J. T., Reisfeld, R. A., Hirsch, P. F., Wasthed, A. B., Voelkel, E. F., and Munson, P. L. 1967. Purification of porcine thyrocalcitonin. Proc. Natl. Acad. Sci. U.S.A. 58:328–335.

Quint, J., Hardy, M. A., and Monaco, A. P. 1969. Modification of the immunosuppressive effects of rabbit antimouse lymphocyte serum by a thymic humoral factor: Thymosin. Surg. Forum 20:252–254.

Ralph, F., Kampschmidt, R., Thomas, A., and McCoy, A. 1960. Effect of tumor cell fractions upon plasma iron, liver catalase and organ weight of rats. Proc. Soc. Exptl. Biol. and Med. 103:869–872.

Rassmussen, H. 1970. Cell communication, calcium ion, and cyclic adenosine monophosphate. Science 170:404–411.

Ratti, P. 1930. Beitrage zur Physiologie der Drusen; die wachstumsregulierende Funktion der Thymusdrusse. Biochem. Z. 233:100–119.

Read, C. P. 1970. Parasitism and symbiology. The Ronald Press, New York. 316 p.

Reimann, E. M., Brostrom, C. O., Corbin, J. D., King, C. A., and Knebo, E. G., 1971. Separation of regulatory and catalytic subunits of the cyclic 3′,5′-adenosine monophosphate-dependent protein kinase(s) of rabbit skeletal muscle. Biochem. Biophys. Res. Comm. 42:187–194.

Reinhardt, W. O. 1945. Effect of thymectomy in rats on lymph nodes and spleen. Anat. Rec. 91:295.

Reinhardt, W. O., and Yoffey. 1956. Thoracic duct lymph and lymphocytes in the guinea pig. Am. J. Physiol. 187:493–500.

Rixon, R. H., Whitfield, J. F., and MacManus, J. P. 1970. Stimulation of mitotic activity in rat bone marrow and thymus by exogenous adenosine 3′,5′-monophosphate (cyclic AMP). Exp. Cell. Res. 63:110–116.

Roberts, S., and White, A. 1949. Biochemical characterization of lymphoid tissue proteins. J. Biol. Chem. 178:151–156.

Robey, W. G., Campbell, B. J., and Luckey, T. D. 1972. Isolation and characterization of a thymic hormone. Infection and Immunity 6:682–688.

Robey, W. G., Ceglowsky, W., Luckey, T. D., and Friedman, H. 1972. Thymus factors and immunity: enhancement of immunologic maturation by a purified calf thymus extract. Proc. Fourth International Congress on Immune Reactions. Dubrovnik, in press.

Rockey, J. H., Hanson, L. A., Heremans, J. F., and Kunkel, H. G. 1964. Beta-2-aglobulinemia in two healthy men. J. Lab. Clin. Med. 63:205–212.

Roitt, I. M., Greaves, M. F., Torrigiani, G., Brostoff, J., and Playfair, J. H. L. 1969. The cellular basis of immunological responses. A synthesis of some current views. Lancet 2:367–371.

Romeis, B. 1915. Experimentelle Untersuchungen uber die Wirkung innersekretorischer Organe. IV. Z. Ges. Exp. Med. 5:99–124.

Romeis, B. 1926. Weitere versuche uber den Einflub der Thymusfutterung auf Froschlarven. Klin. Wochenschr. 5:975–977.

Rosemann, H. U. 1933. Uber die wirkung von Thymusextrakten auf den isolierte Froschumuskel. Z. Biol. 94:74–77.

Rosen, F. S., Gottoff, S. P., Craig, J. M., Ritchie, J., and Janeway, C. A. 1966. Further observations on the Swiss type of agammaglobulinaemia (alymphocytosis). The effect of syngeneic bone marrow cells. New Engl. J. Med. 274:18–21.

Rosen, F. S., and Janeway, C. A. 1966. The gamma globulins. III. The antibody deficiency syndromes. New Engl. J. Med. 275:769–775.

Rosenthal, M. 1969. Zur Erholung des Immunsapparates nach Thymectomie and Bestrahlung. Strahlentherapie 137:596–611.

Rowntree, L. G., Clark, J. H., and Hanson, A. M. P. 1934. Biologic effects of thymus extract (Hanson), accruing acceleration in growth and development in successive generation of rats under continuous treatment with thymic extract. J.A.M.A. 103:1425–1430.

Ruhenstroth-Bauer, G., and Lucke-Huhle, C. 1968. Two populations of small lymphocytes. J. Cell Biol. 37:196–198.

Rusescu, A. D., Germaneanu, M., Stanescu, V., Florea, I., and Ionescu, V. 1964. Timusul. Editura Academiei Republicii Populare, Bucharesti, Romine. 249 p.

Rushing, D. R. 1968. Factors affecting amino acid incorporation by rat spleen ribosomes. Ph.D. thesis, University of Missouri, Columbia, Missouri.

Ruvalcaba, R. H. A., and Thuline, H. C. 1969. IgA absence associated with short arm deletion of chromosome No. 18. J. Pediat. 74:964–965.

Sainte-Marie, G. and Leblond, C. P. 1964. Cytologic features and cellular migration in the cortex and medulla of thymus in the young adult rat. Blood, 23:275–299.

Salkind, J. 1915. Contributions histologiques a la biologie comparee du thymus Arch. Zool. Exp. Gen. 55:81–322.

Salvin, S. B., Peterson, R. D. A., and Good, R. A. 1965. The role of the thymus in resistance to infection and endotoxin toxicity. J. Lab. Clin. Med. 65:1004–1022.

Sampson, M. M., and Korenchevsky, V. 1932. Influence of vitamin A deficiency on male rats in pair feeding experiments. Biochem. J. 26:1322–1339.

Sandberg, M., Perla, D., and Holly, O. M. 1940. The metabolism of nitrogen, sulphur and glutathione in thymectomized albino rats. Endocrinology 26:102–106.

Sanders, A. G. and Florey, H. W. 1940. The effect of the removal of lymphoid tissue. Brit. J. Exp. Path. 21:275–287.

Schimke, R. N., Bolano, C., and Kirkpatrick, C. H. 1969. Immunologic deficiency in the congenital rubella syndrome. Amer. J. Dis. Child. 118:626–633.

Schmitt, F. O., Samson, F. E. J., and Irwin, L. N. 1970. Brain cell microenvironment. In Neorosciences Research Symposium summaries, Schmidtt, F. O., Melnechuk, T., Qwarton, G. C., and Adelman, G. (eds.). Cambridge, MIT Press. pp. 191–325.

Schneiberg, K., Joneko, A., and Bartnikowa, W. 1968. Der thymus ein hamato-poetisches Organ. Der Einfluss von Thymus-gewebe in Diffusionskam-mern auf das Uberleben und des blutbildenoe system von Mausen nach subletaeeb Ganzkorperbestrahlung. Folia Haematol. 89:265–282.

Schneider, L. 1957. Beeinflussung des wachstums durch in thymus enthaltene stoffa. Arch. Entwicklungmech. 149:644—645.

Schockaert, J. 1930. Action specifique des extraits prehypophysaires de boeuf sur le poids du thymus du jeune canard. C. R. Soc. Biol. 105:226–227.

Scholtz, H. G. 1932. Beeinflussung von experimentellem Hyperparathyroidismus durch Thymuspraparate. Zentr. Albl. Exp. Med. 85:547.

Scholtz, H. G. 1933. Thymusextrakt und Blutkalkspiegel. Bemerkungen zu der Arbeit. Fortgesetzte Untersuchungen uber Thymocresin. Biochem. Z. 259:384–386.

Schooley, J. C., and Kelly, L. S. 1958. Univ. Cal. Rad. Lab. 8513.

Schooley, J. C., and Kelly, L. S. 1961. The thymus in lymphocyte production. Fed. Proc. 20:71.

Schooley, J. C., Kelly, L. S., Dobson, F. L. Finney, C. R., Havens, V. W., and Cantor, L. N. 1965. Reticuloendothelial activity in neonatally thymecto-mized mice and irradiated mice thymectomized in adult life. J. Reticuloen-dothel. Soc. 2:396–405.

Schulze, Hanna, 1933. Das Verhalten des Thymus in experimenteller Thyroxin-vergiftung gepruft an verschildenen Saugetieren. Beitr. Pathol. Anat. Allg. Pathol. 92:329–346.

Schumacher, D. R., and Roth, D. 1912. Thymektomie bei einem Fall von Morbus Basedowi mit Myasthenie. Mitt. Grenzgeb. Med. chir. 25: 746–765.

Schwab, R. S. and Viets, H. R., 1960. In Thymectomy for myasthenia gravis, Viets, H. R., and Schwab, R. S. (eds.). C. C Thomas, Springfield, Ill.

Schwarz, H., Madar, L., and Kis, Z. 1959. Exectul inhibitor al cortico steroizilor, extractului timic si al pantoponului asupra secretiei de ACTH. Stud. Cercet. Med. Interna. 10. (Romanian, Summarized in French.)

Schwarz, H., Price, M., and O'Dell, C. A. 1953. Effect of lyophilized thymic extracts on serum calcium and phosphorus. Metabolism 2:261–267.

Schwartz, R. H., Schenke, E. A., Bermann, J., and Ellis, B. A., 1969. Hereditary nonlymphopenic agammaglobulinemia with splenomegaly: A family study. J. Lab. Clin. Med. 74:203–211.

Segaloff, A. 1949. Thymectomy. *In* The rat, Farris, E. J., and Griffith, J. Q., Lippincott, Philadelphia. pp. 443–444.

Segaloff, A., and Nelson, W. O. 1940. Growth and development of six generations of thymectomized albino rats. Am. J. Physiol. 130:671–674.

Selye, H. 1950. The physiology and pathology of exposure to stress; A treatise based on the concepts of the general adaptation syndrome and the diseases of adaptation. Stress. Montreal: Acta., Inc. 822 pp.

Selye, H. 1952. Prevention of cortisone overdosage effects with the somatotrophic hormone (STH). Am. J. Physiol. 171:381–384.

Selye, H., and Albert, S. 1942. Age factor in responsiveness of pituitary and adrenals to folliculoids. Proc. Soc. Exp. Biol. Med. 50:159–161.

Selye, H., Harlow, C. M., and Collip, J. B. 1936. Auslosung der Alarmreaktion mit Follikelhormon. Endokrinologie 18:81–85.

Selye, H., and Masson, G. 1939. The effect of estrogens as modified by adrenal insufficiency. Endocrinology 25:211–215.

Selye, H., Selgado, E., and Procopio, J. 1952. Effect of somatotrophic hormone (STH) upon resistance to ionizing rays. Acta Endocr. 9:337–341.

Shaw, R. K., Szwed, C., Boggs, D. R., Fahey, J. L., Frei, E., Morrison, E., and Utz, J. P. 1960. Infection and immunity in chronic lymphocytic leukemia. Arch. Intern. Med. 106:467–478.

Shearer, G. M., Cudkowicz, G., and Wallberg, H. E. 1969. Hemolytic plaque-forming cells and antigen-senstive units in spleens of germfree and conventional mice. *In* Germfree biology, Mirand, E. A., and Black, N. (eds.). Plenum Press, New York. pp. 269–275.

Sherman, J. D., Adner, M. M., and Dameshek, W. 1963. Effect of thymectomy on the golden hamster (*Mesocricetus auratus*). I. Wasting disease. Blood 22:252–271.

Sherman, J. D., Adner, M. M., and Dameshek, W. 1964. Effect of thymectomy on the golden hamster (*Mesocricetus auratus*). II. Studies of the immune response in thymectomized and splenectomized nonwasted animals. Blood 23:375–388.

Sherman, J. D., and Dameshek, W. 1963. Wasting disease following thymectomy in the hamster. Nature 197:469–471.

Shewell J. 1957. The activity of different steroids in producing thymic involution. Brit. J. Pharm. 12:133–139.

Shibata, K. 1953a. Effect of thymectomy on the adrenal gland. Gunma J. Med. Sci. 2:331.

Shibata, K. 1953b. Relation of thymus to growth and development. Gunma J. Med. Sci. 2:273.

Shortman, K., Diener, E., Russell, P., and Armstrong, W. D. 1970. The role of nonlymphoid accessory cells in the immune response to different antigens. J. Exp. Med. 131:461–482.

Silverstein, A. M. 1964. Ontogeny of the immune response, Science, 144: 1423–1428.

Silverstein, A. M., and Kraner, K. L. 1965. Studies on the ontogenesis of the immune response. *In* Molecular and cellular basis of antibody formation, Sterzl, J. (ed.). Academic Press, New York. pp. 341–348.

Silverstein, A. M., Parshall, C. J., Jr., and Uhr, J. W. 1966. Immunologic maturation *in utero*: Kinetics of the primary antibody response in the fetal lamb. Science 154:1675–1677.

Simonsen, M. 1962. Graft *versus* host reactions. Their natural history and applicability as tools of research. Progr. Allergy 6:349–467.

Simpson, C. L., and Hempelmann, L. H. 1957. The association of tumors and roentgen-ray treatment of the thorax in infancy. Cancer 10:42–56.

Simpson, C. L., Hempelmann, L. H., and Fuller, L. M. 1955. Neoplasia in children treated with x-rays in infancy for thymic enlargement. Radiology 64:840–845.

Simpson, J. A. 1956. The value of thymectomy. Proc. Roy. Soc. Med. 49:795–798.

Simpson, J. A. 1958. An evaluation of thymectomy in myasthenia gravis. Brain 81:112–144.

Sklower, A. 1926. Beziehungen zwischen Schilddreuse und Thymus. Zool. Ana. Suppl. 2:177.

Sklower, A. 1927. Uber Beziehungen zwischen Shildruse und Thymus. Z. Vergle. Physiol. 6:150–166.

Sloan, H. E., Jr. 1943. The thymus in myasthenia gravis with observations on the normal anatomy and histology of the thymus. Surgery 13:154–174.

Small, M., and Trainin, N. 1967. Increase in antibody-forming cells of neonatally thymectomized mice receiving calf thymus extract. Nature 216:377–379.

Small, M., and Trainin, N. 1971. Contribution of a thymic humoral factor to the development of an immunologically competent population from cells of mouse bone marrow. J. Exp. Med. 134:786–800.

Smith, K. C., and Kaplan, H. S. 1961. A chromatographic comparison of nucleic acids from isologous newborn, adult and neoplastic thymus. Cancer Res. 21:1148–1153.

Smith, K. C., and Thomas, F. C. 1950. Studies on the thymus of the mammal. III. Glycogen in the cortical cells of the thymus. Anat. Rec. 106:17–27.

Smith, P. E. 1930. The effect of hypophysectomy upon the involution of the thymus in the rat. Anat. Rec. 47:119–129.

Sokal, J. E., and Aungst, C. W. 1969. Response to BCG vaccination and survival in advanced Hodgkin's disease. Cancer 24:128–134.

Sokal, J. E., and Primikirios, N. 1961. The delayed skin test response in Hodgkin's disease and lymphosarcoma. Effect of disease activity. Cancer 14:597–607.

Solomon, J. 1971. Model mothers. The Sciences 11:12–14.

Soothill, J. F. 1968. Immunity deficiency states. *In* Clinical aspects of immunology, Gell, P. G. H., and R. R. A. Coombs (eds.). F. A. Davis, Philadelphia. p. 540.

Soutter, L., and Emerson, C. P. 1960. Elective thymectomy in the treatment of aregenerative anemia associated with monocytic leukaemia. Am. J. Med. 28:609–614.

Stanescu, V., Florea, I., and Dinulescu, E. 1961a. Efectele timectomiei asupra unor modificari metabolice produse prin administrarea acuta de cortizon. Stud. Cercet. Endocr. 12:38–41.

Stanescu, V., Florea, I., and Dinulescu, E. 1961b. Efectele timectomiei asupra modificarilor de pH si N urinar, produse de administrarea de cortizon. Stud. Cercet. Endocr. 12:41–45.

Starzl, T. E., Groth, C. G., Terasaki, P. I., Putnam, C. W., Brettschneider, I., and Marchioro, T; L. 1968. Heterologous antilymphocyte globulin, histocompatibility matching, and human renal homotransplantation. Surg. Gynecol. Obstet. 126:1023–1035.

Starzl, T. E., Marchioro, T. L. Terasaki, P. I., Porter, K. A., Faris, T. D., Herrman, T. J., Vredevoe, D. L., Hutt, M. P., Ogden, D. A., and Waddell, W. R. 1965. Chronic survival after human renal transplantation. Lymphocyte-antigen matching, pathology and influence of thymectomy. Ann. Surg. 162:749–787.

Sterzl, J. 1967. Factors determining the differential pathways of immunocompetent cells. Cold Spring Harbor Symp. Quant. Biol. 32:493–506.

Sterzl, J., and Riha, I. 1970. Developmental aspects of antibody formation, Vols. 1 and 2. Academic Press, New York.

Steward, J. P. 1971. Immunologic responses of neonatally thymectomized rats to sheep red blood cells and to flagellin from *Salmonella adepaide*. Proc. Soc. Exp. Biol. Med. 138:702–708.

Stiehm, E. R., and Fundenberg, H. H. 1966. Clinical and immunologic features of dysgammaglobulinemia type I: Report of a case diagnosed in first year of life. Amer. J. Med. 40:805–815.

Stoclinga, G. B. A., van Munster, P. J. J., and Slooff, J. P. 1969. Antibody deficiency syndrome and autoimmune hemolytic anemia in a boy with isolated IgM deficiency dysimmunoglobulinemia type 5. Acta Paediat. Scandinav. 58:352.

Strack, E., Fuchs, U., and Rotzsch, W. 1961. Der Einfluss von Carnitine und Throxin auf Maüse-Ascites-Tumor. Acta Biol. Med. Germ. 7:563–576.

Strauss, A. J. L., Smith, C. W., Cage, G. W., van der Geld, H. W. R., McFarlin, D. E., and Barlow, M. 1966. Further studies in the specificity of presumed immune associations of myasthenia gravis and consideration of possible pathogenic implications. Ann. N.Y. Acad. Sci. 135:557–579.

Strauss, A. J. L., van der Geld, H. W. R., Kemp, P. G., Jr., Exum, E. D., and Goodman, H. C. 1965. Immunological concomitants of myasthenia gravis. Ann. N.Y. Acad. Sci. 124:744–766.

Stutzman, L., Mittleman, A., Ohkochi, T., and Ambrus, J. L. 1971. Fetal thymus transplantation in Hodgkin's disease. Proc. Am. Assoc. Cancer Res. 12:101.

Sussdorf, D. H. 1971. Restoration of antibody response to sheep erythrocytes in thymectomized mice following grafting of rabbit appendix. Proc. Soc. Exp. Biol. Med. 137:82–86.

Sutherland, D. E. R., Archer, O. K., and Good, R. A. 1964. The role of the appendix in development of immunologic capacity. Proc. Soc. Exp. Biol. Med. 115:673–676.

Szent-Gyorgyi, A. 1957. Bioenergetics. Academic Press, New York. 143 p.

Szent-Gyorgyi, A. 1966. Growth and organization. Biochem. J. 98:641–644.

Szent-Gyorgyi, A., Együd, D., and McLaughlin, J. 1967 Keto-aldehydes and cell division. Glyoxal derivatives may be regulators of cell division and open a new approach to cancer. Science 155:539–541.

Szent-Gyorgyi, A., Hegyeli, A., and McLaughlin, J. 1962. Constituents of the thymus gland and their relation to growth, fertility, muscle and cancer. Proc. Natl. Acad. Sci. U.S.A. 48:1439–1442.

Takada. A., Takada. Y., Ambrus, C. M., and Ambrus. J. L. 1970. Effects of various thymus preparations on restoration of impaired immunological function in mice. Res. Com. Chem. Path. Pharm. 1:278–287.

Takada, A., Takada, Y., and Ambrus. J. L. 1969. Effects of thymectomy and X-irradiation on the immune response of mice to sheep erythrocytes. Radiat. Res. 40:341–350.

Takada, A., Takada. Y., and Ambrus, J. L. 1971. Effects of intraperitoneal thymus graft on hemolytic plaque formation. J. Immunol. 107:1185–1188.

Takada, A., Takada, Y., Huang, C. C., and Ambrus, J. L. 1969. Biphasic pattern of thymus regeneration after whole-body irradiation. J. Exper. Med. 129:445–457.

Takada, A., Takada, Y., Munson, B., and Ambrus, J. L. 1971a. Shielding the thymus area during X-irradiation: effects on hemolysis formation in mice. J. Reticuloendothel. Soc. 9:147–167.

Takada, A., Takada, Y., Kim, Y., and Ambrus, J. L. 1971b. Bone marrow, spleen, and thymus regeneration patterns in mice after whole-body irradiation. Radiat. Res. 45:522–523.

Takada, Y., Takada, A., and Ambrus, J. L. 1970a. Strain and substrain differences in the recovery of thymus function after whole-body X-irradiation of mice. Proc. Soc. Exp. Biol. Med. 135:473–477.

Takao, T; 1926. Antagonismus schilddruse-thymus. Pfluegers Arch. 213:192–197.

Taliaferro, W. H., and Talmage, D. W. 1955. Absence of amino acid incorporation into antibody during the induction period. J. Infect. Dis. 97:88–98.

Tallberg, T., and Kosunen, T. U. 1968. Detection of an organ specific protein in the rat thymus. Ann. Med. Exp. Fenn. 44:24–48.

Tallberg, T., Kosunen, T. U., and Ruoslahti, E. 1966. Detection of an organ specific protein in the human thymus. Ann. Med. Exp. Fenn. 44:221–226.

Tallberg, T., Linder, E. and Hjelt, L. 1966. Further studies on a human thymus specific protein. I. Immunological purification of the thymus specific antigen lacking in patients with lymphatic leukemia and the detection of an ileo-jejunal protein antigen in the thymus. Ann. Med. Exp. Fen. 44:221.

Tallberg, T., Nordling, S. and Cautell, K. 1968. On the biological activity of human thymus protein. Scand. J. Clin. Lab. Invest. 21:36.

Talmage, D. W; 1969. The nature of the immunological response. Immunology and development, M. Adinolfi and J. Humphrey (eds) Immunology and development. London: Spastics International Medical Publications, pp. 1–26.

Taylor, R. B. 1963. Immunological competence of thymus cells after transfer to thymectomized recipients. Nature 199:873–74.

Taylor, R. R. 1965. Decay of immunological responsiveness after thymectomy in adult life. Nature (London) 208:1334–1335.

Taylor, R. B. 1969. Cellular cooperation in the antibody responses of mice to two cerum albumins: specific function of thymus cells. Transplant. Rev. 1:114–149.

Telegdy, G., and Endroczy, J. 1959. Effect of progesterone treatment and castration on adrenal cortical secretion. Acta Physiol. Acad. Sci. Hung. 16:23–25.

Tepperman, J. 1968. Metabolic and endocrine physiology, 2nd ed. Yearbook Medical Publishers, Inc. Chicago.

Thomas, P., and Reymond, D. 1958. Techniques de biochimie. J. B. Bailliere, Paris. 182 p.

Thurner, K. 1924. Uber den Einflub von Thymusextrakten auf die Leistungsfahigkeit und Ermudbarkeit des Saugetiermuskels. Pfluegers Arch. 202: 444–467.

Tiedemann, H. 1967. Biochemical aspects of primary induction and determination. In The biochemistry of animal development, Weber, R. (ed.). Academic Press, New York. pp. 3–53.

Tilney, N. L., Beattie, E. J., and Economou, S. G. 1956. The effect of neonatal thymectomy in the dog. J. Sur. Res. 5:23–30.

Tobler, R., and Cottier, H. 1958. Familare Lymphopenie mit Agammaglobulinamie und schwerer Moniliasis. Helv. Paediat. Acta. 13:313–338.

Todd, J. H. 1971. The chemical languages of fishes. Sci. Amer. 224:99–108.

Toma, V. 1961. Observatti asupra rolului timusului in cresterea pasarilor domestice. St. Univ. Babes-Bolyai, Biologie, Ser. II, Fasc. 2:371.

Toma, V., and Roman, H. 1969. Actinuni cardiovasculare ale extractului de timus (TP). Lucrari stiintifice, Oradea, Sera A. p. 371.

Torda, C. and Wolff, H. G. 1944. Effect of ether extract of the thymus and pancreas on synthesis of acetylcholine. Proc. Soc. Exp. Biol. Med. 57:69–72.

Torda, C., and Wolff, H. G. 1947. Effect of organ extracts and their fractions on acetylcholine synthesis. Am. J. Physiol. 148:417–423.

Toro, J. 1957. Contribution a l'histophysiologie du thymus. Bull. Ass. Anat. 92:1312.

Toro, J., Bacsy, E., and Oros, I. 1968. Postirradiation changes in ultrastructure and enzyme cytochemistry or rat thymus. Acta Med. Acad. Sci. Hung. 25:355–356.

Townsend, J. F., and Luckey, T. D. 1960. Hormoligosis in pharmocology. J.A.M.A. 173:44–48.

Traggis, D. G., Ruthig, D., Smith, G., and Cleveland, W. 1961. Hypogammaglo-bulinemia in a young girl. Amer. J. Dis. Child. 102:8–16.

Trainin, N., Bejerano, A., Strahilevitch, M., Goldring, D., and Small, M. 1966. A thymic factor preventing wasting and influencing lymphopoisis in mice. Isr. J. Med. Sci. 2:549–559.

Trainin, N., Burger, M., and Kaye, A. M. 1967. Some characteristics of a thymic humoral factor determined by assay *in vivo* of DNA synthesis in lymph nodes of thymectomized mice. Biochem. Pharmocol. 16:711–720.

Trainin, N., Burger, M., and Linker-Israeli, M. 1967. Restoration of homograft response in neonatally thymectomized mice by a thymic humoral factor (THF) Advances in transplantation, Proceedings of the First International Congress of Transplantation Society. Paris, 1967. Williams and Wilkins, Baltimore, pp. 91–97.

Trainin, N., and Linker-Israeli, M. 1967. Restoration of immunologic reactivity of thymectomized mice by calf thymus extract. Cancer Res. 27:308–313.

Trainin, N., and Small, M. 1970a. Studies on some physicochemical properties of a thymus humoral factor conferring immunocompetence on lymphoid cells. J. Exp. Med. 132:885–897.

Trainin, N., and Small, M. 1970b. Conferment of immunocompetence on lymphoid cells by a thymus humoral factor. CIBA Foundation Study Group No. 36. *In* G. E. W. Wolstenholme and D. Knight (eds.), Hormones and the immune response. Churchill, London, pp. 24–41.

Trainin, M., Small, M., and Globerson, A. 1969. Immunocompetence of spleen cells from neonatally thymectomized mice conferred *in vitro* by a syngeric thymus extract. J. Exp. Med. 130:765–775.

Trench, C. A. H., Watson, J. W., Walker, F. C., Gardner, P. S., and Green, C. A. 1966. Evidence for a humoral thymic factor in rabbits. Immunology 10:187–191.

Trethewie, E. R., and Wright, R. D. 1944. Acetylcholine synthesis and myasthenia gravis. Aust. N. Z. J. Surg. 13:244–246.

Tripp, M. R. 1966. Hemagglutin in the blood of the oyster *Crossostrea virginim*. J. Invertebr. Pathol. 8:478–484.

Unanue, E. R. 1970. Thymus dependency of the immune response to hemocyanin: An evaluation of the role on macrophages in thymectomized mice. J. Immunol. 105:1339–1343.

Ungar, G., and Fjerdingstad, E. J. 1971. Chemical nature of the transfer factors: RNA or protein. *In* Adam, G. (ed.), Biology of memory. Plenum Press, New York.

Utterstrom, E. 1910. Contribution a l'etude de l'hyperthyroidsation. Arch. Med. Exp. Anat. Pathol. 22:550–559.

Van Bekkum, D. W., and Vos, O. 1957. Immunological aspects of homo- and heterologous bone marrow transplantation in irradiated animals. J. Cell. Comp. Physiol. 50:139–156.

Vanderputte, M. 1967. Failure of thymoma grafts to restore the immunological competence in thymectomized mice. Pathol. Eur. 2:55–68.

Van Putten, L. M. 1964. Thymectomy: Effect on secondary disease in radiation chimeras. Science 145:935–936.

Verzar, F., and Wenner, V. 1949. The action of steroids on glycogen breakdown in surviving muscle. Biochem. J. 42:48–51.

Vessey, M. P., and Doll, R. 1972. Thymectomy and cancer—a follow-up study. Brit. J. Cancer 26:53–58.

Viets, H. R. Myasthenia gravis. 1945. J.A.M.A. 127:1089–1096.

Viets, H. R. 1950. Thymectomy in myasthenia gravis. Brit. Med. J. 1:139–147.

Viets, H. R., and Schwab, R. S. (eds.). 1960. Thymectomy for myasthenia gravis. A record of experience at the Massachusetts General Hospital. Charles C Thomas, Sprinfield, Ill.

Vojtiskova, M., Masnerova, M., and Viklicky, J. 1963. Homograft response in ducks after thymectomy and/or bursectomy and with or without transplanted homologous thymus and/or bursa of Fabricius. Folia Biol. 9:424–431.

Vojtiskova, M., and Nouza, K. 1965. White blood cell levels and homograft response in thymectomized pigeons. Folia Biol. 11:406–409.

Waddington, C. H. 1966. Principles of development and differentiation. Macmillan Co., New York.

Waksman, B. H., Arnason, B. G., and Jankovic, B. D. 1962. The role of the thymus in immune reaction in rats. III. Changes in the lymphoid organs of thymectomized rats. J. Exp. Med. 116:187–206.

Walford, R. L., and Yunis, E. J. 1971. Immunologic aging and lymphoid involution. In Amos, B. (ed.), Progress in immunology. Academic Press, New York. pp. 1223–1225.

Walters, M. N–I., and Willoughby, D. A. 1965. The effect of tissue extracts on vascular permeability and leukocyte emigration. J. Path. Bact. 89:255.

Warner, N. L., and Szenberg, A. 1962. Effect of neonatal thymectomy on the immune response in the chicken. Nature 196:754–785.

Warner, N. L., and Szenberg, A. 1964. Immunologic studies on hormonally bursectomized and surgically thymectomized chickens: Dissociation of immunologic responsiveness. In The thymus in immunology: Structure, function, and role in disease, Good, R. A., Hoeber-Harper, and Gabrielsen, A. E. (eds.). Hoeber-Harper, New York. pp. 395–413.

Weill-Malherbe, H. 1955. Mechanism of insulin action. Ergeb. Physiol. 48:55–111.

Weissman, I. L. 1967. Thymus cell migration. J. Exptl. Med. 126:291–304.

Wells, B. B., and Kendall, E. C. 1940. Qualitative differences in effect of compounds separated from adrenal cortex on gluconeogenesis. Proc. Staff Meet. Mayo Clin. 15:133–139.

White, A., Goldstein, A. L. 1968. Is the thymus an endocrine gland? Old problem, new data. Perspect. Biol. Med. 11:475–489.

White, A., and Goldstein, A. L. 1970. The role of the thymus gland in the hormonal regulation of host resistance. CIBA Found. Symp. Control processes in multicellular organisms, Wolstenholme, G. G. W., and Knight, J. (eds.). Churchill, London. pp. 210–237.

White, R. G. 1963. Functional recognition of immunologically competent cells by means of the flourescent antibody technique. *In* The Immunologically competent cell, Wolstenholme, G. E. W. (ed.). Little, Brown and Co., Boston.

Whitfield J. F., MacManus, J. P., Franks, D. J., Gillan, D. J., and Youdale, T. 1971. The possible mediation by cyclic AMP of the stimulation of thymic proliferation by cyclic GMP. Proc. Soc. Exp. Biol. Med. 137:453–457.

Whitfield, J. F., MacManus, J. P., and Rixon, R. H. 1970. Cyclic AMP-mediated stimulation of thymocyte proliferation by low concentrations of cortisol. Proc. Soc. Exp. Biol. Med. 134:1170–1174.

Whittaker, R. H., and Feeny, R. R. 1971. Allelochemics: Chemical interactions between species. Science 171:757–770.

Williams, C. M. 1971. Cited in: Insect hormones use requires caution. Chem. Engin. News 49:39–40.

Williams, W. L, Hale, W. M., and Stoner, R. D. 1958. The histogenesis of antibody-producing intraocular transplants of thymus in mice. Arch Pathol. 66:225–233.

Wilson, A., and Wilson, H. 1955. Thymus and myasthenia gravis. Amer. J. Med. 697–702.

Wilson, D. B., Silvers, W. K., and Nowell, P. C. 1967. Qunatitative studies on the mixed lymphocyte interaction in rats. II. Relationship of the proliferative response to the immunologic status of the donors. J. Exp. Med. 126: 655–665.

Wilson, D. B., and Weissman, G. 1971. Lymphocyte activation. I. *In* Progress in immunology, Amos, B. (ed.). Academic Press, New York. pp. 1143–1146.

Wilson, R., Sjopin, K., and Bealmear, M. 1964. The absence of wasting in thymectomized germfree mice. Proc. Soc. Exp. Biol. Med. 117:237–239.

Wiskott. A. 1937. Familiarer angeborener Morbus Werlhofii? Monatschr. Kinderheilk. 68:212–216.

Wolf, J. K., Goken, M., and Good, R. A. 1963. Heredo-familial disease of the mesenchymal tissues: Clinical and laboratory study of one family. J. Lab. Clin. Med. 61:230–248.

Wong, F. M., Taub, R. N., Sherman, J. D., and Dameshek, W. 1966. Effect of thymus enclosed in millipore diffusion envelopes on thymectomized hamsters. Blood 28:40–53.

Wyssmann, K. 1929. Chemische Untersuchung uber den Einflub von Thymus auf den respiratorischen Arbeitsstoffuechsel bei Ratten. Biochem. Z. 216:66–84.

Yamada, T., and Ohyama, H. 1968. Accumulation of fructose-1,6-diphosphate in X-irradiated rat thymocytes. Int. J. Radiat. Biol. 14:169–174.

Yamada, T., Ohyama, H., and Kumatori, T. 1969. Changes in glycolysis of rat thymocytes after a whole-body irradiation. Int. J. Radiat. Biol. 15:497–506.

Yasuhira, K. 1969. Suspicious influence of thymectomy on skin papilloma induction. Gann 60:57–64.

Yphantis, D. A. 1964. Equilibrium ultracentrifugation of dilute solutions. Biochemistry 3:297–316.

Yunis, E. J., Martinez, C., Smith, J., Stutman, O., and Good, R. A. 1969. Spontaneous mammary adenocarcinoma in mice: Influence of thymectomy and reconstitution with thymus grafts or spleen cells. Cancer Res. 29: 174–178.

Zisblatt, M., Goldstein, A. L., Lilly, F., and White, A. 1970. Acceleration by thymosin of the development of resistance to murine sarcoma virus-induced tumor in mice. Proc. Natl. Acad. Sci. U.S.A. 66:1170–1174.

Zondek, B., and Burstein, S. 1952. The relationship of corticoid excretion to ovarian hormones in the guinea pig. Endocrinology 50:419–428.

Note: The proceedings of the Symposium on the Thymus held at Cluj, Romania, in 1969, were published in *Roumanian Review of Endocrinology* 8(1), 1971. This volume did not reach us in time to be incorporated into the present volume, so we present the following list of contents in the interest of making this information available to the reader.

Introduction. **Morphological and clinical aspects of the thymus**. Experimental investigations on thymocyte structure, *A. Muresan and I. Caluser.* Investigations on thymus structure and function in man, *I. Caluser and A. Muresan.* A pneumo-mediastinographic and histopathologic study of the thymus in sucklings, *A. Rusescu, M. Geormaneanu, I. Balaban, and S. Cotovu.* Morphological changes of the thymus in premature newborns under different pathological conditions, *Maria Bedivan and F. Pascu.* Treatment of myasthenia by thymectomy, *I. Juvara, D. Motomancea, Sanda Bossy-Bibicescu, and M. Cristea.* The diagnosis and the surgical therapy of thymic tumors, *L. Hica, G. Cornea, and D. Cristoloveanu.* Observations on the large thymus and on the immunological conditions in infants between zero and two years of age, *Eugenia Mihalca and Dana Ghet.* Immunological changes in infants with acute infections and thymus hypertrophy, *Iuliana Tirlea, A. Chisu, Lidia Marian, and A. Biclesanu.* **Physiological and biochemical aspects of the thymus**. Physiology of the thymus, *J. Comsa.* Biology of thymus involution, *E. A. Pora and V. Toma.* Experimental contributions to the question of thymus involution in tumor-bearing hosts, *I. Kiricuta, G. Simu, and V. Toma.* Thymus behavior during shock due to burns in animals with stimulated reticulo-histiocytic system, *I. Kiricuta and G. Simu.* Relations between the thymus and the striated musculature, *E. A. Pora and V. Toma.* An antiblastic factor of the thymus, *S. M. Milcu and Isabela Potop.* Evidence of steroid biosynthesis in the thymus of white rats using (1-^{14}C) acetate and (4-^{14}C) cholesterol as precursors, *A. D. Abraham.* Stimulating and inhibiting effects of the bovine thymus extract, *K. Bedo, M. Horvath, Viorica L. Losonczi, J. Laszlo, A. Szollos, and E. Balint.* **Bursa Fabricii**. Morphophysiological relations between bursa Fabricii and the lymphoid organs and some endocrine glands, *A. Pintea.* Studies of bursa Fabricii, *E. A. Pora and R. Giurgea-Iacob.*

Index